Christopher Phelps, DMD

The Complete Book on Dental Marketing

edra
PUBLISHING

This edition first published 2022

ISBN: 978-1-957260-03-7
eISBN: 978-1-957260-02-0

edra
PUBLISHING

Edra Publishing US LLC
3309 Northlake Boulevard,
Suite 203,
Palm Beach Gardens,
FL, 33403
EIN: 844113980

info@edrapublishing.com
www.edrapublishing.com

Printed by Graphicscalve Spa, in September 2022

This book is dedicated to my wife Amber and my sons, Riley and Liam. Thank you for giving up our time together so that I could make this dream a reality.

Table of Contents

Introduction

1. WHY THIS BOOK WAS WRITTEN FOR YOU

Dental practices have always relied on a constant stream of new patients to sustain their growth and vitality. In days long past, one could just hang a shingle with their name just outside of their practice and use that to attract enough new patients to thrive. Unfortunately, times have changed and dentists are seeing an increased need to find alternative means to attract new prospects to their offices. There's just one problem. A problem many such as the successful Philadelphia retail merchant John Wanamaker discovered. Mr. Wanamaker is famously credited as saying, "Half of my advertising spend is wasted; the trouble is, I don't know which half." A profound statement from a pioneer in marketing, yet it speaks to the challenge many of us in the dental industry have faced. Marketing for most is considered more of a mystery instead of a science. When it remains a mystery to us it ultimately ends in wasted efforts, poor results, and tens of thousands of lost dollars.

The good news is that it doesn't have to remain a mystery. The goal of this book is to help dentists who are looking to demystify the dental marketing process, those in need of more new patients, regardless of whether you are a marketing director for a current practice or a dentist yourself, a solo practitioner or one in a group practice, or someone who is in network with dental insurance companies or completely out of network with them.

To help those identify and understand the two main areas in dental marketing, you'll need to turn your focus, creating more new patient leads, followed by maximizing those opportunities. In doing so, this can teach you how to be the CEO of your marketing department, a concept none of us were trained on in dental school. As the CEO, you'll be able to turn all of your marketing efforts into an investment, providing a significant and consistent return while allowing you to reach whatever new patient goals you need to grow and creating new opportunities to generate revenue instead of those that might constantly consume it.

While I have personally used and had success with all of the different marketing options I lay out in this book, I realize that some of these may not specifically apply to your practice. I also understand that in some circumstances you won't be able to follow every step or detail that I map out. Despite this, I encourage you to think about the overarching concepts from each section and amend them to fit your practice and your situation.

2. NECESSITY IS THE MOTHER OF INVENTION

I graduated from dental school in May of 2003. I was fortunate to buy the dental practice of Dr. Thomas Grimes, who resided in Matthews, North Carolina. I met Dr. Grimes through my wife as she had been a patient of his since she was age 14. After graduating dental school in 1989, Dr. Grimes had created a dental practice out of renovating an old house. In his day, the main means of marketing to attract new patients was demonstrated by two main facets: signing up to be an in-network provider for many dental insurance plans and the shingle that signified his name and that he was a dentist that sat on the roadside, just out front of his office. Around 1996, Dr. Grimes discovered that the insurance companies he participated with for 8 years owed him over $400,000 in accounts receivable. After many failed efforts to collect what they owed him, he made a bold choice and went out of network with them all.

The bad news for Dr. Grimes was that when his existing patients found out that he no longer participated with their insurance plan, about half of them chose to leave and find an office that did work in their network. The good news for him was that even though he lost half of his patients in that moment, at the end of the year he profited the same amount of money that he had the year prior. Truly working smarter, not harder, he was able to increase his capacity to see more patients. Over the next seven years he turned his marketing efforts to increasing referrals from those patients who stayed and had rebuilt his patient base when I joined him as a partner in the practice in early 2004.

Being fresh out of dental school, I had big ideas and a vision for where I wanted our practice to be. Dr. Grimes was very supportive and willing to invest the practice's resources into my marketing ideas to help us grow—and grow we did. The revenue for the practice doubled that first year, going from $600,000 in collections in the previous year to collecting over $1,200,000. With this success we decided to expand to a new location and started a second satellite office about 9 miles away in a growing part of Charlotte, North Carolina. Utilizing radio and direct mail advertising efforts, that satellite office collected over $1,000,000 in its first year and over $2,000,000 its third year.

From there Dr. Grimes and I diversified and allowed two of our associate dentists to buy in as partners. This gave us the capital and resources to expand to our third location, a rural practice that we purchased from a retiring dentist about one and a half hours north of us. With success attained at this location, we added a fourth location, another practice we opened from scratch, which was located about 8 miles south of our second location. Over a seven-year period, we leveraged dental marketing to grow from one location to four locations, from $600,000 to over $6,500,000 in annual revenue collected. At this point, dental marketing was still a mystery to us, but it was all working, so I didn't ask many questions. But like the popular idiom says, all good things must come to an end.

In 2010, Dr. Grimes and I decided to divest from our other two partners. Nothing against them, but it was more of a decision for Dr. Grimes and me to simplify our life and get back to our roots. To do so, we had to come to an amicable agreement to separate the assets that we had built. When the dust settled, the assets were split in a way that many thought was risky. You see, Dr. Grimes and I sold our two best offices to our partners; those offices were the ones that had the highest production, lowest debt, and highest cash flow. In return, we took over the two worst offices, the ones with the highest debt and lowest production. One was the original office he and I built together, and the second was the newest satellite office our group had built.

It was during this time that I really started to understand the words found in Plato's Republic where it says, "Our need will be the real creator," which a popular translation rendered loosely as, "The true creator is necessity, who is the mother of our invention." It was also a time when I experienced our first real challenges in dental marketing. You see, I found myself spending over $36,000 a month in dental marketing while only gaining 60 new patients per month for those efforts, 30 new patients at one of our offices and 30 at the other. This was a time that led me to the same frustrations John Wanamaker experienced. Tens of thousands of dollars spent, yet no real idea on what was working and what was not working.

It was this struggle that created a real need for me to understand and define the dental marketing process, which helped me:

- increase our new patient count from 60 per month to averaging over 300 per month, 130 per month at one office and 170 per month at the other;
- decrease my marketing costs by 74 percent;
- turn my overall marketing expense into a 6:1 return on investment (ROI).

The lessons I learned throughout this process make up the two core components of this book. Two halves of the same marketing coin, if you will. First and foremost, it's about understanding how to attract the patients' attention and drive them to your practice. But we're not done. What happens if we bungle that opportunity? You see, it's not enough to focus on attraction alone. We also need to have strategies to maximize these new patient opportunities. If we don't, then we're doomed to spend more marketing dollars to overcome this lost opportunity. My hope is that you can take the lessons learned here and avoid the mistakes and pitfalls I've made along the way. But to do so, it all starts with your marketing mindset.

3. MARKETING MINDSETS: HUNTING VERSUS FISHING

"There's not one thing you can do in dental marketing that will get you 100 new patients, but there are probably four areas you could focus on that will get you 25 new patients each." This was one of the most important lessons I learned marketing my dental practices these last 17 years. In computer science, it's called a "divide and conquer" algorithm, one that works by recursively breaking down a problem into two or more subproblems of the same or related type, until these become simple enough to be solved directly. The solutions to the subproblems are then combined to give a solution to the original problem. In dental marketing, one action won't get you 100 new patients but maybe four or five different ones could. On the surface it seems so simple, yet it's a solution that is poorly understood or utilized in the dental space.

A. Dentists Have a Hunter's Mindset

Growing up, my father was a big hunter. Fish, ducks, and deer were his passion. I remember many mornings being awoken at 4 a.m., darkness and cold being the main elements present. My dad would get us out into the woods and up onto a deer stand in what seemed like the middle of nowhere. Our goal? To wait patiently, sometimes for four or five hours, sitting in that deer stand until one deer happened upon our path. Then, we raised our weapon to fire, hoping we had the skill to hit our target with one shot. If we hit it, then we'd be victorious and enjoy the spoils. If we missed, it meant that all our efforts for the day were wasted as the sound of the gun shot would send any other deer in the area well away from our position. The good news is those hours spent on deer stands did teach me a few lessons about hunting.

- **Hunting requires money**. It takes a large investment of cash to purchase the camouflage gear you wear, to buy the deer stand you sit in, for the rifle you'll need to shoot with, and the high-powered scope you'll need to see your prey.
- **Hunting requires luck**. You're hoping the deer you seek happens to be in your area and just happens to wander through your path.
- **Hunting requires time**. This is not a 20- or 30-minute event. It's something that typically takes up your entire day.
- **Hunting requires skill**. You have one chance with your shot, a shot that has to be good enough to hit that deer in the right spot to put it down. Miss your shot, and the deer is gone for good. Hit it in the wrong spot, and the deer will take off running to the point that when it does finally succumb to its injury, it will be so far away from you that you'll never find it. Either way you're left empty-handed with the time, money, and effort invested being a waste.

When I talk with dentists around the country, there is typically one question that always comes up. "What's the one thing in marketing I can do to reach my new patient goals?" I know what they are really asking, but what I'm hearing is this:

- Where is the best place to hunt for a deer?
- Where should I put my deer stand?
- Will I see a deer?
- Can you tell me when and where I should shoot?

The truth is I can't give you a definitive answer for any of these questions when it comes to the amount and type of marketing you need to do to hit your new patient goals, not with this hunter's mindset.

B. Dentists Need a Fisherman's Mindset

In addition to deer hunting, growing up I remember lots of fishing trips with my dad. One thing fishing did teach me was patience. I'd spend hours with him on the side of a pond. Lure in the water. A hook with bait connected to a fish bobber that would float at the top of the water. Watching, staring, waiting for that bobber to move, signifying that a fish had taken my bait so I could reel it in.

After many outings, I felt like the lessons I was learning from fishing in this manner were starting to mirror the ones I learned hunting for deer. That is until an important event changed my perspective on fishing and eventual marketing strategies moving forward.

One day my dad I both threw our fishing lines into the water, and both instantly had fish grab our hooks. Usually waiting hours to get our first nibble, we both were shocked. We reeled in those fish, rebaited our hooks, and threw them right back out again. Immediately, we both had another pair of fish hooked. The next round I didn't even put bait on my hook, I just threw it right back out there into the water and amazingly had another fish on the line.

This was the most excited I had ever been fishing, not realizing that we had stumbled upon a natural spawning bed, an area where fish come to reproduce. It's this reproductive act that makes the fish ravenous for food and willing to bite a hook that had no bait. Excited by this newfound ability to catch fish, I got an idea. If with this new approach it was so easy to catch fish, why can't I multiply my efforts? I set my fishing rod down and ran to our truck and grabbed our backup fishing pole. Now equipped with two fishing poles, one for each hand, I was catching fish at twice the rate I had before.

When it comes to dental marketing, dentists should divide and conquer their new patient problem by fishing with multiple fishing poles. To be an effective dental marketer, you can use this fisherman's mindset and understand that marketing is a trial-and-error process, not done by "hunting for deer," spending all of your marketing budget hoping your one marketing attempt will solve all of your new patient problems. Instead, it's done by "fishing with multiple fishing poles," investing small amounts of money that is spread out over several different types of media, each one tracked well enough to establish what is providing you with a 3:1 or higher ROI and which ones are not.

Lessons learned by taking a "fishing with multiple fishing poles" approach to marketing:

- **Corrections can be made earlier**: This method allows you to correct any inefficiencies found in those media that aren't achieving acceptable ROIs and redirect your efforts as needed.
- **Avoid hunting mistakes**: Instead of spending all of your money in one area and hoping for the best, it sets the stage for you to find four or five solid channels that will help you reach your new patient goals.
- **Avoid marketing expenses**: Not only will you reach your new patient goals, but you'll collect back more of a return than what you invested.
- **Get confidence to do more**: You'll turn marketing into more of a science and avoid wasted marketing efforts and dollars. This will give you more confidence to fish in new marketing streams and take your practice to the next level.

C. How the Quantity and Quality of New Patients You Attract Can Affect the ROI

Once you have a "fishing with multiple fishing poles" mindset, you can now turn your attention to answering this. What do you need more of? Do you need more quantity of new patients? Do you need a better quality of new patients?

Let's start with the first one. The goal of your marketing attempt is to attract enough quantity of new patients to reach your practice goals. The greater the number of new patients that come into the practice, the more likely you are to see a return on your marketing investment.

Application example: You've spent $5000 to run a marketing campaign for one duration. The new patients who were attracted to your marketing efforts each spend $150 during their first visit at your practice. Which is better? A marketing attempt that brings in 10 new patients or one that brings in 50 new patients?

- **10 new patients**: With 10 new patients attracted, each of whom spends $150 in their first visit, that allows you to collect $1500 in revenue, which divided by $5000 spent gives us a negative ROI, or 70 percent loss of the marketing dollars you've spent.
- **50 new patients**: With 50 new patients attracted, each of whom spend $150 in their first visit, you've now collected $7500, which compared to $5000 invested is a 1.5:1 ROI. You've covered the cost of your marketing expense and made some on top of that. Especially if you factor in your ability to retain these patients. When they return for future restorative and preventative oral health care treatments, your ROI from that original investment will only continue to rise.

From this example, we see that attracting a certain quantity of new patient opportunities is an important goal that we should strive for, but we also need to factor in the quality of new patient opportunities we're attracting. Let's define a high-quality new patient as one who:

- **pays your full fee in some capacity**, which includes supplemental aides such as dental insurance or them utilizing a dental membership plan discount;
- **returns for future appointments**, in other words, repeat customers, those who will return every six months for their next preventative cleanings but not someone who came in for the "dental special" you offered today only to leave you tomorrow to go to a different office that offers them the same discounted special you once did;
- **says yes to your treatment recommendations**, not someone who is a price shopper and will compare your fees to every dental office in the area before choosing the lowest price office for their care.

The better quality of new patients you attract, the more they return and the more they spend. This increases their patient lifetime value (PLV) for all time periods measured and allows you to see a greater ROI for your marketing dollars spent.

Application example: Let's look at two scenarios. For both, you've spent $5000 to run a marketing campaign for one duration. Each example yields 20 new patients.

In the first scenario, you offered a discounted new patient special and reduce the potential new patient exam, cleaning, and x-ray fee collected from $199 to $99. The new patients who were attracted to your marketing efforts each spend $99 during their first visit at your practice, but only three returns to your office for a second visit, each spending an average of $1000 in the first year as your patient.

In the second scenario, you did not offer a discounted new patient special. Instead, you offered something to attract better-quality new patients. This allows you to charge your full $199 initial visit fee. Of those 20 patients attracted, 15 returns for future care and appointments, each spending an average of $1000 in the first year as your patient. Which is better?

- **$99 new patient special**: 20 new patients came in and spent $99 for their first visit, which provides $1980 in total revenue collected. Of those, three returned for additional treatment recommended, allowing you to collect an additional $3000. Your total revenue collected from this marketing campaign is $4980. Divide that by our $5000 spent on the marketing campaign and it gives us an ROI of about 1:1, or breaking even at best.
- **Attracting better-quality patients**: Twenty new patients came in, and each spend $199 for their first visit, which provided $3980 in total revenue collected. Of those,

> 15 return for additional treatment recommended, allowing you to collect an additional $15,000 over the next year. Your total revenue collected from this marketing campaign is $18,980. Divide that by the $5000 spent on the marketing campaign, and it gives us an ROI of about 3.8:1, covering all the expense plus returning more on top of that.

To turn your marketing dollars spent into an investment, you have to be in the right mindset, someone willing to "fish with multiple fishing poles," who'll create marketing pieces that not only bring in a good quantity of new patients but also attracts the right quality. In doing so, you should be able to achieve a minimum of a 3:1 ROI in the first six months following your marketing expenditure. To accomplish this, we now have to turn our attention on how to create these new patient opportunities, and that starts with attracting the patient's attention.

Part 1

Attracting the Patient's Attention

If your advertisement can't attract the attention of a potential new patient, then you have no chance of them coming into your practice and thus no chance of getting a return for the marketing dollars you've invested. To change this outcome, you'll need to build a brand they'd want to be a part of, craft a message that resonates with their situation, and define a call to action that will motivate and influence them to make an appointment. Let's go through each of these areas in more detail.

Chapter 1
Building Your Brand: Four Practice Identifiers That Make Up Your Brand

The first step in creating more new patient opportunities comes from attracting the potential new patient's attention. To be able to draw their focus your direction, you need to have a solid brand to put in front of them.

A brand is a name, term, design, symbol, or any other feature that identifies one seller's good or service as distinct from those of other sellers. It helps patients, and potential patients, more quickly know, like, and trust you—which helps them make more frequent purchasing decisions. Branding encompasses all the ways you establish an image of your dental practice in the eyes of your patients and gives them a reason to choose you over another dentist and a reason to continue to choose you over going to a different dental office. Understanding the four practice identifiers that make up a brand will help you create one that will resonate with current and future patients.

- **Name**
- **Logo**
- **Website**
- **Office interior**

1. NAME

One of the main sticking points dentists face when naming their office is to decide whether to use their own/family name or to come up with a unique practice name. There are pros and cons to both approaches, so let's look at some situations that may direct your decision. Perhaps one of your parents or grandparents practiced dentistry in the town where you are setting up your office. Maybe your family ran a successful local business in the same town. If you have an established and respected family name in the community, you can leverage that to benefit your dental office. Leveraging a well-established family name can give you an advantage over other dental practice names out there. If you're part of a minority group and your target market is to attract patients of the same ethnicity, then using your own name could provide an advantage to attract more of these patients. At the same time, it might influence some patients to not choose your office.

Another important consideration for using your actual name is the marketability of your practice to potential buyers. If you have goals of one day retiring from the profession, then you may want to avoid using your personal name to brand your office. This will make all your branding including, logos, Google business profile listing, marketing materials, brochures, website, patient reviews, stationery, staff uniforms, and so forth, transferable to the new owner, making your dental practice a turnkey solution for potential buyers. Another point to consider is how you plan to run the office not just in the present but in the future. Do you plan on bringing associate dentists into the practice? If so, then having a brand that is not associated with your personal name would be the preferred route you should take.

When I joined Dr. Grimes in 2003, he had branded the practice name around his own name. Thomas D. Grimes, DDS. To keep things simple, my name was added to the monument sign just out front of our space and any marketing materials we had created. This worked well for us during our first couple of years in partnership, but when it came time for us to open a second location, adding two more associate dentists, we quickly realized that we couldn't rely on our names alone. The second location was 8 miles from our home location, so to save money on shared expense items such as letterhead, signage, appointment cards, and marketing materials, we decided a shared, unique name made more sense than creating two separate practice names.

To create a unique practice name, I recommend a combination of authority cues and specifics of your location to position your practice as a local or regional first choice. Authority cues are words, places, or things that signify that you are an expert in any given area. Words that convey authority include:

- Advanced: Defined as modern or recently developed, far on or ahead of others in development or progress. Ex., Advanced Dentistry;
- Center: The point from which an activity or process is directed or on which it is focused. Occurs mainly in or around or placed in the middle of a specified area. Ex., Center for Dentistry;
- Solutions: A means of solving a problem or dealing with a difficult situation. Ex., Dental Solutions.

When it comes to having your location in your name, it should give patients an idea on where to find you. Using our examples above, we could modify those names accordingly. Since I lived in Charlotte, North Carolina, a recommended name would be Advanced Dentistry of Charlotte or Advanced Dental Solutions of Charlotte. If your city is fairly large geographically, you can also try to narrow this down to a more specific geographic area of your city or town to help patients understand where to find you. One of my practices was in a historic part of the Charlotte area, a small town called Matthews. My second location was in an up-and-coming city called Waxhaw, named after the American Indian tribe who inhabited that region. To come up with our name, I combined an authority cue with a more specific marker for our locations, rebranding the practices as Carolinas Dental Center of Matthews and Carolinas Dental Center of Waxhaw.

2. LOGO

Your logo is a graphic, symbol, emblem, or stylized text used to identify your dental practice. Many times your logo will be the most widely recognizable aspect of your brand, only second to your name. Now remember that many say a picture is worth 1000 words. If that is the case, then your logo will not only be recognizable, but it will also tell potential new patients a lot about your brand. Here are some factors to consider when designing our office logo.

- Design: Do a search in your area and look at the logos of those around your location. You can use these as a reference, but ideally your logo should stand out and differentiate you from them.
- Colors: Bright, vibrant tones represent more energy and excitement than softer tones. Understand that there is a psychology of colors and how they impart emotions in people. Blue, for instance, can instill calm, trust, and relaxation. Green can relay being environmentally friendly or growth. Yellow implies youth and happiness. Black represents luxury and sophistication. Red can stand to mean power and excitement, but in the medical world it means blood, an image that could invoke fear in those who see it.
- Legibility: Not only should your design be aesthetic and pleasing to the eye, but the words including your practice name that are shown or featured should be easily read. Font selection is key. Too much cursive or overlap of the lettering may make it difficult for people to read what's in front of them.

3. WEBSITE

Designing a website for your dental practice should not simply be checked off a to-do list by outsourcing its creation to the lowest bidder. Doing so means that you are gearing up for a most atypical marketing journey. Your website is the anchor for your external marketing efforts, your community engagement, converting any traffic you generate into actual patients. How do you create this conversion machine? Focus on the story, building relationships, and evoking emotional responses from potential patients. Do not solely focus on clinical data and financial information.

What makes a great dental website? After 17+ years in the industry and working with great website companies such as the Art of Dental Marketing, I've realized it comes down to five main things. Too many dental web designers ignore these areas and create mass-produced, templated, out-of-date websites. These archaic layouts are accompanied by a vast number of pages, far too much written text, and a never-ending rotation of uninspiring, boring stock photography. This is a classic recipe for underwhelming performance, resulting in wasted time and money. Instead, here are the 5 key areas on which we need to turn our focus:

- Clarity and story
- Ease of use
- Page speed
- Responsive design
- Content strategy

A. Clarity and Story

Your homepage is your first impression, and first impressions matter. In his book *Building a Storybrand*, author Donald Miller lays out a powerful template for a website *wireframe*, or skeletal framework, for your content. The objective is to be simple and unambiguous, focused around a heading that tells the user who you are and what you offer. This sets the tone and creates expectations for the entire patient experience, from the clinical aspects to the culture of your team.

A few examples of a simple heading:

- Modern dentistry for Kansas City families.
- We help create your dream smile.
- Healthier smiles for a healthier future.
- You may also include sub-points beneath each header. These sub-points can focus on affordability, speed of service, or even a dental specialty service that your office provides. It's important not to be clever or "salesy." Keep it simple. Confusion kills conversion.
- Your story is what compels and sells dentistry, not clinical data. Over 60 percent of the US population suffers from some form of dental fear. Telling your story with intention can help ease anxiety by humanizing yourself and your team. How do you do this? That can be a complex answer. However, a great place to start is with video creation.
- A video-driven website provides much needed depth and dimensionality. Video allows patients to see you, your team, the practice, and the clinical setting before they ever actually visit your practice, easing the fear of the unknown. Telling your story (why you became a dentist, your hobbies, etc.) is a great way to provide assurance and establish trust-building connections.

B. Ease of Use

Clear, simple navigation is your friend. The moment a user lands on your homepage, your contact information, address, and hours of operation should be easily available. It is unnecessary to have an exhaustive menu with dozens of pages. Think quality over quantity here. In actuality, you simply need more great content than a lot of content. Remember, visitors have a goal in mind when they reach your site. It's not to read in-depth information about the procedures you provide. It's to find the right dentist for them or a loved one. That dentist should be you!

C. Page Speed

Year over year, user preferences lean toward mobile devices over traditional desktop usage. As we continue to advance, it is imperative for web designers to keep up with evolving technology. Page speed is vital, not only from a conversion standpoint but for a great user experience. What started as a simple metric for measuring website load time has evolved into a key performance indicator on your site's user experience. Put simply, if your site takes too long to load, people will become disinterested and leave. Most users will give you about 5 seconds. Five seconds! That's all it takes for users to leave without site engagement. This is known as **bounce rate**. A high bounce rate tells Google, and other search engines, that your site isn't providing value to the end user. This means your site will fall in the organic search engine optimization (SEO) rankings.

D. Responsive Design

Responsive design is when a website can adjust and stretch, based on the size of the screen it's being viewed on. No matter the device or network, your website should load quickly and adapt seamlessly. This will ensure your end user has an enjoyable experience and will, in theory, keep users engaged and on your site longer. The longer they stay, the lower your bounce rate. Making your site accessible, fast, and easy to use will mean a great experience, better conversion, and better placement in organic search rankings.

E. Content Strategy

Content is still king! The content on your site is the foundation for everything. Content will tell your story. It will resonate with your audience. It will tell search engines what you do and where you do it. Valuable, relevant content is just as important as the design itself. You can develop your content arsenal in a variety of ways including blogs, FAQs, podcasting, videos, and more!

That's it! You are now on your way to avoiding the marketing pitfalls of underwhelming, unfocused web design. Don't settle for a web designer that throws you on autopilot, while providing an ineffective templated website. Web design and how people use the Internet is ever evolving. Future-proof your practice by becoming proactive, staying aware of trends, and adopting new advances in technology.

4. OFFICE INTERIOR

Studies show that it takes less than seven seconds to make a first impression. Once set, people tend to get attached to their initial impressions of others and find it very difficult to change their opinion, even when presented with lots of evidence to the contrary. As a result, it's important to be aware of how we come across to our patients. From our marketing materials, messages, and logo to what their perception will become when they walk through the doors of our practice for the first time. These are some tips to help your office complement the branding work you've created thus far.

- Current but not outdated. Your office doesn't have to always look like it's brand-new, but at the same time it shouldn't look like as something from an old dental museum. Utilize bright, energizing colors and lights. Bright white walls that are accented by fresh and bold colors such as orange, blue, and green are on trend in dental offices right now.
- Incorporate your logo. Reinforce your branding by highlighting or featuring your logo in your office. Either at the check-in area or some prominent place in your reception. Consider incorporating the colors of your logo into the color scheme of your interior.
- It shouldn't smell like a dental office. Studies show that the sights, sounds, and smells of your office can influence your patients' first impressions and mindset. Does your office have that traditional "dental smell" that everyone probably associates with a bad experience? Instead, maybe it should utilize a smell that helps create an impression. ScentAir is a time-released product that can greatly change the smell in your waiting area. One popular scent has been labeled by users of this product as the "Disney smell," a smell that makes people associate to their time spent at the happiest place on earth.

  A dentist I know outside of Ontario, Canada, used this idea of smell to influence more referrals for his three offices. Each day, a team member would arrive early to his offices and fill the place with the smell of fresh baked chocolate chip cookies, a smell most would not expect upon arriving to a dental office for the first time. The cookies were baked all day, with several being bundled up and given to each patient at checkout as a way to thank them for coming in that day. For those who appreciated this gift, they were given a second bundle of cookies and asked if they would pass that bundle on to someone they know might need a good dentist. The result? The smell of the cookies created a mindset of family and encouraged them to refer. In doing so, he attracted

40–50 new patients per month to his offices without spending any other money to market his practice.

- Amenities of home: Waiting rooms should no longer be filled with tables topped with magazines or rows of chairs backed up against one another. Instead, consider having several different seating areas, arranged so that there is no risk of leaning back and accidently touching another person's head or looking up and locking eyes with a complete stranger. Perhaps we'd like our patients to trust us or feel like we're family and that they are at home and not at a scary dental office. If that's the case, then our reception room should look and feel like their home. So bring in large, comfy chairs, sofas, and ottomans or have a fireplace so it looks like you're in someone's living room. Consider having a snack station with sodas, coffee, water, and snacks available.

Chapter 2
Clarify Your Message

Once you have fully defined your brand, you can now turn your attention to clarifying who your potential new patients should be and how to garner their attention. To accomplish this goal, you have to consider who is this target market that you're attempting to influence. Let's look at these in more detail.

1. WHO IS YOUR TARGET MARKET?

In dentistry, our target market is defined as a particular group of patients who want the services that we offer. We can break down this generic concept into more specifics by answering the following questions.

A. Who Do You Want More of in the Practice?

- What type of patient?
- Someone to fill your hygiene chairs?
- Someone to fill your doctor/restorative chairs?
- Someone who needs more traditional dental work such as crowns and fillings?
- Someone who wants more specialized procedures such as dental implants?

B. What Does Your Existing Market Look Like?

- Run a demographic report from your practice management software to see how your current patient base breaks out. Where do they live in relation to your practice? What's the age range? Breakdown based on reported gender?
- Create a list of the top 20 or so people who've spent the most money with you over the last 12 months.
- Look at those existing patients who've referred the most patients to your practice over the last 12 months.

C. Can You Categorize Them?

- Create as many categories as possible.
- What percentage are men vs women?
- Are they younger, working families or older retirees?
- Do they live within a 0–5, 5–10, or a 10+ mile radius of your practice?
- What dental procedures are they having done with you?

D. Can You Interview Them When Present?

When someone you'd identify as your target market is sitting in your dental chair, stop and take some time to talk to them and ask them questions related to:

- What do they like to do locally in the area for fun?
- What are their favorite restaurants?
- Beverages or desserts they enjoy?
- What hobbies they have?
- Any local charities they support?
- Recreational places they visit?
- How do they search for information? Online sources like Google vs print media such as local magazines, direct mail, or the newspaper.

E. What's the Pattern?

Typically, the more information you can compile about your target market, the more likely you are to find a pattern. This could lead to having one specific patient market you'd like to attract or show you that you have numerous patient types you want to target.

Application example: When I followed the sequence outlined above and mapped out who my market was, I noticed an interesting pattern among those interested in sedation dentistry. Given that my average sedation patient spent $3554 in their first year at my practice, I definitely considered them one of my target markets and wanted to attract more of them to our practice. After running a report about the patients who had received sedation dentistry services from us over the last 12 months, I noticed that about half of them lived over 10 miles away from our practice. There is an old adage in dental marketing that states that your average dental patient lives or works within a 3- to 5-mile radius of your practice. Because of this, at that time I was focusing the majority of my marketing efforts with radio and direct mail to cover that 5-mile radius. Once I saw the pattern, I increased my efforts to cover a 15-mile radius around our practice since it was now obvious that people were willing to drive a good distance for our sedation services. Increasing that radius more than tripled the number of new patients we attracted who were seeking sedation services and significantly increased the ROI of the direct mail and radio marketing I was using.

F. "Map Your Market" Worksheet

To aid you in your discovery, use this "map your market" worksheet. By asking yourself these questions and examining who or what your current base is made of, who you've had previous success with, and so forth, you'll gain valuable insights and narrow your focus on who you want your marketing pieces to speak to.

Map Your Market

Instructions: Use this worksheet to help map out who you will target with your marketing efforts. Here are some ways you can identify who is your target market.

Potential Categories to Identify Your Target Market

- Existing patient base

Run a demographic report and attempt to categorize them as much as possible.

Possible criteria to search:

- Age
- Working vs retired
- Radius they live or work from your practice
- Gender
- How did they hear about your office?

- Identify the top 20 patients who have spent the most money with you in the last 18 months.
- Identify the top 20 patients who have referred the most people to your practice in the last 18 months.
- What type of new patient do you want?

- More hygiene patients?
- More patients for hygiene patients doctor treatment?
- If you will be marketing specific services such as sedation, orthodontics, cosmetics, implants, etc., please identify the top 10 patients who have spent the most money with you in these categories.

Existing pt. base	Top 20 spenders	Top 20 referrals	What type of NP?	Top 20 special category

Once you have identified your patients, interview them in person, email, or call them to ask questions to find out how they search for information. Examples you could ask:

- What magazines do you read?
- What newspaper do you read?
- Which section?
- What TV shows do you watch?
- When you need a service, do you look online, prefer to receive information via the mail, find it in a magazine, or some other source?

Identify a pattern. What connects them together?

- Is there a common marketing source?
- Is there a common place they heard about you?
- Is there a common age, gender, or working status?
- Do they live or work within a certain geographic area around your practice?

List your answers here:

____

____

____

____

Say hello to your target market! Now let's figure out how to get more of them!

THE PHELPS® INSTITUTE

1

Figure 1. "Map your market" worksheet. Follow this worksheet to help you define who your market is and what type of procedures you want more of.

2. WHAT'S YOUR HEADLINE OR MAIN MESSAGE?

Once we've identified who is your target market, your next step is to figure out what headline or main message you'll put in front of them. It's been reported that the average patient today receives 15–20 different dental marketing messages a month. Because people are overwhelmed, due to lack of time or real interest, they tend to scan the advertisement, looking for the most important areas first to decide whether they should continue on. That means the main points of your message really act like the headline of your story and they have to stand out, to differentiate you from all others. You need messages that when scanned, grab their attention and will motivate them to want to make an appointment at your office. Let's look at the areas that will help clarify your message.

A. What Your Message *Is Not* About

It's not about what makes you similar to other dental offices

Putting messages about all of the standard, routine dental services that you offer doesn't help you stand out from the crowd. It just makes it harder for patients to decide why they should pick your office over the other dental messages being placed in front of them.

It's not about your price or new patient special

Trying to define your practice based on your price or the discounted special you are offering is a no-win situation, a race to the bottom, as many say.

Case study: For many years, it's been the advice of dental marketing companies to recommend that we offer a $99 new patient special.

In my travels over the last 10 years, I've seen how this new patient special has negatively affected our practices. When you compete on price, you make our services and the care we provide our patients a commodity. A commodity is defined as a basic good or service used in commerce that is interchangeable with other goods of the same type. In essence, a crown is a crown. It doesn't matter who I get my crown from if they are the same. If all things are equal and interchangeable, the patient will then seek to find the office that will do that crown for the cheapest price.

Because more and more dentists began using this offer to attract patients, the effectiveness of the $99 special started to diminish. This led to a significant decrease in the quantity of new patients they received, so they had to do something to stand out again. That's when I started noticing the $99 special had changed to the $79 special. This of course led to the same outcome as seen before. More people offering the same discount led to another reduction in the new patient special. This time to $49.

Where has this led us? To the very bottom, to what's commonly known as a "foot in the door" strategy, where dentists now feel like they have to give away the entire exam, cleaning, and x-rays to attract enough quantity of new patients and hope that they return as paying customers.

Instead of offering a deeply discounted special, why not go the other way? If everyone is offering $99, why not double it and make your offer $200? That was the advice I gave Dr. Christopher Green, who was about to open his first start-up practice in Parker, Colorado. Here's what Dr. Green had to say about his start-up experience and the offer he went with.

"Direct mail for a start-up can be tricky. Dentists tend to think they have to give away all things for free in order to draw new patients to their practice. In my experience, when we advertise free, this often draws a certain type of patient to our practice. Often a 'one and done' or a price shopper. Another advertising technique that is just as bad as the word 'FREE' is the $59 new patient special. As Dr. Phelps would say, this is a race to the bottom. It's true! Our practice started with a $200 new patient special and averaged 100 new patients per month out of the gates. These are quality patients that value what we do and the quality of our work. It worked out great. On the other hand I have a friend who did the $59 new patient special with their start-up, and those patients ended up showing up for the one cheap cleaning and never coming back or accepting recommended treatment. When you put a deal out there it may be worthwhile to consider what might be the second-order consequences of that deal."

B. What Your Message *Is* About

It's about what makes you unique and different

It's about what makes you the scarce resource. We'll discuss Cialdini's principle of scarcity in more detail later on in this book, but for our purposes here, it's about what you or your office do, what you provide your patients that few in your area or industry offer them.

Application example: In my offices, we offered four different levels of sedation dentistry:

- Anxiolysis using nitrous oxide gas and a tranquilizing muscle relaxant like diazepam (Valium);
- Oral conscious sedation, utilizing a benzodiazepine such as triazolam (Halcion) administered by one of our doctors;
- IV sedation, administered by a dental anesthesiologist (DA);
- General sedation, administered by a DA.

Our DA assisted our dental board with all things related to sedation dentistry in our state, things such as licensing, credentialing, and approving sites for the type of sedation they wanted to perform on patients. From our discussion, I discovered that at that time, we were one of only three offices in the entire state of North Carolina that offered all four levels of sedation. When I looked at different dental advertisements that were currently in circulation, I noticed several docs promoting sedation, but they were really only promoting one type of sedation, oral conscious sedation. Here was something that made our offices unique and different, something a patient who was interested in being sedated for their dental care could use to differentiate the 5–10 different dental offices marketing sedation dentistry at that time. So I came up with an analogy and marketing message to describe our uniqueness: "Not all sedation dentistry is equal. Don't be a square peg in a round hole. We're one of only three dental offices in the entire state of North Carolina that offers every level of sedation dentistry. Find out which sedation option is medically right for you."

It's about the solutions to their problems

In most dental marketing advertisements, you may have noticed that the focus seems to be on promoting some piece of dental equipment that the office has purchased. For example, you may have seen headlines such as "Now offering CEREC 3D technology" or "Fotona Laser Therapy." While highlighting that you have invested in technology or equipment such as these does help promote you as an authority in your area, it doesn't do much to grab people's focus and attention to your marketing piece, mostly because the average patient has no idea what the equipment you're promoting is or what benefit it really provides them. Instead, you should reframe your message and focus on how the technology or service you want to promote goes about solving the patient's problem.

Steps to figuring out your message

- Identify the service you want to promote. Example: sedation dentistry;
- Figure out what problem a potential new patient might have that your service might be good for. Example: fear of going to the dentist;
- Define how your service solves their problem. With sedation dentistry, we know that one of the side effects for oral conscious sedation up to general sedation is amnesia. Patients will have little to no memory of their visit. With no memory of their visit, they are less likely to fear it going into it.
- That's the headline or message your marketing piece should highlight to grab a potential new patient's attention and encourage them to read what else you have to say. Choose messages such as: "Relax Your Way through Your Dental Visit," "Forget You Were Ever Here," "Dentistry That's a Breeze."

Differentiating messages that I've had success with

1. **Never miss work or school to visit the dentist**. The unique feature I wanted to promote was that our offices were open extended hours and days of the week. We were open from 7 a.m. to 7 p.m., Monday through Wednesday, and we were open on Saturdays from 8 a.m. to 2 p.m. One of the problems I noticed potential new patients had to visit the dental office was that there was more and more pressure for them to not take time off work for routine dental care during the workday. What's more, because they often took their kids out of school for numerous days to attend family vacations, they were less likely to schedule their children during the bulk portion most dental practices were open. With my expanded hours/days I had the perfect solution to their problem, which gave me a great differentiating headline.

2. **No dental insurance? We got your back!** In my book *Grow Your Dental Membership Plan*, I discuss what a membership plan is, the psychology of why patients are attracted to it, and how I used it to grow my dental practices by attracting more noninsured fee-for-service patients. Since there were no other dental offices in my area that offered these dental membership plans, I knew this was a unique feature I wanted to promote. From my grassroots marketing efforts, I discovered one of the problems keeping potential new patients from going to the dentist was this mindset that occurs after they retire from working and they lose their dental insurance plan. Because most are on a fixed budget, they decide against purchasing a private dental insurance plan because they feel it's too expensive. Since they don't carry dental insurance anymore, they feel like they can't go to see a dentist unless they are in discomfort or pain. With my dental membership plan, I had the perfect solution to their problem, which gave me a great differentiating headline that showed them that we offered a solution to their problem.

3. **Call today, get in today!** At our offices, we always budgeted some chair time and capacity to see emergency patients. Because of this, I wanted to fill our open chair time and promote our capacity to get someone in who had an immediate or urgent dental need. Having developed a call tracking system that tracked dental marketing efforts for dentists in the US, Canada, Australia, and the UK, I knew this was a problem for patients because the overwhelming majority of dental offices we tracked struggled to get these patients scheduled in a timely manner. In fact, it took an average of 4–5 days before most offices were able to see a patient with an immediate or urgent dental need. As you can imagine, that didn't sit well with those with an immediate dental need, so they continued calling around until they could find an office that could get them in sooner for an evaluation. In contrast to what most were able to offer, my philosophy was that if someone called with an immediate or urgent dental need, we'd do everything we could to get them in for an evaluation that day. Since we budgeted to have that capability, I knew I had the perfect solution to their problem, which gave me a great differentiating headline.
4. **Can't get to us? We'll pick you up!** Here, the unique feature I wanted to promote was that transportation did not have to be a barrier to coming to the dental office. One of my target markets I'll discuss in the grassroots marketing section of this book is the active, independent living retiree. From my discussions with these patients in my chair and at educational seminars I put on at their community, I discovered that many of them are afraid to drive outside of a certain radius from where they live, where they are most comfortable. As a result, they tend to shop, eat, visit doctors, and so forth, within that radius. With the advent of transportation companies such as Uber, I realized that I could attract more of these patients if I took away that fear of them driving to see us for their dental visit. So I started using Uber to pick them up and take them back home from their dental visits. For me the ROI was simple. An average round trip cost for me to offer my patient transport through Uber was approximately $20. The average amount spent by that patient for a cleaning was $150 or for dental work it was usually $1000 or more, money we would not have collected if we hadn't solved their problem.

Patient example: Even if your service doesn't solve a problem they have today, they may be attracted to it because it could solve a problem they have tomorrow. I once asked a new patient how they heard about us, and she responded that she saw our advertisement in their community magazine. I then asked her what about the ad did she like or influenced her to choose us for her dental care. She told me that she loved that we offered to pick people up who didn't feel comfortable driving on their own to see us. She stated that while she didn't need that service today, as she drove herself to her visit, she was glad to know that we'd already thought about what she might need in the future and that we had options for her. Lesson: When our market speaks, we need to listen as they are giving us great messages to use for the future.

C. "Map Your Message" Worksheet

Use this worksheet to help you craft your unique, differentiating messages, to identify what dental service you want to promote, what problem the patient has, and how your service solves their problem. With these defined, you'll have a much greater chance to grab your potential new patient's attention and persuade them to want an appointment at your office.

Map Your Message

Instructions: Now it's time to craft your message or the headline of your story. Start by asking yourself these questions:

1. What makes you unique or different?
2. What do you do that few, if any others, do in your town, city, or state?

Your message can also come from the solutions your services create for your patients. Here are some examples:

Services offered or would like to promote	Problem it will solve for the patient	Solution aka message
We are open from 7 a.m. to 2 p.m. on Saturdays	Can't get off work or school to make it to the dentist	Never miss school or work to get the dental care you need!
Uber partnership	Can't get transportation to the office	Can't get to us? We'll pick you up!
Sedation	Afraid of the dentist / bad experience	Forget you were ever here! Relax your way through the best dental visit you've ever had.
Same-day appointments	They are in pain and need an appointment now	Call today, get in today! Call before noon today, get in today!
Dental $avings Plan	Don't have dental insurance, so they think they can't come unless they are in pain.	No insurance, no problem. Ask about our Dental $avings Plan.

Now it's your turn. List out the services you want to promote and determine how they solve your patients' problem. This will lead you to your ideal message to grab their attention and want to learn more.

Services offered or would like to promote	Problem it will solve for the patient	Solution aka message
We are open from 7 a.m. to 2 p.m. on Saturdays	Can't get off work or school to make it to the dentist	Never miss school or work to get the dental care you need!

THE PHELPS® INSTITUTE

2

Figure 2. Map your message. Use this worksheet to help you define the headlines of your advertisement. Choose those that will grab the patients' attention and make them want to learn more.

3. CONTENT

At this point, you have thoroughly defined who your target market is and crafted some unique messages to act as headlines to grab their attention. It's time to clarify how the content of the advertisement should be chosen. To start, ask yourself these questions:

- What visual content is available? Consider images, video, and other formats available for you to use.
- How much written content or detail will you need? The answer here depends on whether your target market skews toward a certain gender. Studies show that each side has a different preference to how much detail is provided in your content.
- Are there certain emotions you're trying to invoke? Utilizing content that creates emotions can capture people's attention and can motivate them to have interest or a desire to learn more about you and your services.
- What colors need to be featured in your pictures, graphics, and font type to have the most impact on your target market?
- What stage of the buying cycle journey is your target market in? Will your content focus on building more awareness or education about a certain dental procedure or service? Will it focus on those in the evaluation stage, those confident that they need that procedure but who are unsure about who is going to be the best dentist or dental office to help them? Will it be targeted for those in the buying stage, those ready to say yes and move forward with this treatment with you?

Once you're clear about the answers to these questions, you can start to detail out what factors you'll need to embed into your marketing piece and how to properly structure them to get the best response from your target market. Let's break these areas out into more detail.

A. Visual Content

There is an old adage that says that a picture is worth 1000 words. With the rise of smart phones and our unlimited access to information at the palms of our hands, pictures are now worth 1,000,001 words. Studies show that 65 percent of the world's population are visual learners. Take into account that 90 percent of the information that comes into our brain is visual in nature, and it makes sense that in our marketing attempts we must incorporate different visual content types as a way to engage with our target market. Let's look at a few different visual content types:

Images

Provided your images are of a high resolution and contextually relevant to the topic at hand, when you split up the body of marketing text with images, people are more likely to finish reading what you've written. In fact, marketer Jeff Bullas cites that advertisements with images get 94 percent more views than advertisements without. A big advantage they have over other visual types is that they can be utilized in both online and off-line media.

Given how much influence they can have, where should we get these pictures? First, the images that seem to have the biggest impact to draw potential new patients' attention are those that you've taken yourself. People view these images as being more real and genuine than standard stock photos. If you don't have the time or resources to acquire these types of photos, you can look to popular photo-sharing sites such as Flickr or Morguefile, which offer a large library of inexpensive yet high-quality images.

With all of the picture and image choices available to you, how do you decide what are the best ones to use in your marketing pieces? My recommendation is to use pictures that tap into some of the six principles of influence and persuasion described by Dr. Robert Cialdini in his pioneer work, *Influence: The Psychology of Persuasion.*

Liking

In its simplest form, this principle states that people like to do business with those who are like them, those who show them that they like them and have some type of commonality or similarity. An easy way to show patients that you like them is to ask them to take a picture with you. The act of taking a picture with someone automatically shows that person that you like them since we normally take photos with friends and not enemies.

By incorporating creative graphics within our pictures, our images can serve two purposes. They showcase just how much we like our patients and by their smiling faces, just how much they like us. It also creates an opportunity to highlight other similarities that potential new patients may have with those at our office. For example, they may find some connection if they are of the same age, race, or gender of the people in the photo or at a basic level, they can connect in that they would be a new patient to our practice, just as this person was.

By seeing a photo such as this and now knowing about the positive experience on their first outing, it should influence this person to feel more confident about what their experience at our office might look like vs looking at other dental ads that don't show pictures or photos of their patients' experience.

Social proof

This principle states that in times of uncertainty, people look to what those around them are doing or have done to give them insights into what they should do, especially the closer to home that evidence becomes.

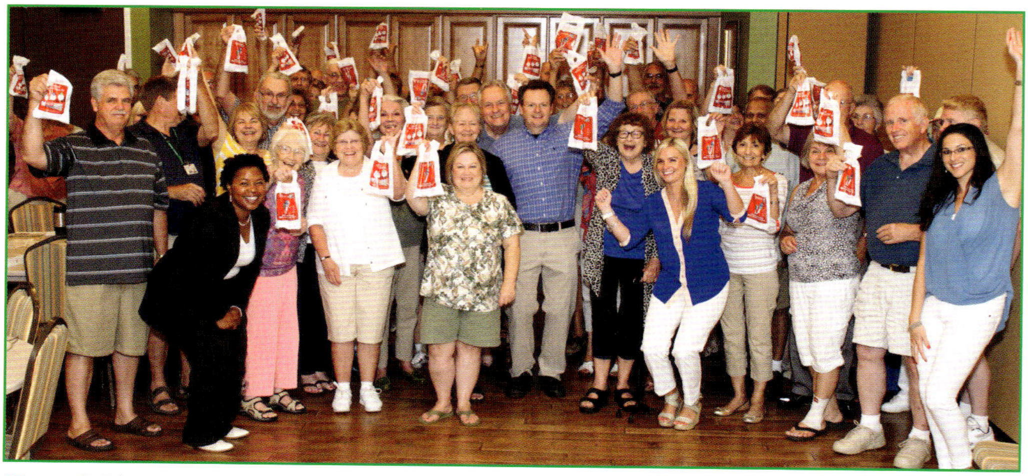

Figure 3. **Photo example to show the social proof principle.**

This photo (Fig. 3) was taken at a large active, independent living retirement community near my practice and concluded a large promotional event that I used as a new patient attraction tool. Each of the people in the photograph had taken the time to become patients at my practice. Once taken, I placed this photo as the main focal point in a one-page advertisement in their community magazine. By taking this photo with them as a group, it sends a powerful social proof message to others who live in that community. While they may know nothing about our office, this photo shows them two things. It shows them that a large number of people, just like them, who live in their own community chose me as their dentist. At the same time, it tells them that if this many people trust me with their dental care, maybe they'll be safe trusting me with their care as well.

Authority

This principle speaks to the influence of an expert's opinion. Because we don't have time to become an expert in everything, many times we look for trustworthy, credible experts to tell us what we should do. One of the cues that signify that you are an expert and one who is successful at your craft is to showcase the technology and equipment you've invested in. This could be Dental CBCTs, 3D printers, CAD/CAM units, lasers, or intraoral scanners. While patients may not fully understand the detail surrounding these items, they do perceive medical equipment and technology as being expensive. By showing that you have one or more of these units it tells others that you must be well trained and educated to use them and that you must be successful to be able to afford them.

Scarcity

People care more about what they stand to lose or what they've already lost than what they stand to gain. Using this principle, we can showcase photos that highlight specific patient pain points, problems they have for which they may be searching for solutions. For instance, imagine a person biting into an apple, but their dentures get lodged onto the apple when they pull it away from their mouth. Clearly, this type of photo would show someone who's lost the ability to eat the foods they want without their teeth falling out.

Without ever showing a picture of a dental implant, whose screw-like appearance could intimidate or scare someone viewing it, you can highlight that you understand the problem they are having and let them know you have options to counter their issue.

Mindsets

In Dr. Cialdini's book *Pre-suasion*, he talks about mindsets and how influential they can be when we make our decisions. All kinds of things can affect and create our mindset. The sights, sounds, smells of our environment, the words of items we've recently read, to the pictures or images that are put in front of us, all influence our potential decisions.

Selecting images that create mindsets that are symbiotic with your messaging is a powerful influence technique to grab people's focus and attention. Images like one of an hourglass showing the level of sand in the upper portion about to run out can create a mindset of urgency. Showing a picture of a caterpillar turning into a butterfly can relay a mindset of renovation or metamorphosis, much like you could give a patient with cosmetic dentistry. An image of the sun rising can impart a mindset of change. A new day dawning could pair well with messages of how your dental service can effect a change in their life.

Videos

Videos are incredibly useful for presenting common problems and then showing the solutions that your product can offer. While there are much cheaper types of visual content available, a great video serves as extra clout for your marketing piece by demonstrating that you're prepared to go the extra mile for quality. One study showed that including a video on a landing page increased conversions by 86 percent.

The challenge with using video is that it is limited by the medium you're using. Most off-line marketing and online marketing media use a static format to present their content. Billboards for instance aren't usually dynamic but feature the same picture and words until the entire advertisement is changed and updated. Pay-per-click advertising still utilizes a static banner or link to relay their information. One thing you can do in both media to bring the power of video into play is to host videos and embed them to a dedicated section of your website. Another way you can accomplish this is by creating a landing page, a special website address that you've created just for this promotional purpose. Utilizing the static nature of online and off-line marketing media, you can focus your messaging to encourage potential new patients to take one step and visit your dedicated page about that topic. Here they can watch and be influenced by the videos you've utilized.

There are many types of video content you can use in your marketing efforts such as making them "how to" or instructional videos such as "how to floss correctly." They can be more informational videos, providing basic information about a product or service you offer and the options available to those interested.

Your videos can be more educational in nature, teaching others about the root cause of their dental condition in a way that not only sets you up as the expert in this area but also gives them good actionable advice they can use to change their daily habits and improve their oral health.

Lastly, you can use patient testimonial videos that show people can trust you. When people are uncertain about a decision that needs to be made, such as which dentist will they select for their oral health care, studies show they look to two of Cialdini's principles for guidance, authority and social proof. As described above, in these situations in particular, we look to find a credible, trustworthy expert who can tell us what we need to do and one who has the support of multiple others like us.

Each individual patient testimonial video you share with potential new patients shows them that someone trusted you and had a great experience. When we can accumulate four or more of these videos, we invoke more social proof to show just how many others trust you and had a great experience with you.

Memes

The term "meme" was first coined by Richard Dawkins in 1976 to describe a concept or idea that has the capacity to replicate itself into different meanings from person to person. Today, memes are commonly known as images that are accompanied by humorous captions. Not many people envisaged that memes would play a role in content marketing when they first started to gain traction online, as they were primarily shared and made popular by college students as a form of entertainment. However, they now represent an easy-to-create, quirky form of visual content.

Creating your own meme is a great way to evoke positive emotions and set yourself apart from your competitors. They also can be utilized in online and off-line marketing media. Another unique benefit of memes is that they allow you to create inside jokes about your industry, which is a great way to make people laugh and build a community around your brand. When deciding whether a meme might be a good visual to use in your marketing piece, go back and think about your target market. If that person is from generation X, a millennial, or younger, then this just may be the visual you are looking for to stand out and grab this market's attention.

B. Written Content

While visual content is important to grab people's attention, we can't forget to consider what text-based content we'll use to hold that attention and create interest about our practice or service. But how much detail should we include in our advertisement? Should it be bullet points that just focus on the most important aspects of the service or procedure we're trying to promote? Should it be more detailed, laid out like a newspaper article or story? While many things can be considered to help you answer these questions, the most significant factor to consider is the gender of your target market.

In her book *Gender, Design and Marketing: How Gender Drives Our Perception of Design and Marketing*, Gloria Moss offers some valuable information about how differences in gender preference can affect your marketing effectiveness. One study Moss performed showed that there are distinct differences between the perceptions of the sexes in nearly every creative area: size, color, detail, dimensionality, and subject matter. Let's look at some of these differences separately.

According to Moss, men tend to look at a product's usefulness, it's technical specifications, or how it works. They prefer pictures over the written word, but when there's written information, they prefer as few details to read as possible, focusing instead on the headlines, top priorities, or most important aspects of your practice or service. Men value outcomes and ultimate solutions to the problem, so they may respond more readily to an advertisement that shows a solution that gets them to their ultimate goal.

Women, as Moss points out in a 2004 study, make up 80 percent of consumer buying decisions. They want to know what a product will do and how it will affect their life in a functional and social way. They want all of the information, not just the highlights, and won't make a decision until they've exhausted their search and are satisfied. They prefer the written word to be laid out like a story that builds to an ultimate conclusion. Telling a story also helps to create emotion, which is an important content type that we'll get to shortly.

Instead of being only solutions-focused, women tend to engage more readily to value propositions of belonging and community. This is why they may respond to messages and text about becoming part of your dental family and seeing evidence of others doing the same. They enjoy researching your patients' stories by looking at reviews and testimonials to get a sense of what their experience may be like.

C. Emotional Content

Emotional marketing refers to marketing and advertising efforts that primarily use emotion to make your audience notice, remember, share, and buy. Typically, this type of marketing targets one specific type of emotion such as happiness, desire, or fear to elicit a consumer response. One way or another, it makes a first impression.

Picture you were exposed to two different advertisements for a new business you were considering, one that simply talked about that business products or services and one that made you laugh or cry. Which one do you think would stand out and stick with you longer? Most likely it would be the one that created some emotion. First impressions are critical from an advertising perspective because you have just seconds to grab your potential new patient's attention. If the impression goes well, then they'll continue reading on, giving your messages a chance to have an influence. If the impression goes poorly, you've lost them and your marketing ROI drops significantly.

Let's think of this in another way. Do we tend to make our decisions with our head, using logic and reason as our decision determinants, or do we tend to decide with our heart? All things being equal, when it comes down to having our marketing piece motivate someone to pick up the phone and call us to make an appointment, the heart tends to win out over the head. Out of 1,400 successful advertising campaigns tested, those with purely emotional content performed twice as well, 31 percent vs 16 percent, as those with only rational or fact-driven content. Thus, when it comes to this battle of fact over emotion, studies show that people actually rely more on their emotions to make their decisions.

While there is a literal "wheel of emotions" that are available for us to tap into, I tend to focus my efforts on happiness, trust, sadness, and fear.

Happiness

Happiness makes us share, and sharing leads to increased brand awareness. Studies show that good news and positive content spreads faster on social media than any other type of content. Why? When someone is happy, we tend to mirror that emotion and want others to feel the same. An example of this might be getting a video testimonial from someone who has just received their new smile makeover and then hosting that video on your website or by sharing it on your Facebook, Instagram, and other social media accounts. Typically, people are overwhelmed with joy from their new smile, and you see this enthusiasm come through on these videos—enthusiasm that is sure to spread to all who view this video.

Trust

While people may think of you as being smart, educated, or successful, if they don't trust you, then they won't do business with you. Using images and videos to create a feeling of trust is key to move patients past their uncertainty and motivate them to pick up the phone and call. Patient reviews and testimonials do just that. Each review and testimonial, whether in text or video form, shows how much that particular patient trusted you. It presents you as the authority that you are. Adding social proof by displaying four or more of these adds even more influence by showing a potential new patient how numerous others trusted you for their dental care, reinforcing the emotion that they had begun to feel.

Sadness

Sadness makes us connect and empathize. Empathy leads to increased giving and increases the motivation to act on behalf of others. It's no surprise that organizations that support animals feature sad photos of those animals in need and moving songs while asking you for a donation.

Feelings of sadness inspire us to act and help, typically translating into fiscal giving. I realized how true this was when I began posting photos and stories following our "Dentistry from the Heart" event. One day a year we offer free cleanings and extractions to those in our community who can't afford it.

After six-plus years we've been able to have a significant impact and increase access to care for those around us, donating hundreds of thousands of dollars in free care as a result. While it created a significant amount of goodwill with my existing patients, I noticed that when I started featuring the events in my advertisements, it started drawing in new patients. When I asked a new patient how they heard about us, countless numbers of them told me that they had learned about our event and how they really empathized with the people we helped and wanted to support a dental office like ours that supported those in their community. In essence, by supporting us, they were playing a role in actively supporting those people in need.

Fear

Fear makes us cling to what's comfortable, what's safe, and what's sure. While you may be afraid to leverage fear in your advertisements because you are afraid that potential new patients may associate negative feelings with your practice and brand, the opposite is in fact true.

Studies show that eliciting fear allows your brand to be seen as the "one good thing" in a dark world. That means when their dental issues take a turn for the worse, potential new patients will look to you for help and for solutions to the problem at hand. Of all the things we could be afraid of, it's the fear created from Cialdini's scarcity principle and of what we stand to lose or have recently lost that really motivates people to take action today. For example, picture an image of a couple lying next to each other in bed, one spouse sleeping deeply and snoring their head off while the other lies wide awake as a result. That reminder of the loss of sleep can be a powerful motivator to influence that potential new patient to seek out an answer to their problem, for fear that they may never have a restful night of sleep again. Now they'll look to you and your sleep apnea therapies to solve their problem.

D. Color Content

While images and written text can make up the majority of our content, we can't forget color. Color plays an integral role in the way we comprehend the world around us. It saturates our language and has created a never-ending list of idioms such as "feeling blue," "caught red-handed," "black sheep of the family," or "little white lie." We use color to describe complex ideas such as emotions and character traits. It influences how we organize, identify, and interpret sensory information to help us form a better understanding of the world around us. Let's look at some facts behind the psychology of color.

- While a customer's assessment of a product is shaped in less than 90 seconds, between 62 and 90 percent of their judgment is based on color alone.
- Color impression is responsible for 60 percent of the acceptance or rejection of a product and comprises 80 percent of brand recognition.

- For 84.7 percent of consumers, color is the main reason for buying a particular product. For example, two-thirds of shoppers will not buy a large appliance if it doesn't come in their preferred color.
- Gender roles play a major part in color preferences, women being more receptive to tints, specific shades, and softer colors such as aqua blue while men tend to prefer more bold colors such as a dark navy blue.

What do the colors themselves represent to us?

- **Red:** It is the most emotional color. It increases your heart rate and creates urgency. That's why it's commonly used in clearance sales. In the medical world, red is associated with blood and danger. Ideal if your practice caters to patients having a dental emergency and in immediate need of care but not ideal if you're trying to promote a family-friendly mindset.
- **Blue:** The most commonly used color in today's branding and website design. From the dental world, Oral B's logo comes to mind. It's favored by 57 percent of men and 35 percent of women. It has come to stand for loyalty, wisdom, intelligence, and trust.
- **Green:** The color of nature. It symbolizes growth, harmony, freshness, and tranquility. It can be a popular color to use in a dental office whose focus is on getting patients to relax or to feel at ease.
- **Orange:** Combines the energy of red with the happiness of yellow. It implies ambition, enthusiasm, and confidence, which is why it's popular in health care marketing to highlight or accent your call-to-action offer.
- **Yellow:** The color of sunshine. It is associated with joy, happiness, intellect, and energy, which is why it's often used by brands to evoke cheerful feelings.
- **Black:** While popular in promoting technology, clothing, and cars, it's underutilized in health care marketing. When seen, it invokes a sense of power, authority, and elegance, making it a popular choice for marketing luxury products and services.
- **White/silver:** It is often associated with light, goodness, innocence, and perfection. It symbolizes safety and purity. Popular in health care marketing, this color is often associated with coolness and cleanliness. One of the most well-known brands that had success with this color is Apple.
- **Purple:** A popular color often used in health care marketing, this color combines the stability of blue and the energy of red. It's often associated with royalty and can symbolize power, nobility, luxury, and ambition.

Use the tips above to decide what colors will have the most impact on your target market by bringing their attention and focus to your messages, influencing them to want to respond.

E. Timing Their Stage of the Buying Cycle Journey

Now that you've put some thought into what visual, written, emotional, and color content can make up the body of your advertisement, you should add content that speaks to what stage your potential clients are in their buying cycle process. Think of it this way, unless there is some pressing emergency need, most potential new patients don't wake up in the morning and decide, "I'm going to find a new dentist today." Instead, they go through a process or journey that includes research and evaluation before committing and picking up that phone to make an appointment. In the marketing world, they call this the "buyer's journey." By understanding the three main stages of this buying cycle, we can tailor our content to better resonate to where our target market is on their path.

Awareness stage

The majority of potential new patients begin their journey here. While they most likely fit our target demographic, they are not usually aware of our office or the services we provide. At some point, something triggers a change in their mindset to where they become focused and aware of a problem that needs to be solved. It could be an immediate need such as a toothache that brings finding dental services top of mind. It could be something as simple as someone who has recently moved to your area, but six months have passed since their visit with their dentist back home, and they now realize they are overdue and focus their attention on finding a new dental office to call home.

If your marketing goal is to find those in this stage, you should tailor your content to provide answers to commonly asked dental questions about the service you're trying to promote or share research data and studies around the implications of poor oral health. For example, you could focus content on the oral systemic link and how the mouth, being the gateway to the body, can have a big impact on people's overall systemic health. Once your target market is aware of their problem and your content has let them know that you have potential solutions to that problem, they then move into the next stage of the buying cycle.

Consideration stage

At this stage, potential new patients are aware of a problem and know that you have a solution to address it, but they are unsure about whether you're the best option to help them solve it or not. At this point, people will begin doing heavy research into all of the available providers of the product or service. Questions they must satisfy before they'll schedule include: Will they like you? Do you have the expertise and training to solve their problem? Can they trust you?

Showing pictures of you with your satisfied, smiling patients while they hold signs that say, "I love my dentist" can go a long way to show them that people do like you, so maybe they will too. Highlighting the number of years you've been practicing, mentioning the different degrees, certifications, and dental academies you have memberships or fellowships in go a long way to show patients you have the expertise, training, and experience they may be looking for. Having Google, Facebook, Yelp, and other similar types of reviews and featuring those reviews in your content becomes important to help show them that people trust you. The more reviews you can showcase, the more you stand out over others they may be investigating. Showing before and after photos on patients who had similar problems to them can also go a long way to satisfy a potential new patient's comparison search of providers.

Decision Stage

At this stage, your potential new patient is ready to pick up the phone or get online to make an appointment at your office. Here is where it's critical to provide content that gives them enough detail on how they can do that. It should feature your office hours and days you're open for business. It should promote as many channels as you have available for them to make their appointment: by calling you, talking to you through a web chat portal, texting and emailing you, or going to your website to book their own appointment through an online scheduling tool. We have to let people communicate with us in the way they want to communicate with us, not the way we tend to force them, which is by only one way—calling our office to make their appointment.

F. "Map Your Content" Worksheet

Creating great marketing content starts with understanding your target market. You then shape your content through the use of different visual means, through written word or text, using color strategically, by adding items that elicit an emotional response and by providing information that connects with your potential new patient at every step of their buyer's journey. Use this worksheet to map out how your marketing content will look.

Map Your Content

Instructions: Use this worksheet to map out what content needs to be included with your advertisement.

- Written content
- Visual content
- Emotional content
- Color content
- Stage of buying cycle

Written Content

How much detail does your content need to contain?

1. Circle one: Which do you think your target market would prefer? Bullet points and pictures or headlines with more story-driven content and detail?

2. Circle one: Is your target market male, female, or both?

Video Content

What images, video, and/or memes can you use to:

- Create the ideal marketing mindset, e.g., a photo of a sunrise can create a mindset of change or symbolize a desire to try something new.
- Show/demonstrate social proof, e.g., before and after photos.
- Promote your authority, i.e., a logo or graphic of the number of years you've been in practice.
- Enhance your likeability, i.e., photos of yourself, your family, your hobbies, and interests.

Emotional Content

Your visual and written content should help you generate emotions. Check all that apply:

- [ ] Happiness
- [ ] Trust
- [ ] Sadness
- [ ] Fear
- [ ] Loss
- [ ] Anger
- [ ] Other: ____________

Color Content

Check all that apply:

- [ ] Red
- [ ] Blue
- [ ] Sadness
- [ ] Yellow
- [ ] Green
- [ ] Orange
- [ ] Black
- [ ] Silver/White
- [ ] Other: ____________

Stage of Buying Cycle

At what stage is your target market? Check all that apply:

- [ ] Awareness stage
- [ ] Consideration stage
- [ ] Decision stage

THE PHELPS® INSTITUTE

3

Figure 4. "Map your content" worksheet. Use this worksheet to help you define the content of your marketing piece. What text, images, video will you use? What colors and emotions to tap into? What stage of the buying cycle you are targeting that all speak to your target market?

Chapter 3
Define Your Call to Action

Once you have made decisions concerning the type of content you want in your marketing piece, it's now time to decide how to motivate people to respond. Your first option is to rely on your messaging and content to actively attract those with a top-of-mind awareness about a dental need or issue they are experiencing. Someone who has a toothache, for instance, is very aware of a problem they are having and doesn't usually need more motivation to seek care.

This is great if you run an emergency dental clinic and your target market is aware of their issue and actively seeking a solution to it. But what about the rest of the market? What about those who may be overdue for a preventative prophylaxis appointment, those who may not know they have a dental issue or who are aware of an issue but aren't actively seeking dental care at this time? For situations like these, you may want to consider using a call-to-action offer.

1. OFFERS

A call to action is the copy or graphic you use to entice and influence your readers to act. Including a persuasive call to action in your marketing efforts can help drive potential new patients to respond immediately. A call to action urges your readers and online visitors to do something at once, such as click a button, submit an email address, or call for an appointment. Some of the best calls to action come with placing an enticing offer they'll receive in exchange for taking a desired action. An example of this would be offering a new patient special or promotion that discounts the amount they'd normally spend at their first visit.

Why use a call-to-action offer? Numerous studies show that advertisements with call-to-action offers get higher response rates than those focused more on top-of-mind awareness. They motivate a broader audience by appealing both to those with an immediate awareness of their dental condition and those who are not aware. Let's look at some tips to maximize the responsiveness your offer can create.

- **Make it beneficial to your patients**: Most people enjoy getting something for doing what they know they need to do anyway. For example, my wife was in need of some gasoline/petrol to fill up her car and she had multiple stations in her area to choose from. While shopping for groceries, she learned that the grocery store had recently built a new gas station on-site for its customers. Because she was a loyal shopper, she had stacked up a significant number of loyalty points, which she found out she could use at this new gas station. In doing so, they offered to let her use her points in exchange for discounting the price of the fuel $1 per gallon, saving her $18 compared to paying full price for that fuel elsewhere. Because of this offer, she is more committed to shopping at this grocery store and has decreased her frequency at their competitive stores. Why? This store now brings more value. She gets something for doing what she was going to do anyway. Not only can she buy the food our family needs, but now she can buy that same food and save on gasoline. By offering them an incentive to choose your office over others, you're tapping into this same mindset.

- **Make it something they want**: Unless it's a life-or-death situation, people care more about acquiring the things they want versus the things they need. In our minds, our patients need dental care, but they may not necessarily want it. By offering them things they do want, we might be able to change their mindset and motivate more people to call your office to make their appointment today.

Let's look at a few different types of offers that tap into what patients want and what part they'll play in attracting both quantity and a better quality of new patients to your practice.

A. Monetary Discount

Overwhelmingly, this is the most popular offer used in US dental marketing today and is called the "$99 New Patient Special." Instead of collecting your full fee, say $265, for a comprehensive new patient exam, cleaning/prophylaxis, and bitewing x-rays, you offer these same services to new patients for only $99. This offer is targeted to patients who do not have dental insurance and thus would be paying out of pocket for these preventative services. In contrast, this seems like a great deal from the patient's perspective and usually motivates a significant quantity of people to pick up the phone and call to make an appointment. Unfortunately, there seems to be some challenges with the mindset of those who respond to this type of offer.

Price shopper

By focusing their attention on your discounted price instead of the relationship they could have with you and your team, you attract those who'll use price as their main criterion for making their purchases. When it comes to presenting any dental treatment that is needed, this could be a problem, one that manifests in two ways. The patient trying to negotiate with your team to get the price of your treatment down as much as possible or it will motivate them to call around to other dental offices and price-shop your treatment plan. The office that will do it for cheaper tends to be the one who gets their business.

Poor-quality new patient

While this special may generate a significant quantity of potential new patient calls, they are not generally of good quality. Quality to me means someone who pays my full fee, either through the use of dental insurance, a dental membership plan, or with cash, and it means that when they're due for their next cleaning in six months, they will be a repeat customer, not someone we've lost and now have to replace. With so many dental offices offering this $99 "New Patient Special," there are too many options available for patients to go elsewhere, so the patient attrition rates (PARs) tend to be extremely high as a result. A constant, high turnover means less ROI for your marketing dollars spent and more money required to replace these lost patients.

A loss leader that keeps losing

The patient attrition this type of special causes means that you still have to drive a significant number of new patients into the practice to maintain your marketing ROI and grow your practice. With every dentist in town offering the same special, patients start to look at dentistry and dental services as commodities like a hamburger. If all dental offices are essentially the same, that means that a crown is a crown or that a cleaning is a cleaning, anywhere they go. So why not look for the cheapest price to get these services?

To capture new patients, dentists and dental marketers have started competing on the price of their new patient special, continuing to decrease the amount so that they stand out from the crowd. As mentioned earlier, this is a race to the bottom that no one wins from. The $99 special suddenly dropped down and became a $79 special. The $79 special then became the $49 special. I've even seen this trend bottom out completely in some markets where the dentist is offering the exam, cleaning, and x-rays for free, giving away $265 in services and hoping that this person appreciates the deal and hoping that they return for their next cleaning or recommended dental services, only to find out that the challenges these monetary discounts create only grow the further down the commodity trail you go.

Too good to be true

The steeper these discounted specials become, the more they turn off a better-quality new patient, one who would pay your full fee in some capacity and who would return in six months for their next preventative treatment. These are people who tend to be turned off by these discounted specials because they seem too good to be true or have learned through time and experience that you get what you pay for. So if this offer seems like too good of a deal, there must be a catch, in a poor quality of service they'll receive, in their experience, or both.

To counter these mindset challenges and attract a better-quality new patient yet still use the power of monetary discounts to attract a significant quantity of callers, we should do the opposite of what everyone else is doing. If those in your market are offering a $99 special, then you should offer a $199 special. The better-quality patients prefer to receive a little something off the dental treatment that they know they need. They don't necessarily need or want half off or to have it for free. In contrast of our full fee of $265, getting all of that treatment for $199 will still be perceived as a good deal yet won't trigger the "too good to be true" mindset.

B. "Gift with Purchase" Offers

"Gift with purchase" offers have been around in the US marketing world since they were first introduced by Loreal cosmetics in 1946. The popular promotions offer the consumer a "free gift" upon completing a certain purchase. Many of you may be familiar with this technique and have seen it used by popular food franchises such as McDonalds who offer a free toy upon purchase of a Happy Meal. This type of offer is still popular today because they have a powerful influence to motivate customers to come your direction.

In the dental world, we've participated in this type of promotion by offering free tooth whitening to anyone who comes in to receive a new patient exam, cleaning, and x-ray. In comparison to the monetary discount offer, this type of promotion has some big advantages.

- Unlike monetary discounts, which are limited to patients without dental insurance, this offer is available to patients with or without dental insurance.
- It taps into the mindset of those who want to get a little something in exchange for getting the dental care they know they need. Instead of a monetary discount, they're getting some type of free gift with their purchase at your practice.
- You may end up giving away less than you would have by just discounting your treatment. If our full fee is $265 and you offer a $99 special, that means you're missing out on $166 of revenue. By offering a free tooth whitening package, your hard costs for the tray materials and whitening gel may cost you around $50. Assuming you collect the full $265 for your services, when you factor in the $50 cost of your offer, you're gaining $116 more in revenue that you would have missed out on by going the monetary discount route.

I have used "gifts with purchase" offers in my practices since its inception in 2003. In my first seven years of practice we offered free tooth whitening as the *Extreme Makeover* television show was at its height of popularity in the US and demand for tooth whitening was at an all-time high as a result. Once that demand diminished and the dental marketing market got saturated by every dentist offering some type of free tooth whitening, I changed my strategy and looked for something else I could give my patients that they might find value in. One of the most popular and one I still use to this day is offering a free Sonicare electric toothbrush with any paid dental exam, cleaning, and x-rays. Considered a luxury purchase item, these brushes would cost patients $100–$150 to purchase online or at a local retail store. By buying them in bulk, I was able to get the per-unit cost on these same toothbrushes to $44 each, still collecting my full fee but in essence only giving a $44 discount off the total visit.

C. Convenience Offers

A 2019 study reported that 81 percent of Americans have a smartphone, a statistic that has risen from 34 percent in 2011. With the rise of smartphone usage, the market has shifted its focus to making their purchasing decisions based on convenience. A report released by the National Retail Federation in January 2020 showed that 83 percent of consumers say convenience while shopping is more important to them now than it was 5 years ago. The report also found that 97 percent of respondents had backed out of a purchase because it was inconvenient for them. This explains the rise of popular services such as Amazon Prime, Instacart, and Uber Eats. If our potential new patients are using convenience as one of their factors to make a decision, then why don't we factor this into the offers we give them? In essence, help them "scratch two things off their to-do list."

One of the most popular convenience offers I've ever used revolved around a task that most of us have to deal with at some point but few actually have the time for, much less enjoy doing: washing our cars. The idea came to me when I was getting out of my car and walking up to the practice one day and a man stopped me and asked me if he could wash my car. He told me that he had a mobile car wash business and was set up with everything he needed to wash and detail my car right there in my parking lot. The price he wanted to charge seemed fair, so I thought I would help the man out and let him wash my car.

After a long day, it was time to head out to my car. Given how hectic that day had been, I completely forgot that this man had washed my car that morning. When I got to my car I was instantly reminded as my car had not been washed in well over six months, and thanks to the wondrous pollen of spring, it had a nice yellow color to it. My first instinct when I saw my car was amazement at how clean it looked as I'd almost forgotten the original color. My second thought was how much I appreciated the fact that it was now washed since I didn't really feel like I had the time to get this done, neither to wash it myself nor to go to a car wash facility and spend 20–30 minutes having someone else do it while I wait. This gave me the idea. If I appreciated the convenience of having my car washed while I was working, would potential new patients appreciate me taking this task off their plate?

Thus began what I now call my "Clean Teeth, Clean Car" promotion. With any paid new patient exam, necessary cleaning, and x-rays, I'd offer to wash and detail their car during their visit. I targeted days that had the largest open capacity at our practices, which were Tuesday, Wednesday, and Thursday. I negotiated a discounted rate with the owner of the mobile car wash business. Because of the volume of consistent business I was able to provide him, I was able to reduce the cost of washing a car and SUV by $10.

While I couldn't guarantee I'd have enough new patients each day to support him during this promotion, I could guarantee that I had someone who could get their car washed. My first priority was to give the car wash to any new patient who came in for the promotion. If we didn't have someone who specifically came in for this, then we'd offer it as a reciprocity gift to a different new patient who came in through other means. If there were no new patients that hour, then I'd offer it to one of our existing patients. If there were no takers from our existing patient pool, then I'd offer it to one of my team members. Ultimately, I guaranteed him 8 cars a day, which was two times what his best day usually averaged. I decided this was more of a seasonal promotion and chose those high pollen times of the spring and fall when people's mindsets might appreciate scratching this task off their to-do list.

When patients looked at other dental marketing pieces in our area, they all looked the same. When they looked at my advertisement and convenience offer, I wanted to give my target market something else to use to make their decision. "I can go to this office and get my teeth cleaned. Or I can go to this office, get my teeth cleaned as well as get my car washed and detailed! I'm going to do that."

With that mindset as my goal, I chose to try this promotion out in my newspaper insert ad as I could send it out one time and measure the response before committing to this offer for a longer period of time, which I would have to do in a billboard ad. We had over 35 new patients respond to this ad, specifically mentioning the car wash when they scheduled, an increase of 15 new patients from previous insert ads I'd used with offers such as free tooth whitening, which gave us a 10:1 ROI from these patients for this single campaign during a two-month time frame. We collected 100 percent of our preventative visit fee from these patients with the car wash costing me about $15 on average.

Of the 20 other new patients we gave the car wash too who did not come in through this promotion directly, 18 of the 20 moved forward with the recommended treatment given to them that day. Of the existing patients who received the car wash, over 90 percent reciprocated and left us a 5-star Google review that day about their experience with our practice.

People really appreciate it when you help them scratch things off their to-do list. I was reminded of this during that first campaign when one of the new patients received the car wash. After checking out at the front desk, she returned to her car and was so pleased that she came back into the office and asked if she could use our telephone since her cell phone had ran out of power. Curious about who she was calling, I asked her if everything was okay, to which she responded, "Everything is great. Remember we were talking earlier about my young children? Well I can tell you right now that my car has not been that clean in some time. I'm so happy that I'm going to call three of my friends and tell them that they have to come to this dental office. You guys are amazing!" Our offer led to three on-the-spot referrals. Convenience sells and is a powerful force we should not overlook in our marketing offers.

D. Reciprocity Offers

"Let other people's giveaways be your gift or offer." There are a vast amount of businesses offering deep monetary discounts to try to incentivize new customers to use their services. Many of these businesses have competed for price for so long, they now have to give away their service for free as a "foot in the door" strategy to try to attract new customers. One example that comes to mind is the maid or house/apartment cleaning industry here in the United States.

Many of these businesses are offering to spend 1–2 hours cleaning your residence for free in an effort to influence you to continue to use their paid service. Given how popular convenience offers such as these have been, the response they get has served many of them well but because of a poor conversion rate on retaining customers, they continually have to make this offer. Since these companies are committed to giving away this service, I decided to approach one and ask them if I could give their service away for them as well. I offered to promote their free home cleaning offer to all of my active patients as well as in my advertisements. All I asked them to do was to provide my patients with a great service and protect them from having a bad experience.

This is a great deal for the business as it extends their promotional network and increases the chances of attracting new customers but without it really costing them more to their marketing budget. This was a win for our advertising as I now had a new and unique offer I could make to attract more potential new patients my way. Thus began my "Clean Teeth, Clean House" promotion. Much like with the car wash, more patients chose to visit our practice to scratch another thing off their to-do list, only this time it didn't cost my practice anything for this offer. Timing wise, I pick times of the year where a person's mindset might better appreciate this type of gift I'd give them. Typically, during spring cleaning season as well as holiday times such as November, December, or January, when people's schedules are at their busiest and things like cleaning their home may fall through the cracks.

I once worked with a dentist in Kansas who was looking for advice on how to attract more implant patients. When I talked to him about letting other people's giveaways be your offer, he remembered an advertisement he had recently received at his home offering a percentage discount off your first meal at a newly opened Brazilian steakhouse. After our talk, he reached out to the manager of the restaurant and offered to promote their offer to his existing and potential new patients. While their offer was a percentage discount off their meal, I encouraged him to put a monetary value to it. In this case, that was $10 off their meal. Looking for any promotional opportunities, the manager eagerly accepted. After a few months of running this direct mail campaign and offer, I followed up with the dentist about the results. He reported that it had been the most successful offer and advertisement that he had done to attract more dental implant patients to his practice, working for him on two levels. First, for those who used the $10 off gift at the restaurant, they reciprocated by coming in as new patients. Secondly, for those who had dental issues that prevented them from eating the plentiful meats offered at the Brazilian steakhouse, they were touched that the doc offered them the $10 off and came in for consultations to see what it would take to get their teeth in a position that they could enjoy his offer and the fine meats at the steakhouse.

To find more of these potential opportunities, think about different services that you might appreciate if someone took care of most or all of the expense for you, those that have a convenience factor to them. Something that if you offered it to your potential new patients as a choice between getting their teeth cleaned elsewhere vs getting their teeth cleaned with you plus this other item, it might influence them to pay your full fee and choose your office instead. Once identified, look these businesses up online, look for their direct mail marketing pieces, and identify what they are currently giving away in their offers.

E. Offers: Rules of Thumb

a. **Give it to them when they want it**: Make sure your offer lines up with what your potential new patient is looking for today, not tomorrow or yesterday. Giving away free popsicles or ice cream treats to any child who comes in for a dental visit might be a great offer for parents to bring their child to see you during the warm summer months but may not be as enticing if you're trying to give this away when it's freezing cold outside. Not only what we offer is important but the timing of that offer can be just as important as well. Offering free tooth whitening as our offer made sense when you understand the demand for tooth whitening was at an all-time high in our country. Once that demand had passed, that meant it was time to shift my focus to find the next item that people might want to receive.

   Another factor to consider with timing is not only the current target market demand for an item, like we saw with tooth whitening, but also consider any seasonal aspect of your appeal. In my town, I found that the car wash offer worked really well at certain parts of the year, times when people's mindsets were more focused on keeping their car clean. Typically, this was during the spring months of March, April, and May as well as the fall months of August, September, and October. In the spring, there was a yellowish pollen, originating from the various pine trees that dominate our area. For months this pollen would continually cover cars, leaving them with a nice yellow hue. In the fall, ragweed pollen saturates the air, clinging to our vehicles to give them a light greenish color.

b. **Give people a choice of offers**: Different people may respond to different types of offers. Some may want a monetary discount like a free examination or consultation while others may be motivated by a gift with purchase such as receiving free tooth whitening when they come in for a new patient appointment. By giving people some choices, you're broadening the appeal and setting the stage for more people overall to respond to your marketing piece. My advice would be to have two or three offers at the most. Some could be focused on acquiring more hygiene patients while others may focus more on niche-type procedures such as dental implants or sedation dentistry. For example, with hygiene patients, I like to offer a choice of a nice Sonicare electric toothbrush or a Sonicare Airflosser when they come in for their new patient exam, cleaning, and x-rays.

c. **Make sure it's fresh**: With proper tracking, you'll know how effective your offers have been to attract new patients to your practice. Inevitably, if you market to a certain list or group of people long enough, they will become desensitized to the offers you're giving. Those who would have responded because of that offer, probably have already responded to that offer. To overcome this saturation, consider changing your offers with some type of regular frequency that makes sense for the medium you're marketing in. I prefer to change my offers quarterly because most of my direct mail campaigns will only be received by my target market one time during that three-month period.

   On the next go around, I may run with the same offer as I did before. Mostly to give those who didn't see the advertisement a second chance to see it and then hopefully respond to the offer in front of them. When it's time for them to receive my piece for a third time, I'd consider replacing those offers with something different. Keeping it fresh and changing gives you a chance to appeal to those who weren't attracted to your offer originally and increases your chances to incentivize them to respond during this next marketing cycle. The more who respond overall means the higher your ROI will be in return.

d. **Create urgency**: Cialdini's principle of scarcity teaches us that when resources are dwindling, limited, or about to disappear, it motivates us to want that item more and spend considerably more resources to get it. In marketing, we can leverage the scarcity principle in two ways: by limiting the amount of time people have to take action, for example, having a one-day sale, or by limiting the quantity of offers we're willing to share with people, with a message such as "Only five remaining spots". Both will motivate more patients to respond to your offer than if you didn't tap into this principle, but the first one does have more influence than the second one.

F. "Map Your Offer" Worksheet

Using what we've discussed thus far, you can use the worksheet below to map out what call to action offers you'd like to use in your marketing pieces, whether it be monetary discounts, "gifts with purchase" offers, offers of convenience, or items others are already giving away so that you can use them to motivate more of your target market to respond.

Map Your Offer

Instructions: Use this worksheet to choose what offer or offers you plan to use. Remember, the offer can affect the quantity and quality of the new patient you attract. Ultimately, your offer's goal should be to:

- Make it beneficial to your patient
- Make it something they want
- Give them a choice
- Create urgency

Which offer will you choose? Circle all that apply.

- Monetary offer
- Gift with purchase offer
- Convenience offer
- Reciprocity offer
- Authority offer

Monetary Offers:
1. $99-type discount special: Note: This is not recommended for those with little open chair time available as it can attract the "price shopper" mindset and lead to higher turnover rates.

2. Double everyone else's discount special: Instead of a $99 special, you might offer a $198 new-patient special. This Offer tends to attract a higher-quality patient and satisfies the "too good to be true" mindset discussed in the book.

3. Other:____

Gift With Purchase Offers:
Attracts someone with a "two-for-one" mindset "I can get my teeth cleaned and get XYZ as well!"

Examples:

1. Free tooth whitening
2. Free WaterPik®
3. Free Sonicare air flosser
4. Free Sonicare electric toothbrush
5. Free Oral-B® electric toothbrush
6. Other:____

As discussed in the book, remember to add this disclaimer to gift with purchase offers: *Offer good with any paid exam and necessary cleaning and x-rays.*

Convenience Offers:
Attracts those with a "scratch two things off my list" mindset: "I can go to that dental office and just get my teeth cleaned, but here I can get my teeth cleaned and get my car washed! That takes two things off of my to-do list."

Examples:

1. Free on-site car wash
2. Free pizza (dinner is on us!)
3. Other:____

Reciprocity Offers:
These are gifts they can receive but they don't actually have to come into your office to receive them. Those who use these offers will tend to reciprocate and become your patient. Remember, look for opportunities to let other people's giveaways be your offer!

THE PHELPS® INSTITUTE

4

Figure 5. "Map your offer" worksheets. Your offer can help determine the quantity and overall quality of the new patients who respond to your advertisements. Use this worksheet to help you choose what type of call to action you'll choose.

Cont'd

Map Your Offer

1. Free home-cleaning service
2. Free gift card at a local restaurant
3. Other:____

Authority Offers:
By default, these help promote you as an authority or as an additional expert from whom they are seeking advice and counsel.

1. Free/complimentary second opinion
2. Other:____

Create Urgency:
How can you create urgency with your offers?

1. Limit the time they have to get the offer, e.g., this month only or today only.
2. Limit the quantity of the offers you'll make available, e.g., offer available to the first 5 who respond and schedule an appointment.

If you limit the quantity, what ethical concession can you make to others who respond after the fact?

For ex., offering a free Sonicare electric toothbrush to the first 5 who respond and then you offer an Oral-B® electric toothbrush to the 6th, 7th, 8th+ patient who respond.

What will your ethical concession be when you give away all of the main offer?

THE PHELPS® INSTITUTE

5

Figure 5. Cont'd

Chapter 4
Make Your Marketing More Effective

A research study once showed that the average American is bombarded with over three million marketing messages a year. This was a study done before the age of the smartphone, and current studies put that number of exposures above 10 million per year. On top of these thousands of daily exposures, think of all of the decisions you have to make on a daily basis. 100, 1000? That's during the workday. It doesn't count all of the family decisions you have to make when you get home. Now, how many things are on your to-do list right now?

How does our brain process all of this information and stimuli? The short answer is that it doesn't. In a popular research study by Dan Simons and Christopher Chabris at Harvard University, they found that 75 percent of the information that comes in through our eyes and ears is completely ignored by the brain, meaning it doesn't reach the logic center of rational, conscious thought. With too many things to absorb and focus on, the brain has learned to become very selective about what grabs its attention and what it lets in.

The lessons learned from their findings are simple. What grabs and holds our attention, we see. What doesn't, we don't see. That's why the goal of your marketing is to first grab your potential new patient's attention and then have your message motivate them to want to schedule an appointment at your office. Without that attention, your marketing has little chance to be effective. So what other elements can we incorporate into our advertising to set the stage that our marketing efforts grab people's attention?

1. CIALDINI'S PRINCIPLES TO ADD INFLUENCE TO YOUR MARKETING

To aid us in this area, we can lean on the behavioral science research of Dr. Robert Cialdini. Dr. Cialdini is Regents' Professor Emeritus of Psychology and Marketing at Arizona State University. As mentioned earlier, he is the author of the *New York Times* best-selling books *Influence: The Science & Practice*, *Influence: The Psychology of Persuasion*, and *Pre-suasion*, which collectively have sold over 5 million copies worldwide. He is known globally as the foundational expert in the science of influence and how to apply it ethically in business.

I first met Dr. Cialdini after attending a two-day seminar in Arizona that centered on his research. Learning about the behavioral science research that went into his discovery and being able to apply those teachings to my dental practices was invaluable. After a year of study under him, I was awarded the title Cialdini Method Certified Trainer, which you may have noted is the CMCT credentials you'll see listed after my name and dental degree.

One of the main lessons I learned by working with Dr. Cialdini and understanding his six principles of persuasion is that they are powerful tools to consciously and unconsciously grab people's attention and guide them to say yes to any request made. In short, the busier we become, the more distracted we are by the technology available to us at our fingertips, and the more we lean on Cialdini's six principles to make our decisions. By incorporating these principles into our marketing efforts we're now more likely than ever to capture people's attention, reduce their uncertainty about what dentist they should choose, and motivate them to want to schedule an appointment with us. Let's look at some ways we can use these principles to add more influence to our marketing.

A. Principle of Reciprocity

This principle states that we feel obligated to give back to those who've given to us. It's not about giving people conditional items such as rewards or incentives. Our new patient toothbrush offer is a great example of this. While we call it a new patient "gift," it's actually a reward. They first have to perform a task, and then they get the reward. With our toothbrush offer, to receive it, they have to come into our office and get a new patient exam, cleaning, and x-rays.

A true gift is given on the front end of an interaction with someone, and there are no strings attached. With gifts, I want you to think about some tangible gifts you could give to potential new patients. When we discussed letting other people's giveaways be your gift or offer, these are true examples of reciprocity in action. Your potential new patient doesn't have to come into your office to receive the gift certificate for $10 off at the Brazilian steakhouse. Instead, the gift is right there in the advertising piece. All they have to do is clip it off, take it into the restaurant, and use it, but because you were the one who gave it to them, those who appreciated it will feel the need to reciprocate. That means when it's time for them to seek out dental care, you'll come top of mind in their search and are now likely to attract them to your office.

While physical, tangible gifts such as gift cards and certificates can work well to create the reciprocity effect, so too can indirect gifts, things you may have already given to others that someone might appreciate or find value in and want to be a part of. I mentioned earlier that my offices host an annual day of free dental care for our community, offering free extractions and gross debridement cleanings to those who can't afford it. Over the years of doing these events at my offices, the amount of dental care we donated to our community continued to rise. This was a gift we gave to our community, but I was surprised at how much pride our existing patient base took from our efforts. Time after time I'd hear them thank us for doing those events for the community and how they were glad that indirectly supporting us a patient helped to support those in need as well.

As I've said before, when your market speaks, you need to listen. If my existing patient felt this way, how many more potential new patients could we attract who might feel the same? So as part of my messaging in my direct mail campaigns, I'd use the headline: "Carolinas Dental Center (CDC) Continues to Give to Our Community." In the content I'd show pictures of the people standing in long lines for these events, waiting to get the free care. I'd share with them how much money we'd donated over the years to those in need and then invite them to be a part of that giving. "We've donated over, $600,000 in dental care to our community on behalf of the doctors, our team, and our patients. If you'd like to be a part of this continued gift, we invite you to become one of our patients. Supporting us means you're playing a part in supporting our community."

Countless times when I talked to new patients at the chair and asked them how they heard about us, I'd hear them tell me how moved they were by our free dental care day and how they wanted to be a part of supporting their community. Think about what gifts you can give your potential new patients in your marketing efforts to grab their attention and influence them your direction.

B. Principle of Liking

As stated earlier, people like to do business with people they like. More specifically, they like to do business with those who are like them, who have similarities, commonalities, or other shared interests. It helps build a connection between two parties who are unfamiliar with one another. The more connections we have established, the more likely they are to say yes to our requests.

In marketing, there can be a challenge to establish these connections as the person isn't directly in front of you, limiting the number of questions that you could ask to identify those shared interests. Our only option at this point is put as much information about ourselves and our teams into our marketing pieces that we feel comfortable sharing. This could be a video hosted on our website, lead generation landing page, or social media channels. It could be in written form as biographies or show pictures of the doctor and team.

Your goal is to highlight as many areas as you can so that whoever is reading might be able to find a connection with you. For instance, I may share that I have two boys, that I enjoy playing tennis, and that we have a family dog. Someone who has kids, plays tennis, or has a dog and reads this or hears it in a video message will discover that we have some commonality. It will influence them to like us more automatically compared to other dental advertisements that chose instead to solely focus on the products and services they offer.

If you take your staff out for team-building events in your community, there may be opportunities to leverage this principle. On several occasions, I purchased tickets to our local professional football team, called the Carolina Panthers. I'd hire a group that would set up a staging area for us, and we'd tailgate by enjoying food and beverages before the game started. We had custom signs made up detailing how our dental office supports our local team, and throughout the event and game we'd record video and take photos as a group.

Often, I'd place the videos on our website and social media pages while substituting the standard profile photos of our doctors or team members in our advertisements for these more fun team outing event shots. These photos were unique and unlike anything others in our market were using in their marketing pieces. It showed patients that our office supports our local team and that we like to have a good time together. When talking with new patients about why they chose us, I'd often hear them say how they really liked our photos at these games, how they were fans of that team, and these pictures showed them that we weren't going to be the kind of office that was cold, unwelcoming, and sterile like most dental offices they had encountered. Instead, it showed them that we were just the opposite, that we liked to have a good time and that this was the type of office they wanted to be a part of.

By putting yourself out there, sharing the hobbies, interests, and family stories of you and your team, you're allowing potential new patients to find a connection with you. When you connect, you grab their attention and set the stage for more to respond to your advertisement. It's these small little things we do that sometimes can stack up and make a huge difference in the results our marketing can deliver.

C. Principle of Authority

One of the most popular general dentists on Instagram today is Amanda Seay, DDS, FAGD, FAACD. Dr. Seay graduated from dental school in 2002 and is a multi-practice owner near Charleston, South Carolina. She is founder of the imP.R.E.S. dental training institute and a clinical instructor at the world-famous Kois Center. She is the director of outreach for the Seattle Study Club and is a board member, examiner, and accredited fellow at the American Academy of Cosmetic Dentistry. In the world of cosmetic dentistry, it's hard to find someone who she hasn't had an influence on, having spoken both nationally and internationally on cosmetic dentistry and residing as editor of the restorative section of the magazine *Inside Dentistry*. Combined, these media reach over 20,000 dentists nationwide.

While having a significant presence on Facebook and LinkedIn, she has built a following of over 15,000 dentists on Instagram, all looking to Dr. Seay for her expert opinion and advice in dental photography techniques, cosmetic dentistry, dental materials, and how she balances her distinguished career with a successful home life as she is also a mother of four children. Through her actions, articles published, podcast interviews, Instagram posts, and mentoring of young dentists over the years, she's earned the respect of her colleagues and is viewed as a true authority that dentists around the world look to for advice. But why is that? Why do we look to people like Dr. Seay for advice and mentorship?

The reality is that while we are all smart, educated people, we don't have time to become experts in every subject or area we come across. That's why we look at trustworthy experts such as Dr. Seay as our authorities for advice, to tell us what we should do in that given situation or circumstance. So translating this into the dental marketing space, our goal is to use certain words, phrases, and pictures that signify that we have expertise in the subject matter being discussed and that we can be trusted.

Here are some ways you can highlight your expertise:

- **Years in practice**: Notice in Dr. Seay's biography, I mentioned that she'd been practicing for over 18 years. By highlighting how many years you've been in dentistry, you're telling patients that you have experience. The longer you've been practicing implies you have more experience and wisdom than those who haven't been practicing as long. Create a badge or logo to promote that fact. A logo that can be used on all of your advertising media, website, social media channels, and other influence touch points such as your appointment cards. To keep from having to update this logo annually, I like reporting it in 5-year increments. "5+, 10+, 25+ years serving this community."

- **Credentials**: Christopher Phelps, DMD, CMCT. Amanda Seay, DDS, FAGD, FAACD. Dr. XYZ DDS, MAGD, MAACD. These are all examples of highlighting your degrees, fellowships, or masterships in different dental academies and certifications, all of which show you've had a higher level of training than those who don't have these credentials.
- **Awards**: In 2016, I was nominated by one of my colleagues for the Doctor's Choice National Dental Award. Out of 6000 other dentists who were nominated, I was selected as the winner. Given this award was voted on by my fellow dental colleagues, I was truly honored. In 2018, they honored me again as the national dental award winner. In 2021 I was selected as one of the top 100 dentists in the world. I don't bring these awards up to brag or boast about my accomplishments but instead to highlight that these awards do have influence in the eyes of our potential new patients. Maybe you've been nominated for awards similar to these or for some local consumer voted awards such as a "Top Doc" in your city. If so, you're missing an influence opportunity by not highlighting this fact in your marketing pieces.

By highlighting your years of experience, your training, certificates, and other credentials along with any awards you've achieved, you're using these items to present you as a dental expert in your region, a true dental authority, one that patients may choose for their care over other dentists and dental ads that don't highlight these features. While all of these aspects are important to influencing more new patients your direction, patients still need to know they can trust you.

In marketing, this is not an easy thing to accomplish as trust is usually one of those things that is built in person and over time. Let's look at some ways you can overcome this trust hurdle:

- **Years in practice**: Pointing out the number of years you've been practicing does help as the longer you've been practicing typically implies you are good, honest, trustworthy company. You've stood the test of time because you could be trusted.
- **Celebrity endorsements**: People look to certain celebrities as a trusted source for information and advice. So if a celebrity is endorsing you and your practice, it shows the community that they trust you, influencing more of their fans to then trust you as well. Let's look at a nationwide celebrity example such as Oprah. Do you know who Dr. Phil is? Well, Dr. Phil wouldn't be the most followed psychologist on Twitter today or have had the career he had without Oprah endorsing him as her authority in the area of psychology and counseling on her popular television show. You could also use local celebrities to tap into this principle like I did with two popular local radio hosts, Matt and Ramona. Countless patients told me they selected our practice because of the recommendations they gave out on their radio program. Another example might be paying to sponsor a local or professional sports team. "Dentist for the Charlotte Hornets Basketball Team," for example. Even though these are paid endorsements, they still have influence on attracting the attention and trust of potential new patients.
- **Patient reviews**: When patients give their review, they are testifying about why they trusted you as their dentist and are taking a stand on why others should trust you as well. That's why it's imperative to create a great customer experience to influence people to want to give you these reviews. Each one is fuel you can add to amplify the influence of all of your marketing endeavors.

- **Professional patient reviews**: To take these reviews a step further on the influence scale, highlight reviews or testimonials from other medical/dental colleagues. When a patient reads a review from Dr. XYZ MD, it tells them that there is someone who is educated at a similar level as you are who trusts you for their dental care. This signifies that not only does someone trust you, but this is someone with real expertise in that area who trusts you as well. When it comes from another professional within your industry, people tend to put more emphasis and importance on it as a result.

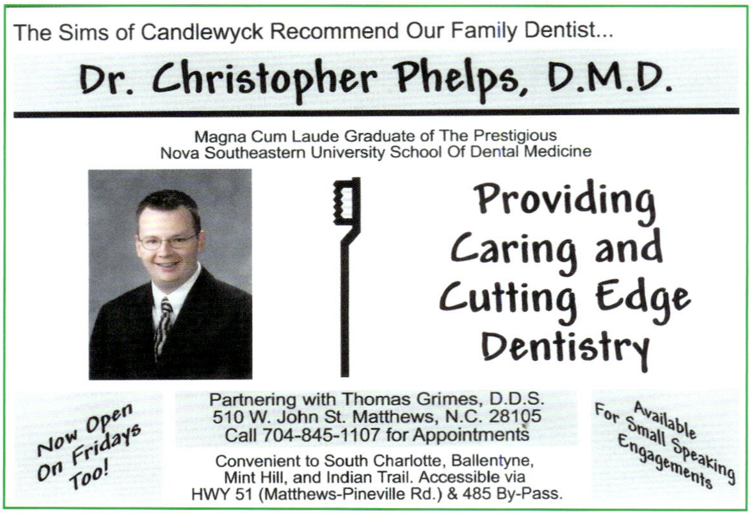
The Sims of Candlewyck Recommend Our Family Dentist...
Dr. Christopher Phelps, D.M.D.
Magna Cum Laude Graduate of The Prestigious
Nova Southeastern University School Of Dental Medicine
Providing Caring and Cutting Edge Dentistry
Now Open On Fridays Too!
Partnering with Thomas Grimes, D.D.S.
510 W. John St. Matthews, N.C. 28105
Call 704-845-1107 for Appointments
Convenient to South Charlotte, Ballentyne,
Mint Hill, and Indian Trail. Accessible via
HWY 51 (Matthews-Pineville Rd.) & 485 By-Pass.
Available For Small Speaking Engagements

Figure 6. **My first self-designed dental advertisement.**

In Figure 6, you'll find the first advertisement I ever produced back in 2003. I designed it myself on Microsoft Publisher and submitted it as a paid advertisement in the monthly neighborhood newsletter where my wife's parents lived. As a recent graduate of dental school, I need to create some authority triggers to build trust with potential new patients, hopefully allowing them to overcome the fact that I was right out of school and had limited patient experience at that point.

Note that I mention the name of my in-laws at the top of the ad. Given this was their community and were well known and liked, I wanted to draw on that association. I put the only award and real credential I had at the time, which was that I graduated in the top 5 percent of my dental school class. I put it out there that I was available for speaking engagements, a fact that got me several speaking opportunities in my local community and started to show me the power of how these grassroots efforts can attract more new patient to the practice. I also highlighted some scarcity or uniqueness that we were open up on Fridays. In that time, we were only one of two offices in a 10-mile radius who were open on this day.

While this piece may look and seem simple in its design, because it leveraged several of the principles of persuasion, it produced a very successful outcome, helping me attract enough new patients that year to help double the revenue of the practice.

D. Principle of Social Proof

Sometimes called the consensus principle, this one is all about the masses. Social media has become a huge part of our daily lives and focus. We are constantly checking sites such as Facebook, Twitter, and Instagram to see what others are up to. That's why social proof information is one of the strongest influencers in marketing today. We can't help but be persuaded by what others around us are doing.

When I left for work this morning, it was cloudy and rainy outside. When I headed out, I did not have my headlights turned on because there was little rain happening in that moment and it was light enough that I didn't feel like I needed them to see properly. During the drive I noticed that every car around me had their headlights turned on. Those going my direction and those going the opposite way as well, and by the time I got to work I noticed that I had unconsciously turned my lights on as well. Why did I do this?

It was because of this principle, which states that many times we look to the behavior of others to tell us or show us what we should be doing as well. Evolutionarily, it's so engrained in our unconscious decision-making because it's a protective mechanism. If the majority of those around us are doing something, then it could mean a danger situation is present. Like fish schooling and moving in unison for safety, if one stands out from the group it could set them up to be injured or eaten by a predator. This is why many don't like to be the first to step out and try something new, something few have done before because it's unknown what could happen.

Even though our brains have developed and we've become more educated, we are still heavily influenced by what others around us are doing. This fact is especially true in times of uncertainty. You've pulled up to an area where you want to eat. You see two restaurants that on the surface have a lot in common. Same location, same type of food and drinks offered, yet one restaurant has a line of people outside waiting to get in, and the other is empty. Which one do you think you might choose?

When we have questions or doubts about a situation or decision to be made, we look to the evidence of what those around us are thinking or have done to guide us. Choosing a new dentist or dental home can be an extremely difficult decision for patients to make. "Will they like me? Will I like them? Are they the best one to take care of my smile?" These are the thoughts running through our potential new patients' minds when making their decisions. If they don't see evidence that others are frequenting or have frequented our office, then it may make them question whether they should as well.

That's where we can leverage social proof to change that mindset, by sharing information that highlights that people have frequented our office, they are engaging in our social media posts, and are actively choosing us for their dental care. But what information can we share?

Pictures

I love getting my patients together and taking pictures with them. First, I love doing this because it strengthens my relationship with them. It shows them that we like them, are proud they are our patient, and want to showcase that fact. Second, I love it because the more pictures we have, the more people we can show in those pictures and the more social proof evidence we have to use in our marketing materials.

I may have a single picture of a new patient with their hygienist, one where the hygienist has a sign that states she's with a new patient and where the patient is holding up a sign that states how much they love their new hygienist. When I group 4 or 5 of these photos together in an advertisement, it speaks two truths to a potential new patient who sees it. First, they will see a connection. Here is a new patient, just like they'd be if they came to our practice, and look how much this person already loves their hygienist. Second, when they see multiple examples of this, it further reduces their uncertainty by saying, "Look how many new patients that go there love their new hygienist. Maybe I'll have a great experience here and love them too!"

When I can group lots of patients together, it only serves to magnify the influence social proof will have. This could be during one of my many patient appreciation parties or on days when we provided free dental care for our community and the demand for our services was a line that was wrapped around our building. Earlier I spoke of one of the most successful ads I ran, which was in an active, independent living retirement community magazine. After holding a contest at this community, I was able to get a large number together who had become my patients (see Fig. 3). With their permission, I made this photo the bulk of my one-page advertisement in this magazine. In doing so it showed potential new patients some important information to grab their attention. "Look how many people, who live right here in this community chose this office for their dental care. Look how happy they are. I need to find a good dental office, and if that many people choose them, maybe I'll be safe choosing them as well."

After a few months of running this version of the advertisement, our new patient numbers from this medium increased by 35 percent. All because the photo was able to capture their attention. Once we had their attention, we had a chance to influence them in our direction.

Numerous testimonials

As we mentioned above, a single testimonial or review, whether in written or video from, speaks to your trustworthiness as a dental care provider. Liking you is one thing, but if patients don't trust you, they don't move your direction. To increase the effect these reviews can offer us, instead of placing a single testimonial on our advertisement, we should try bundling them together into groupings of four or more, depending on the amount of space we have available to use.

If we have a significant number of reviews, we should add them all up and report that number. After each of our patient appointments, we had an automated program that would send out an email request for patients to fill out a review about our office and rate us as to their experience. While these weren't featured on Google, Yelp, or any other popular review site, they were still valuable, so I copied each review and featured them on our website. In addition, I copied and pasted all other reviews we had from Facebook, Google, and Yelp and pasted them on our website as well. In total, we had over 700 five-star reviews on our website, a number I wanted to share to our existing patients to influence more people to give us a review but also in our ads to show people that a large number of patients choose us for their dental care, so maybe they should consider doing so as well.

If we have reviews from multiple trusted sources, we should share that fact as well. People trust review sites such as Google, Yelp, Facebook, and Healthgrades and look to them to gather the information they'll use to make their decision. If you have reviews spread out across several or all of these platforms, you'd be bungling an opportunity to not share that fact with your patients. One office I worked with down in Ft. Lauderdale, Florida, was able to increase their new patient count by 23 percent from a newsletter campaign after they updated it with the following information: To read over 180 five-star reviews found on Google, Yelp, Facebook, and Healthgrades, check out our website. This was a small change that led to a big increase in their new patient count and thus ROI from this medium.

Surveys and other statistics

Many of you may be familiar with Trident gum. Trident is a sugar-free type of chewing gum, and since the 1960s they've successfully used the slogan: "4 out of 5 dentists recommend Trident" as part of their marketing messaging to differentiate themselves against other types of sugar-based chewing gum available in the marketplace. In their original survey, Trident only interviewed 5 dentists. They didn't do a nationwide survey of all dentists, yet the influence impact to the consumer was the same. What people interpreted from this slogan was that when surveyed, the majority of dentists would recommend this gum over others. Not being dental experts but wanting a gum that was safe for them to chew, this consensus information influenced many to choose Trident over their competitors. The fact that Trident still uses this as part of their current day messaging, some 60 years later, is a testament to the power social proof has on our buying decisions.

To leverage this idea in my dental practice, I used an automated program that sent a satisfaction survey to our patients immediately after their visit with us, as I previously mentioned. One of the questions I placed in that survey related to referrals when I asked: "Would you or have you referred someone to our office? Yes or No?" The more surveys returned only served to elevate the influence power. At one time, we had amassed over 697 survey responses with 96.7 percent of people reporting that they would have or had referred patients to our practice.

Armed with this consensus data, I decided to place it on our appointment cards to highlight to those who had not referred to our practice yet that many already have or plan on doing so, influencing them to the next thought of, "If that many others have referred, maybe I should too!"

Another way to leverage this principle comes when you are highlighting your most popular option available for different procedure options in your marketing pieces. Studies show that when you point out what a majority of others have chosen in a similar situation, this influences 14–21 percent more people to choose the same path for themselves. In a newspaper insert ad, for instance, I might highlight the different types of implant-based edentulous arch treatments that are available, from "snap in" implant supported overdentures to "fixed" implant retained appliances, showing pictures of each appliance to demonstrate what all is involved. If the majority of my patients choose a fixed, titanium hybrid solution that I can accentuate by placing a "Most Popular" icon above it, in doing so, I'm more likely to attract patients who want to specifically learn more about that option.

Remember, if people don't have evidence that others have said yes to your request or moved your direction, they may be resistant and feel like they are the first. That uncertainty typically leads to inaction. If you have evidence of what a large number or majority have done or are doing, if it's a behavior you want to see more of, then you should share that information with others like them and counter that inaction. In doing so, you'll leverage the principle of social proof, grab your potential new patients' attention, and guide more of them your direction.

E. Principle of Consistency

In *Influence: The Science & Practice*, Dr. Cialdini described an experiment done at a horse racing facility. In this study, they surveyed participants and asked them how confident they were that the horse they were about to place a wager or bet on was going to win the race. After they had placed their bet, a different group of researchers interviewed them and asked them the same question they had before placing their wager: "How confident are you that the horse you selected is going to win the race?" Despite the short amount of time that passed between when the questions were asked, respondents were significantly more confident that their horse was going to win after they had committed to the bet. Why do you think this occurred?

It turns out that the more committed we are to something, the more value we place on it. That's why this principle states that when people make a real commitment by taking a stand on an issue or putting some type of effort or resources into it, there is a lot of social and internal pressure on them to stay consistent with the commitment they have made. Before the participants had made their wager, they weren't truly committed to believing that their horse would be the winner. They thought it might be, they hoped it could win, but they weren't really committed to the idea that it would win. Once they had made their wager, making that small commitment to this ideal, it changed their mindset and their belief system, influencing them to be more confident with the decision they had made. Otherwise, why would they have put real money down if they weren't committed to the idea that their horse was going to win?

In dental marketing, this is probably the most difficult principle to engage. To initiate this principle, you have to get the person to commit to something, to take an action within the dynamic of the ad itself. For static advertisements such as a direct mail piece, radio, or TV ads, this is next to impossible to accomplish. With digital advertisements, it becomes a little easier. Within your ad you could have a white paper for patient education on the "Top 5 Dental Issues Affecting Your Teeth" with a call-to-action request to download and read now. By getting them to download your paper and take this one small step, they are now more committed to improving their oral health, a small move that should bring them one step closer to seeking your office for their care.

Another popular way to use this principle in dental marketing, especially with the lead generation medium, is by creating an assessment or quiz for potential new patients to take. The questions asked in this test will further their commitment to improving their oral health with each question answered, ultimately, motivating them to want to take action. Those who commit to take and complete this quiz are now more likely to schedule an appointment with you than those who don't.

Using this principle, we can place small commitment steps for potential new patients to take. For example, "Schedule a virtual consult," "Click here for more info," "Answer these questions to see if you're a candidate," or "Download this e-book." Each action they take changes and increases the perceived value on the subject matter they are committing to, everything leading to them to want to stay consistent and continue on the path that they started to travel down. If staged properly, all paths should lead back to you and scheduling an appointment at your office.

F. Principle of Scarcity

Of all of the principles, this one has been leveraged the most throughout the advertising industry. Why? Because it's a powerful motivator for action. In essence, this principle tells us that things appear more attractive when their availability is limited or we risk losing the opportunity to acquire it. It's a principle that can instill powerful emotions in people, namely fear such as FOMO, or fear of missing out. It's a fear of missing out on resources that has an evolutionary base to it. Running out of food or water could be a life-or-death situation, so we always prefer to have information that these are running out well before they actually do. While time has progressed and our struggle to maintain resources for life have diminished, the anxiety concerning the loss of any resource has persevered.

Let's look at some ways to use this principle in dental marketing:

Promoting dental services

Focus your advertising content and messaging on what they stand to lose or what they've already lost the ability to do. When trying to promote dental implants, instead of showing pictures of the anatomy of a dental implant, which could scare more patients away, you could focus on the problem the patient is facing, a problem that your dental implant services could solve for them.

Maybe there it's a social problem they have, being concerned by how lose their dentures are that they may fall out when talking or eating among friends. Perhaps they have a functional problem you could address? Having less teeth than before has now compromised their ability to eat certain foods.

Perhaps you'd like to do more sleep apnea treatment cases? If so, you could speak to your target market's lack of sleep, showing a picture of a couple in bed, one sleeping soundly while the other one is wide awake due to the loud snoring occurring next to them.

What if that patient had a situation that isn't readily apparent today but is something that would have a consequence if no action or treatment was taken? Early in my career I had a patient who was in the early stages of orthodontic relapse. She had stopped wearing her removable retainer for about a year, and during her exam I noted that she was developing an anterior open bite and her mandibular anterior teeth were starting to shift in their position. When I showed this patient a mirror and pointed out these areas, I asked her if she was concerned about their appearance. To the untrained eye, these changes were small, so her natural response was that it didn't concern her, even though I warned her about the changes that would continue if she didn't move forward with a new retainer.

About 10 years later, this patient was now back in my chair and wanted a consultation about Invisalign's clear aligner system to straighten her teeth. We took photos that day and compared them to photos we had taken of her smile 10 years before. As predicted, her teeth had completely relapsed. At this point, her priorities had shifted. What originally had been a dental need in my mind had now become a want in hers. The plan was simple. She'd need comprehensive aligner treatment with an estimated cost of $5700.00 and approximately two years of time. The patient remarked how she remembered that I had warned her about this happening some years ago and that she wished she had done something sooner to address it. As such, she happily accepted our treatment plan and moved forward with impressions that day to start.

Immediately preceding this interaction, I moved down the hall to complete a new patient comprehensive exam. After completing my exam, I had identified several areas where orthodontic relapse was starting to occur, a situation very similar to what my previous patient had been in years before. With both patients' permission, I decided to introduce them to each other and highlight this fact. After an introduction, I asked the new patient sitting in the operatory chair to smile for us. Right on cue my existing patient spoke up and remarked: "Yes, that's exactly what my smile looked like ten years ago." I then turned to that existing patient and asked her to share her smile today. When she did, I noticed the patient in the chair was taken by surprise at how much her smile had changed over the years.

Thanking them both for allowing me to make the introduction, the existing patient went back to taking impressions for her comprehensive Invisalign treatment. When I sat back down with new patient, using a mirror I pointed out to her some of the relapse issues I saw developing. I let her know that her first option was to do nothing and continue, but in doing so her relapse would worsen, and in 5–10 years it could look like the patients smile she just saw, costing her a significant amount of money and time to treat. I then asked her an important commitment question: "Does this concern you?" Immediately the patient told me that it did and she did not want her teeth to shift and end up like the smile she had just seen. I then reviewed her short-term orthodontic aligner therapy treatment options, and the patient started treatment that day.

From that day on, I've used those before photos showing minor, almost unperceived issues compared to the after photos showing full relapse in all of my marketing efforts moving forward, sharing the patient's testimonial about this cautionary tale. By using the scarcity principle and focusing people's attention to what they could be missing out on in the future, their current smile and tooth positions, I was able to increase the interest and case acceptance of our clear aligner therapy by over 40 percent that year.

Promoting your busy schedule

Sometimes you or your capacity to get patients into your office can be the scarce resource. If you are busy, if you have limited capacity or availability to get patients in the door, you can use the power of scarcity and promote that fact by saying, "We have limited appointments available."

Promoting what makes you the scarce resource

Earlier in the book we talked about finding things that make you unique, things that you do or your team does that few in your office or area perform. For one of my hygienists, that was promoting that she was the only hygienist of the four in our office who had experience using a Prophy Jet to clean people's teeth. Highlighting her unique feature actually led a new patient choosing our office because she was searching for an office or someone who could use that Prophy Jet on her. Earlier, I discussed another example when I discovered that I was only one of three offices in the entire state of North Carolina that offered every level of sedation dentistry, offering laughing gas and valium as an anxiolytic therapy to oral conscious sedation to having an in-office dental anesthesiologist perform IV and general sedation at the practice. Being only one of three such offices meant we were a scarce resource as all others who were promoting sedation dentistry for general dentistry services provided only oral conscious sedation. To showcase this fact in my ads, I used the square peg and the round hole analogy to contrast this difference and what made our office unique and scarce.

Promoting end-of-the-year events

In the United States, one of the busiest times for a dental practice comes at the end of the year. Typically, dental insurance plans will provide an annual allotment of money that they will pay toward a patient's treatment during that calendar year. This amount can range between $1000 to $2000. The good news about this is that when the policy resets around January 1, that total amount they'll pay resets and in theory could be used each year the policy is active if problems continue to occur. The bad news about this policy is that if our patients don't use their insurance allotment in that calendar year, they lose it. It doesn't carry over and add to the next year's benefit. The scarcity of this potential loss is the rationale behind why our chairs are in high demand in those last few weeks of the year. To capture the benefit of this end-of-the-year scarcity effect, you should actively market this fact both internally to your existing patients and externally in whatever marketing media you are using. The is key is not to wait until the end of the year to share this information but instead to get this "Use it or lose it" message out to patients in early September or October, making them aware sooner and giving them time to get into your office and do something about it before it's too late. Doing so, you can use the scarcity effect to expedite the momentum you'd normally see and keep your chairs at maximum capacity for a longer period of time.

Promoting urgency

In the offer section, I talked about how you can use scarcity to motivate more people to take action. You can do this in two ways: Limiting the time period that you make your offer available, with "Only Available For 24 Hours" or "One Day Only," having the most influence compared to those offers available for longer periods of time; otherwise, we can do this by limiting the quantity of the offers you'll make available for interested patients to attain. Let's look at how these two differ.

One I've used with great success is offering a $500 discount off Invisalign clear aligner orthodontic therapy. Instead of offering this discount throughout the whole year, I would limit the offer to a single month of the year. The problem with a limited time offer is that it still implies that people have time. Maybe not a lot of time, but they don't necessarily have to put down what they are doing and act right now. If they don't act now, that means they could get distracted with some other life event or situation that may prevent them from ever responding to your advertisement.

Instead, I decided to limit the quantity of the available offer, to make it a really good deal for small number of people. By limiting the quantity of the offer, you significantly increase the competition element present, further increasing the desire the scarcity effect would have on them for this item. With my standard $500 off Invisalign treatment offer that was limited to a single month, we'd attract 3–5 patients per month who responded. When I modified the offer to say, "Only 4 $500 off Invisalign Specials Available," the number who responded grew to 8–10 on average.

By limiting the quantity of specials available, you'll motivate more those who are truly interested to respond as we showed above, but it could put you in an interesting ethical dilemma. In our example above, you've offered this deal to the first four who respond, but what do you do with the next six who respond to the offer?

Consider the ethics

Let's pause for a moment to consider the ethical implications of what using scarcity in marketing can create. I have spent many summer vacations throughout my life down in Myrtle Beach, South Carolina. Every time I frequent this beach, I'm reminded of a retail store I pass along the way that uses scarcity in their marketing. For the last 20+ years, this store has claimed to be going out of business. When true and ethical, this could imply that there are some really great deals or discounts available off the merchandise they sell because they must get rid of their inventory. It also implies a limited quantity as new stock would not be appearing. That's why retailers tend to see a major spike in sales that leads up until the day they close their doors for good. Yet, 20+ years later, this business still stands. They have not gone out of business, and new stock is available every year that I have passed by.

I've surveyed many people who call Myrtle Beach their permanent home and have asked them what they think about this business. Every local resident I talked with told me that they were aware of the unethical practices of this business and choose not to shop there as a result. Fortunately for this business, Myrtle Beach is a major tourist destination with 80 percent of the people present throughout the year being on vacation. With a constant influx of new potential customers, the scarcity effect has served them well. With people using social media, Google, and Yelp reviews to help them with their purchasing decisions, this business risks having their unethical use of this principle exposed and could dramatically affect their business moving forward.

Whenever we use scarcity, we want to stay on the ethical side of the line. One objective way to do this is by being true in our intentions, efforts, wording, and how we communicate our messaging. In doing so, we can be assured that no one will find our practices misleading and lose trust in our name and brand. Let's look at a more specific dental example of an ethical dilemma I found myself in while using scarcity in marketing an offer to potential new patients.

As I mentioned previously, I have had great success with the Sonicare electric toothbrush "gift with purchase" offer. The first time I ran this promotion, my intent was to tap into the scarcity principle and limit the number of people who could get the offer to a maximum of 15. In my ads, I promoted it as such: "Offer good for the first 15 who respond." In preparation for this campaign we ordered 15 Sonicare toothbrushes and were ready to track the brushes given out to measure the campaigns success. To my surprise, we had given out all 15 toothbrushes within the first two weeks of our advertisement hitting mailboxes.

When my team alerted me that we had given out the 15th electric toothbrush, I made a point to congratulate the patient and make a big celebration of it with them. After walking them to the front desk and watching them leave the office, a new patient walked up to the front desk and told me that they were here because of the free Sonicare offer and were wondering where they could get theirs. I informed them that unfortunately we had given out the very last one just moments before them asking. Just then, my lead assistant happened to be at the front desk and had overheard our conversation. She is in charge of ordering supplies for the practice, and informed me, in front of this patient, that she had noticed a few days ago that we were running low on Sonicare toothbrushes and that she had reordered some to increase our stock. Luckily, she said, the new brushes had just arrived at our office about an hour earlier.

What would you do? The patient was interested in a Sonicare and came to our office because of this offer. I told them we had run out, but then my team member tells them that we actually now have one we could give them. Do you withhold the toothbrush or give it to them? In that moment, I felt like it was more of a customer service issue and didn't want the patient leaving having had a bad experience in our office, so I gave them one of the new toothbrushes that had arrived. They left happy and scheduled for their next visit with us. What's the harm, right? Was there a risk here?

The truth is that from an ethical standpoint, we couldn't say that we were being honest in our efforts, wording, or communication of this offer. We advertised that we'd only give it to 15 people, yet we gave it to 16 people. While this wasn't an issue in this example, imagine for a second that the 15th person to get the toothbrush had gone to the bathroom instead of leaving our office as this exchange occurred. Imagine now, after I just made a big deal about how they got the last toothbrush that they come out of the bathroom and see me giving the 16th toothbrush to this patient. What do you think patient 15 is now thinking about me or my practice? That we can't be trusted. How many people do you think they'd relay that message to? Pretty much all of their friends and family. Perhaps in a review on Google, Yelp, or another social media platform. Regardless, it's never a good idea for people to deem you as being unethical in your actions or for word to spread to that effect.

So how do you combat this? Anytime you limit the quantity or time people have to respond, it will motivate more people to act, which could put you in a similar ethical dilemma. Do you keep giving out more toothbrushes once you pass the number you said you'd give out? Do you allow them to use your offer even though the time frame you gave them has run out? Ultimately, that decision is up to you, but beware there is risk involved, and as practitioners, we can't afford for patients or the community to find our actions as being unethical. To avoid this ethical dilemma, we have another influence tool we can lean on: the principle of reciprocity.

One aspect of reciprocity concerns concessions. Concessions are backup plans, alternative options, a plan B, if you will. People who are the first to give a concession or alternative option after the first request is rejected are likely to see a reciprocal concession returned. What this means is that after the first request is rejected, if we offer something else in exchange, many times we'll set the stage for a yes to this alternative option. I temporarily suspended the use of scarcity in my offer for a free Sonicare toothbrush until I could satisfy this ethical dilemma that I felt would continue to occur if it continued. With each new patient who received a toothbrush moving forward, I wanted to know what part of the offer really captured their focus and motivation to come in. Was it that I was giving them a Sonicare brand of electric toothbrush or something else? From my conversations it became readily apparent that people were focused on getting an electric toothbrush, not so much on the Sonicare brand name itself. That meant I had an opportunity to solve this ethical dilemma.

Using the power of concessions, you can ethically use scarcity to influence more people to respond to your advertisements. Now when I run the toothbrush special and offer a free Sonicare to the first 15 who respond, when we run out of Sonicare, we let the patient know that we've given out our allotment of those but that we could offer them a free Oral B electric toothbrush instead. When we give away all the Sonicare AirFlosser appliances, we can now offer patients a nice Waterpik as an alternative option.

Going back to the Invisalign example we started with, if we have given out all four of the $500 off Invisalign gift card specials, we can offer those other six who responded with a concession of receiving a $200 off gift card instead. By using scarcity, we can motivate more patients to respond to our promotion. At the same time, we can still be ethical in our attempts by being true to how many we said we'd give out of that particular item and then offering those that missed out an alternative option in that category, allowing us to serve an unlimited number who responded above the first couple we targeted. When all is said and done, this will lead to more treatment being performed and with you giving away less of a discount overall than you would have given otherwise.

G. Contrast Effect

While not one of Cialdini's six principles of persuasion, the contrast effect is still an important psychological phenomenon we need to consider as it has a huge impact on attracting the focus and attention of potential new patients. We use contrast as a mechanism to shape our perceptions of the world around us and help us make decisions. Because of this effect, you can change the way people experience anything, by changing what they experience first.

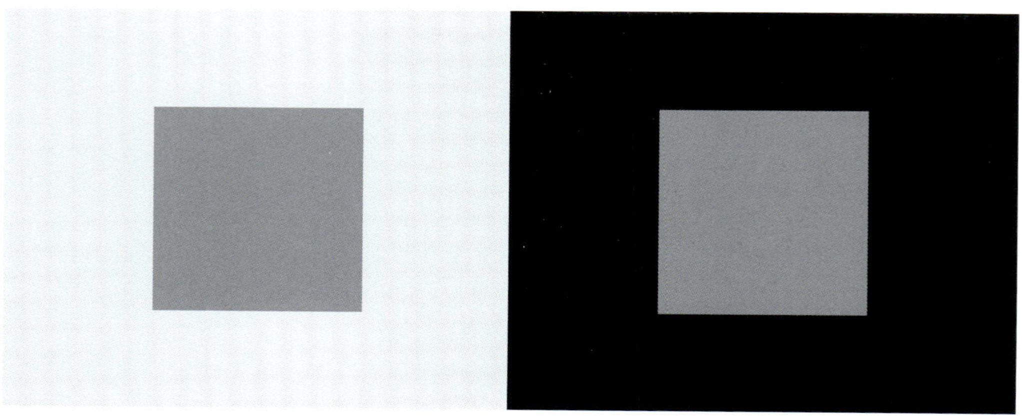

Figure 7. Example of the contrast effect.

For example, in Figure 7, you can make this light gray area in the center appear lighter than it actually is when it's placed up against a dark background vs placing that same gray item up against a lighter background. Despite the gray box being the same color in both examples, our perception of it is altered by what we see in comparison around it.

When making comparisons, what we experience first will tend to change our perception of what we are exposed to next as a result. This comparison can have a positive change on our perception of that item or it may have a negative one, for instance, when you're describing good news and bad news to someone. Starting out by telling someone the good news about a situation means you'll direct more of their focus and attention on the bad news that comes next, making the bad news be perceived as worse than it actually may be. Telling someone the bad news first will have the opposite effect, focusing their attention on the good parts of the news you delivered. Either way, the contrast effect will shape their perception about that matter and ultimately will affect their decision.

In dental marketing, we can use this contrast effect to frame comparisons of our products, services, and even the price of what we'd like to present.

Comparisons of before vs. after

Before and after photos are a great example of how we can use contrast in dental marketing to promote a myriad of services we offer. By starting out with the before, we can draw people's attention to the amazing result a better smile can bring someone.

Comparisons of procedures

In orthodontics, you could show a smile picture of an adult wearing traditional brackets and wires vs a person wearing a clear aligner system. You could show metal brackets and wires compared to cosmetic brackets and tooth-colored wires. I showed an example of this under the scarcity section when I discussed how I showed patients what their smile could look like if they continue to let their relapse.

You can show pictures of traditional dentures vs a "snap in" set of overdentures vs a "fixed" or non-removable appliance. With tooth whitening, you can tell and show differences between Kör whitening vs Zoom 1 hour tooth whitening vs a traditional bleach tray method. Whatever it is you're looking to promote, always frame it in comparison to something else, and in doing so, put more emphasis on the service you'd like to do more of.

Price comparisons

You've seen examples of this when you see an item on sale. Usually you are anchored to the old price, which has now been scratched out. Next you see the current price. By putting these two numbers together, we're using contrast to make that comparison. Seeing the higher priced item first, even though it's not the actual price, now changes our perception on the sale priced item, making it seem more reasonable than it might have seemed had we just been exposed to the actual price today.

In the Invisalign example I discussed in using scarcity to promote dental services, in those advertisements I'd highlight the cost of doing nothing when it came to their current orthodontic relapse situation, with waiting translating into $5700 in treatment and two years of time that would be needed to correct the problem down the road. I then leveraged the contrast effect by showing how saying yes to short-term orthodontics today, at $3700, was significantly less expensive. By first anchoring them to the $5700 price, we've now made that $3700 price seem a lot more reasonable.

Depending on the positive or negative effect we'd like to generate, there is a lot of influence opportunity in dental marketing to frame comparisons for the products and services we offer in a similar way. In doing so, it's sure to grab people's attention and persuade more to come your direction.

While each of Dr. Cialdini's six principles of persuasion and the contrast effect alone can have a powerful influence on our perceptions and the decisions we make, studies show that when we are able to incorporate one or more of them into our marketing messages and content, we can magnify the overall influence effect. For seven straight years I ran a three-panel brochure, direct mail campaign for one of my dental practices, consistently sending this piece out to my ideal patient demographic and using a targeted list a marketing company had created for me. On average this piece produced 22 new patients per month and gave me a 3:1 ROI within the first six months of release, despite being devoid of the influence elements we've discussed thus far.

After going through my influence training with Dr. Cialdini I made small tests with each of the principles and contrast in different marketing media, seeing great success with every principle I added. With this confidence, the day came when I decided to take that consistent direct mail piece and completely redesign it, adding reciprocity, liking, social proof, authority, scarcity, and contrast elements to it. With a long-term baseline of results to compare, I decided to send my influence-designed marketing piece right back out to the same list that I had been mailing for seven years, wondering if adding more influence would have any effect on my results.

Not surprisingly, it did. My new patient numbers from this ad rose from 22 to over 45 per month. The ROI rose from 3:1 to 6:1. Increasing the new patient count meant more revenue to the practice without raising the cost of the advertisement. Despite mailing this to the same list of my target market, the newly updated piece grabbed more attention and caused more people to take notice and then take action.

H. "Map Your Influence" Worksheet

Use the "Map Your Influence" worksheet to discover how you can add more of Dr. Robert Cialdini's six principles of persuasion and the contrast effect to your advertisements.

Map Your Influence

Instructions: Follow along and see how can you add more of Dr. Robert Cialdini's 6 principles of persuasion to your advertisement.

How to add Reciprocity

- Give them a gift they value such as allowing them to be a part of a gift that has already been given, e.g., "This past year we've donated over $100,000 of free dental care to those who couldn't afford it. By supporting our practice as a patient, you're playing a part to support our community."

How to add liking

Providing a small section of your advertisement that shares information about your family, hobbies, and interests can help others find connections to their own family, hobbies, and interests.

- What information do you feel comfortable sharing about your family, hobbies, or interests?
- What information will your team feel comfortable with you sharing with potential new patients?

How to add authority

Adding authority triggers can help highlight your expertise and show that patients trust you.
What authority triggers showcase your expertise?

	What authority triggers show patients that you have experience and expertise?
	Logo with years of expertise
	Credentials
	Academy certifications
	Awards (local or national)
	Other: ____________

	What authority triggers show that patients can trust you?
	Celebrity endorsements
	Patient written reviews
	Patient video testimonials
	Professional patient reviews
	Other: ____________

How to add social proof?

- Pictures
  Ex.: Of you and/or your team with multiple patients present.
  Ex.: Multiple pictures of you and individual patients, collaged together for display.
- Testimonials
  Ex.: Grouping four or more testimonials together for display.
  Ex.: Sharing the total number of reviews you have attained across all platforms, e.g., "To read over 700 reviews, check out our website."
  Ex.: Highlighting multiple trusted platforms that hold your reviews, e.g., "To read over 700 reviews from Google, Yelp, Facebook, and Healthgrades, check out our website."

How to add consistency

This principle is about getting the potential new patient committed to a mindset in that moment and then asking them to schedule an appointment. To gain mindsets and commitments, we need to ask key questions in our advertisements. For example:

THE PHELPS® INSTITUTE

6

Figure 8. "Map your influence" worksheets. Use these worksheets to see which of Cialdini's six principles of persuasion you can incorporate into your advertisement to increase its effectiveness.

Cont'd

Map Your Influence

- Do you prefer to be proactive in your dental health?
- Tired of teeth that constantly breakdown?
- Tired of being in pain?
- Embarrassed about your smile?
- Ready to get out of pain?
- Ready to get a plan for your mouth?

If you answered YES to any or all of these questions, we can help. Give us a call and schedule an appointment to find out what your options could be.

How to add scarcity

- Highlighting what makes you unique or the scarce resource.
  E.g., having a fellowship in the AGD means that less than 1% of dentists achieve that level of certification, or "our office is 1 of 3 in the entire state that offers every level of sedation dentistry."

- Highlighting loss
  What have people lost the ability to do or what are they about to lose if their current condition worsens? E.g., showing a photo with a set of dentures sitting in a glass of water reminds someone of the frustration they feel because they've lost the ability to keep their teeth in their mouth permanently, or showing a picture of a bowl of soup and then a steak while asking, "Are you eating this (pointing to the soup) when you'd rather be eating this (the steak)? We can help."

Document your thoughts and ideas from each principle below.

Remember, you won't always be able to incorporate every principle, but the more you can feature, the more Influence your advertisement will generate.

Reciprocity: ______________________________

Liking: ______________________________

Authority: ______________________________

Social proof: ______________________________

Consistency: ______________________________

Scarcity: ______________________________

THE PHELPS INSTITUTE

7

Figure 8. Cont'd

Part 2

The Basics of Patient Marketing

So far, we've discussed how to identify who your target market is and how to craft headlines and messaging that will grab their attention. We've talked about how to create content that engages the senses and their emotions and reviewed different types of offers that will motivate and influence factors that will persuade them to become a patient in your practice. With these critical areas mapped out, you can now turn your attention to the last two pieces of the puzzle you need to adequately create more new patient opportunities.

First, you'll need to strategically choose a marketing medium to host your headlines, content, and offer, collectively what we'll refer to as your messaging. Choose the wrong medium, and your target market won't even get exposed to this messaging. Choose the right medium, and now your messaging has a chance to be seen. Once chosen, the only thing left is to track its success. Without proper tracking, we have no way of knowing what's working, what's not working, and why. In this section we'll start by diving into the most popular marketing media that are available today.

Chapter 5
External Marketing

1. EXTERNAL MARKETING MEDIA

External marketing is the act of taking your message, transmitting it to a larger audience, one that is outside of your current patient base, and then measuring the response. While not expected to draw in everyone exposed to your message, it's much like throwing a large net off a fishing barge and into the vast sea, hoping that when you reel the net back on board, you've caught some amount of fish. When it comes to external marketing media, they tend to fall into two categories, off-line and online external marketing.

A. Off-line External Marketing Media

Off-line marketing refers to any advertising that is carried out using traditional off-line or non-digital media such as television, billboard ads, and radio. Even though many advertisers are focusing on online, or digital, marketing, these traditional off-line media channels are still utilized with great success today. For our purposes, we'll cover the most popular ones.

- **Direct Mail;**
- **Newspaper Inserts;**
- **Radio;**
- **Television;**
- **Billboards;**
- **Magazines.**

Direct Mail

Direct mail is a type of off-line marketing that's delivered physically to a prospect's mailbox through the United States Postal Service or other delivery service. While many in the marketing arena like to label direct mail as being "dead" and no longer effective, current research says otherwise. On a recent blog post, Neil Patel, an entrepreneur, marketer, and best-selling author, wrote about recent research that investigated the median return on investment (ROI) per marketing medium. One survey showed that direct mail campaigns actually had a higher ROI than both paid search and online display ads. In fact, direct mail was only 1 percentage point behind social media, the second highest ROI medium. Why?

Many attribute this to the advantages direct mail offers over other digital online media:

- **Response rate**: Average between 2.7–4.4 percent, or 27 to 44 potential new patients for every 1000 mailers that went out. This dwarfs the response rate of many digital media like email marketing whose response rate hovers around 0.12 percent.
- **Engages all of your senses**: With direct mail, you can touch it and feel it, thus engaging more of your natural senses, which is why research shows that your messaging in direct mail is 5X more likely to be remembered than through digital platforms.
- **Reach**: It's one of the few marketing routes you can use that guarantees that your message will be reached to every household in your target market list, for instance, if you were targeting everyone who lived in a retirement community. With online marketing, there is no guarantee that everyone in your target market would even see your message.
- **Customizable target list**: Because direct mail is direct, it can be highly targeted to both potential new patients as well as existing ones. This makes using direct mail for on-boarding, re-targeting, and building loyalty extremely effective.

The first step in running a successful direct mail campaign is to decide if you want to target a specific demographic or make sure everyone within a predefined range receives your mailing.

1. Direct Mail Logistics

Your first decision when figuring out your direct mail logistics is to decide if you plan to send your advertisement to everyone who lives or works in a certain radius or zip code, to blanket them all with your messaging or if you'd prefer to narrow your focus to a more targeted list. If you have tons of open chair time, are a start practice, and/or haven't really established who your target market should be, then blanketing everyone in a zip code or area might the route for you. If so, then you want to look at EDDM, or "every door direct mail."

- EDDM is a bulk mailing option offered by the United States Postal Service that allows your business to reach potential customers without knowing their address. With EDDM, your mail piece will be sent to every household on the carrier route you have chosen. With it, you can target larger census demographics such as age range, household income, and zip codes to attract more potential patients. One advantage when using EDDM is that you can do it yourself. You can create and send these out directly through the US Postal Service, meaning you don't really need to employ the services of a direct mail marketing company. Because you're printing and paying for postage in bulk, another big advantage of using EDDM instead of utilizing a more targeted marketing list is the cost savings. Here are some other advantages and things you should consider:
- Since you are sending your mailing out to every business and/or home in an area, you're not spending any money on purchasing a targeted mailing list.
- By using a local or online printer, you can get the costs of your mailers down to 2–4 cents apiece, a 20–30 percent savings over having a direct mail company do this for you.
- The post office requires that you arrange your mailers into 100-piece bundles to aid in their distribution. By sorting and bundling the mailers yourself, you save labor costs by having a direct mail company do this for you.
- Postage for a regular postcard mailing is currently around 36 cents. Through special arrangement with the Post Office's EDDM retail program, postage for bulk mailings is reduced down to 12–16 cents per piece mailed.

- Turn it off or on as needed. There are no contracts with any companies involved here, so it's literally on demand. Send out as many or as few as you'd like. Send it to the whole zip code or just a portion of the zip code, for example, a certain community.

While there are advantages to EDDM, when you have a more established practice that doesn't have as much open chair time to fill, or you are marketing for more specific procedures, then success is often obtained by narrowing your focus and targeting only those who qualify as your defined target market. There are direct mail marketing companies that specialize in this area and can handle the printing, sorting, and mailing of your pieces. They are also eager to help you define your targeted list and segment them into as many categories as possible. Here are a few criteria I apply when using a direct mail marketing company to help me in my advertising campaign:

- **Geography**: Define how large of a radius you'd like your mailers to be distributed in. If your practice is established, look at your current active patient list. Your current patient list will help you answer where more of your likely prospects live. Prioritize the zip codes that have the most patients. If you have a fairly new practice, your target area should be as close to your practice as possible but also should match your budget. For example, if you have $10,000 budgeted for mail over three months, you should reach the closest 20,000 or so prospects with that money. If your practice is in a city, you may be able to find enough quality prospects within 1–3 miles. In rural areas, you may have to go further out, say 7–10 miles. For the majority of practices, targeting people who fit your target market definition and live or work within a 3–5-mile radius around your practice is a great starting point.
- **Age/gender/working status**: Adults vs kids? Age 25–55, 55+? Males vs females? Working or retired? Many of these may already have been answered when you previously defined who was your target.
- **Income range**: A good starting point is to focus on household incomes of at least $75,000. However, $75,000 is an arbitrary household income number. Focus on the prospects with the highest household income that fit your budget. If your practice is in an affluent area, you may have much higher income minimums. If you are in an area with more modest incomes, you may have to go lower than $75,000. Again, let your budget dictate where your income line is.
- **Credit score**: These should be used in conjunction with income ranges. I mentioned earlier that my target market was active, independent living retirees. By this time, most of their major debts are gone, they have been paid off. They're limited in their activities and have reduced their lifestyle expenses to fit a low monthly budget. As a result, many take out less than $50,000 per year in an attempt to avoid paying certain taxes on their social security checks. If we ran our potential new patient list solely on the income range criteria of $75,000 or higher household income, then our list would exclude the majority of our target market. By modifying our list criteria and adding in anyone aged 55 or older with an A or B level credit score, we can change that. Credit modeling lists combined with age and income is a less expensive way to find those most likely to have good credit. A and B modeling is usually equivalent to 700 plus credit scores. Ask your mail vendor to research this for you. Ask your direct mail marketing company to pull names in your area that meet minimum credit criteria.

- **Distribution rate**: How many new patient phone calls can your office handle in a given day? Up to 5, 6–10, 20+? Remember that the average response rate for direct mail pieces is around 2.7–4.4 percent. Let's say you've created your target market list of about 30,000 people and are pulling this list from a seven-mile radius around your practice. If all of your mailers go out at once and you influenced 4.4 percent of those who received it to pick up the phone and call for an appointment, that means you'd have 1320 potential new patient calls, the majority of which will call within 1–2 weeks after receiving your mailing. Do you think your team can answer all of those calls each day? The short answer is that when you factor in all of the other duties such as checking existing patients in and out, verifying dental insurance benefits, confirming future appointments, and other activities, it is impossible to expect them to handle that kind of call volume. Each call that goes unanswered is a wasted opportunity and takes away from your potential marketing ROI.

  To combat this, I recommend breaking up your list and mailing out your direct mail pieces slowly over time. To start, take the radius around your practice that will receive your mailings. Divide that radius into three sections. From our example earlier, let's say our radius had 90,000 potential patients within it. Dividing that out by three means you'll have three areas to mail to, each with 30,000 potential patients residing within. Over a three-month period, everyone on your list will receive your mailing one time. Over a yearlong period they will receive your mailing four times, or once a quarter. Studies

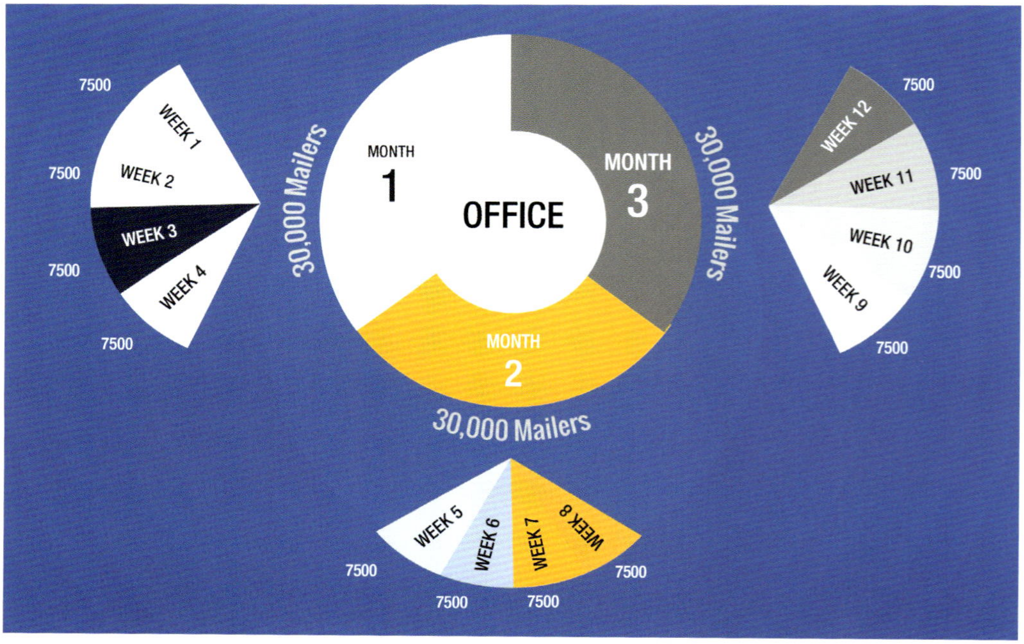

Figure 9. Here is a graphical representation showing how to divide out a mailing list of 90,000 potential new patients from a predefined radius around the dental practice. The radius is divided out into three monthly divisions with each division being divided down into four weekly installments. Each week, 7500 of the total mailers gets mailed out to those in that section. Each week a new set receives the piece until everyone in the 90,000 list has received the piece one time over that three-month period.

show it may take receiving your mailing three or four times to get the best response rate. With 30,000 mailers going out and an average response rate of 4.4 percent, you might expect 1320 potential new patients to call during the first one or two weeks after receiving your mailing. Your team now has a much better chance of answering these calls, but the likelihood that many go unanswered is still high.

What if we divide our list even further? Take each of your one-third sections, and divide that area into fourths, one for each week of the month. Given most months have four weeks in them, that means that each week approximately 7500 mailers will go out, and after three months, everyone in your radius would have received your mailing. With our 4.4 percent expected response rate that equates to 330 potential new patient calls to occur each week. That still amounts to around 66 calls over a five-day workweek, so the total amount of calls that could potentially go unanswered will be significantly less than in the other two mass mailing scenarios. By answering more of these calls, you will have a higher ROI for what you've invested. Worried about your team missing some of these opportunity calls? Contracting with a third-party scheduling service such as Golden Goose Scheduling can also help you answer and schedule more new patient calls from your marketing efforts.

Once you have identified your target market and have decided whether to reach them yourself using EDDM or by enlisting the help of a direct mail marketing company, your next step is to decide what type of direct mail you want to package your message in.

2. Types of Direct Mail

1. *Self-mailer/brochure flyer*

   A self-mailer flyer, commonly called a panel brochure style mailer, is a single sheet of paper, of any size, that is folded one or more times to create a multi-panel flyer. The most common self-mailers are a three- or four-panel piece. The three-panel mailer measures 8 by 15 inches and folds on itself twice to a finished size of 8 by 5 inches. A four-panel mailer typically measures 8 by 20 inches, which folds on itself three times to a finished size of 8 by 5 inches. This brochure style piece may be printed on paper stock or card stock and is mailed on its own, without an envelope.

   The size of the mailer can be as large or as small as you want, as long as it is within some limits from the post office. The finished (folded) size of your brochure style piece will determine your postage rate. Mailers that are no larger than 6 1/8 by 11 1/2 inches qualify for so-called letter rates, which means you'd pay the same as you would pay for regular mail. If the finished size is larger, you will pay a surcharge, which could be double the postage of regular mail. Given that you have 8 by 15 inches of front and back space to utilize, these pieces are ideal for promoting all aspects of your general practice.

2. *Newsletter*

   A print newsletter is a physical piece printed on paper. It has actual weight and feel, giving the reader something to hold as they read. Typical sizes for a print newsletter are either 11" by 17" (four pages) or 8.5" by 11" (two pages). If you're going to mail these to your customers without an envelope, you'll need to fold them down to a final size of 5.5" by 8.5" to meet mailing standards. The two most common paper types to print these on are 70# text or 80# text. The difference in paper selection comes down to thickness (how heavy the paper is), and finish (whether it's glossy or matte).

In 2015, the most extensive neuro-marketing study of its kind proved direct mail was more effective at driving behavior by exceeding the motivation-to-cognitive load threshold when compared to digital media. The standard postcard was the only physical format that didn't outperform digital, finishing slightly behind email on a smartphone. In this study they found that the most effective direct mail formats were large 11" by 17" newsletters. A different test across six million dental consumers in 300 distinct markets revealed newsletters generate a 70 percent increase in new patient calls over other direct mail formats like postcards, despite all having the same brand, content, and offer strategies promoted.

Women make more than 90 percent of all dental buying decisions. This makes them an important criterion we need to consider when defining our target market. They want quality information to make smart decisions for their families. Because a newsletter is significantly larger than a postcard, it offers the necessary "real estate" to educate patients about services dental practices provide and elevates the dentist as a leading authority in the community.

While proving to be a powerful direct mail format to attract new patients, newsletters are excellent tools that you can use to engage existing patients, both to market and promote different services you provide and special offers or promotions you have running. By continuing to communicate with your existing patients through this format, you keep your practice top of mind and will help decrease your patient attrition rate, keeping more of your existing patients from leaving.

CASE STUDY

Dr. Travis Campbell has achieved tremendous success throughout his career. Not only is he part of the country's prestigious group of the top 1 percent of dentists, but he's also an accomplished multi-practice business owner, speaker, dental consultant/coach, and author of many popular dental resources, including his latest book, *Understanding Dental Insurance: A Guide for Dentists and Their Teams*, published in 2021. *The Practice Whisperer*, published in 2019. His practice, 380 Family Dentistry, is in Prosper, Texas. He is co-owner of Choice Dental Associates in Garland, Texas.

At the start of 2020, Dr. Campbell knew he wanted to boost new-patient flow at both practice locations. Following an introduction to Karen Galley, co-owner and president of dental marketing and technology agency Patient NEWS, Dr. Campbell decided to invest in a direct mail program. As part of the campaign, he was introduced to Practice ZEBRA, their proprietary dental software system that tracks key practice performance metrics, marketing results, call conversion and scoring, digital presence, and more. Through the launch process, significant opportunities for growth were uncovered.

1. Each practice was connected to Practice ZEBRA for a diagnostic review of all key metrics and trends, including past and current new-patient flow, average and new-patient values, production, and scheduling. These were compared with industry standard and top-performing practices.

2. Each location received a deep demographic analysis, online audit, current market share report, and competitor review.

3. Following consultation, a plan was set in motion for budget, timing, target distribution, content, and offer strategy development. Results would be highly visible in Practice ZEBRA, and the campaign adjusted accordingly.

To his credit, when many dental offices were curtailing marketing expenditures, Dr. Campbell decided to implement Practice ZEBRA and new-patient newsletters at both locations mid-pandemic in May 2020. He knew there was an opportunity to increase practice awareness and enhance reputation by reaching out to area residents and patients, reassuring them

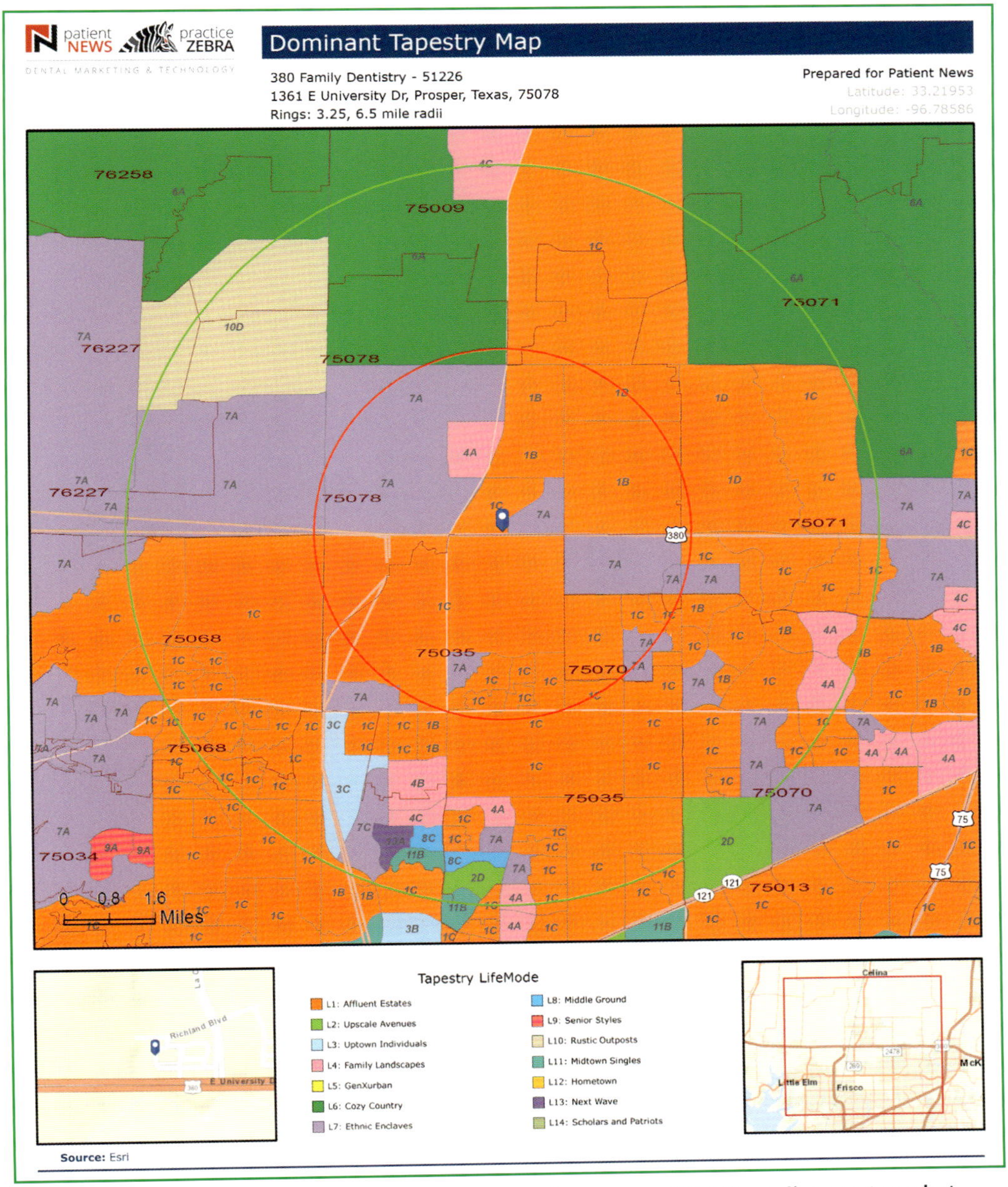

Figure 10. Targeting a radius around the practice to find more of 380 Dental's target market.

of the safety in the dental practice, and by doing so, experienced a surge in new patients and production levels at both locations through the pandemic. Interestingly, one of his practices discontinued their mailings, and the resulting change in new patient flow can be seen from this study.

Target market area analysis

Using a variety of mapping technologies, Patient NEWS determines where a practice's primary target audience is located. No stone is left unturned with the review of high-value existing patient map plotting, patient demographics, socioeconomics, competitive practice data, doctor/patient ratios, and even considerations around drive time and natural boundaries and barriers.

There are 67 different segments that identify common demographics and socioeconomic characteristics to help define targets and inform content decision-making.

380 Family Dentistry in Proper, Texas, is in a mid-level fairly competitive area. The dentist-to-population ratio in the practice's target area is one dentist for 800 families, with 75 competing dentists. 380 Family Dentistry has predominant demographic markets (households that share a common experience) of "boomburbs," "professional pride," and "up-and-coming families." Median ages 30–40, three people per household, and income around $100,000. Very good dental prospects.

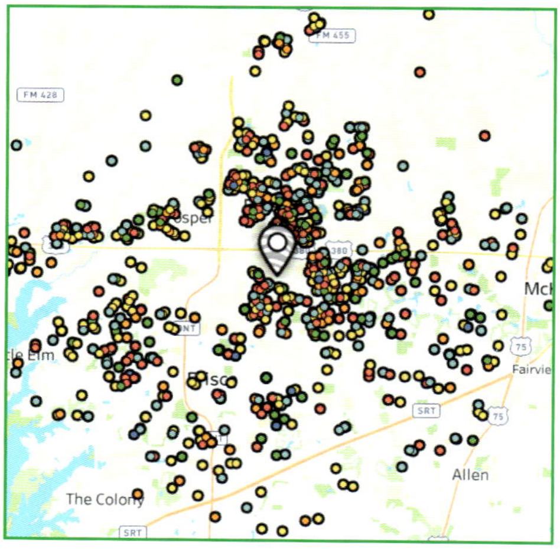

Figure 11. **Discovering where your high-value existing patient lives in relation to 380 Dental's office.**

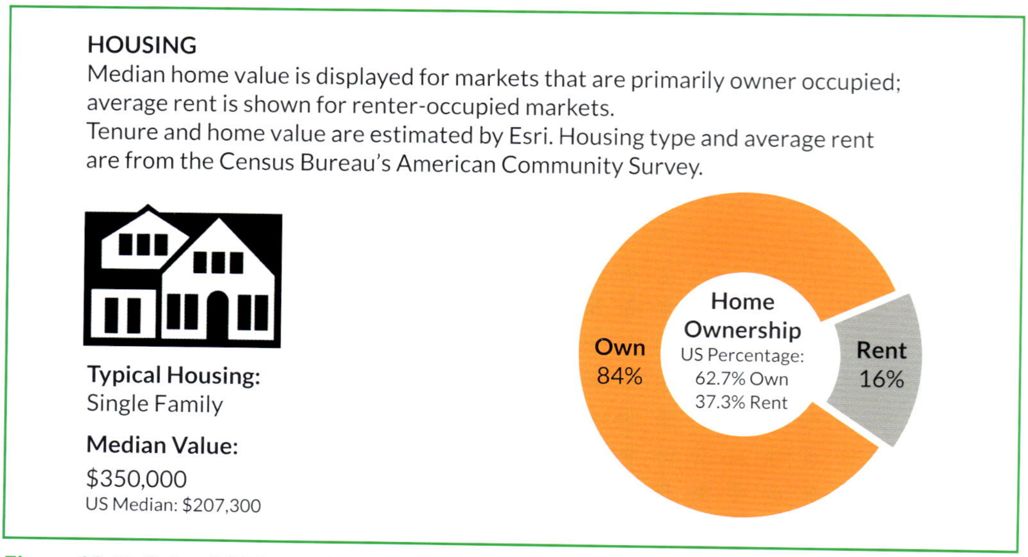

Figure 12. **Defining 380 Dental's median household income in radius search around practice.**

Tapestry overview

Boomburbs

This group has an average household size of 3.25, a median age of 43, and a median household income of $113,400. They are well-educated, young professionals who have opted to trade up to the newest housing in the suburbs. They are big on technology and have their financial affairs in order.

Professional pride

This group consists of consumers who are well-educated career professionals who have flourished through the great recession. The average household size is 3.13. The median age is 40. Median household income is $138,100. Like the boomburbs group, they are well off, intelligent, and have worked hard to get where they are.

Up-and-coming families

In this group, the size of the average household is 3.12. The median age is 31.4, and the median household income is $72,000. People in this group are younger and more mobile and ethnically diverse than the previous generation. They go after their goals, have a strong work ethic, and are willing to take some risks to get ahead. A total of 6 percent have some college education or a degree/degrees.

Choice Dental Associates

In Garland, Texas, is in a much more competitive market, with just 500 families per dentist, 122 dental competitors, and demographics with a slightly different story. While still a positive dental shopper population, it's a younger, much more diverse demographic, heavily populated, including "enterprising professionals," "American dreamers," and "home improvement." Median age in the 30s, households fall short of three people on average, and income levels average $75,000.

Tapestry Overview

Enterprising professionals

These residents are intelligent and advancing in careers that include science, technology, engineering, and mathematics. Because they change jobs frequently, they also move around. They make high-risk investments and enjoy using the Internet and watching TV. The average household size is 2.48. The average age is 35, and the median household income is $86,600 (one-and-a-half times that of the entire country).

American dreamers

This group is family centric and diverse. The majority are married with kids of all ages or they're single parents. Grandparents are also often in these homes. Hard work and sacrifice have made it possible for many American dreamers to improve their economic circumstances. The average household size is 3.19. The median age is about 32, and the median household income $50,900.

Home improvement

Married-couple families make up more than half of these suburban households. Most are single families, and one-fifth of the homes are occupied by renters. Their education and diversity are similar to the rest of the country. These families are usually on the go and frequent restaurants because of it. The average household size is 2.88. The median age is close to 38, and the median household income is $72,100.

Content development

Armed with demographic data and competitive intelligence, Patient NEWS developed content and imagery to resonate with the unique target audience around each dental practice

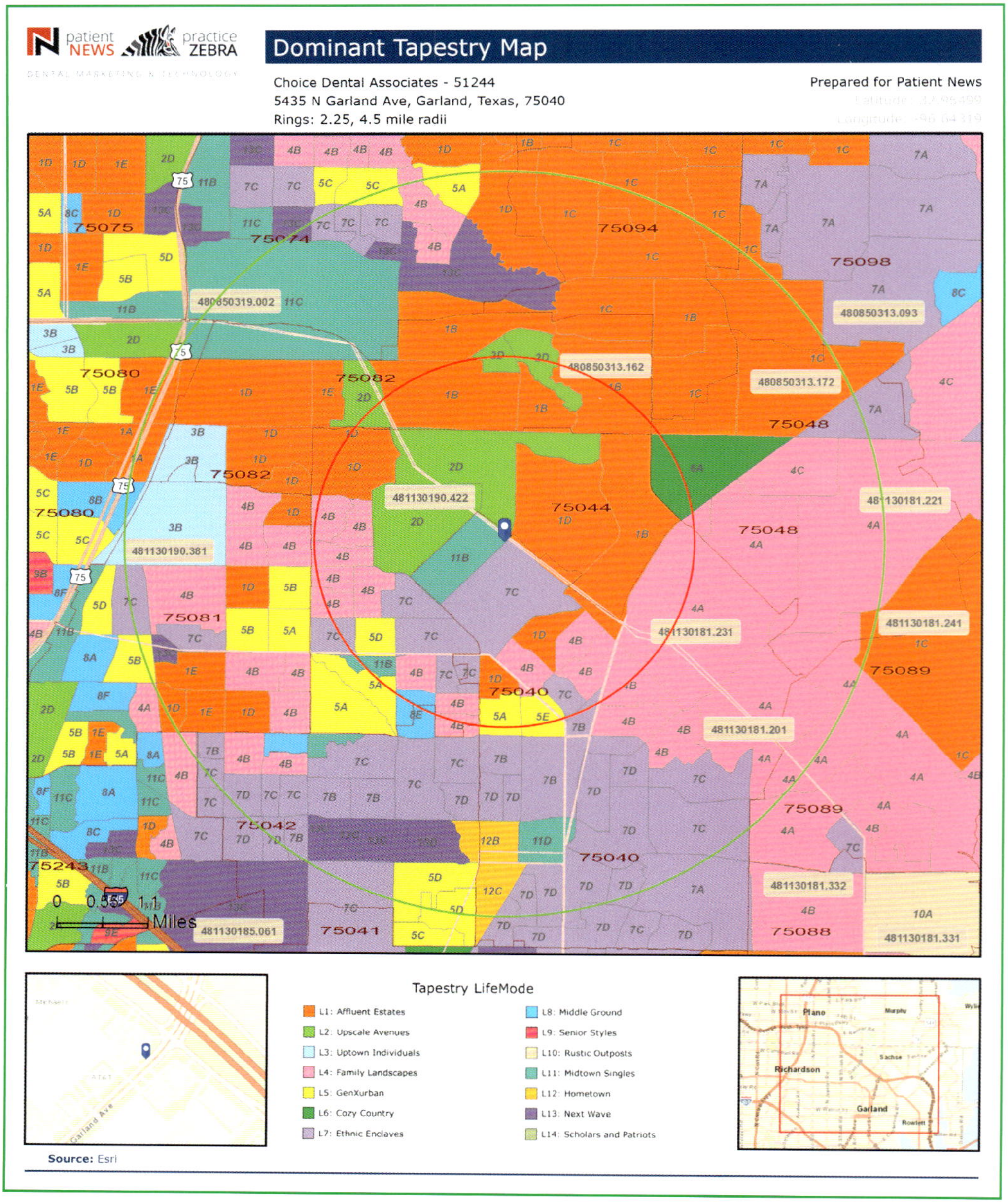

Figure 13. Targeting a radius around the practice to find more of Choice Dental's target market.

to build awareness, build trust with the dentist and team, and inspire action. Studies show that women make more than 90 percent of all health care buying decisions for themselves and for their families. That's not to say that men don't shop—and in particular online—but women want more quality information for study and consideration and do often ultimately drive the family's decisions.

It's sometimes a challenge for marketing companies to get dental practice owners to agree to all the recommendations they make, especially when it comes to offer strategy. But Dr. Campbell was on board with the expert advice he received. Decisions were never made without significant research and comparative analysis.

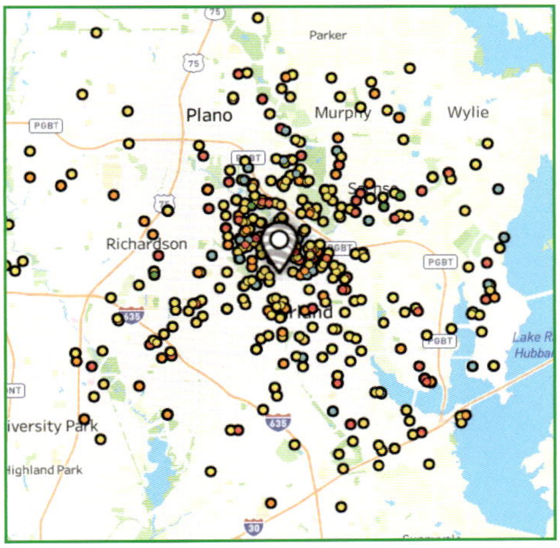

Figure 14. Discovering where your high-value existing patient lives in relation to Choice Dental's office.

As studies have proven, the four-page large-format newsletter is more visible than a postcard promotion. It attracts more attention and a more-educated, high-value patient and supports the dental comprehensive care model. The structure also provides the "real estate" to elevate practice differentiators and build familiarity and trust in the practice's expertise. Female head-of-house decision makers want quality information to make good decisions for their families, and content like a new recipe each month is noticed and appreciated.

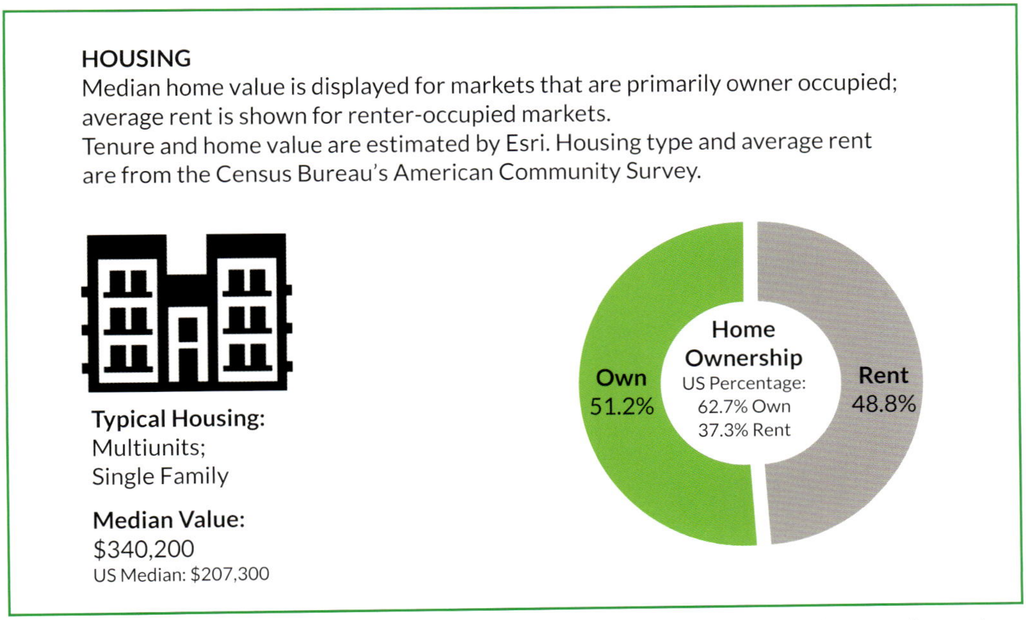

Figure 15. Defining Choice Dental's median household income in radius search around practice.

380 Family Dentistry (Figs. 16 and 17)
1. Prominent branding;
2. Mother-daughter image;
3. Free consultation/second opinion (implants, Invisalign, sedation);
4. $25 new patient special that includes exam and digital x-rays (objective to drive significant new-patient flow as opportunities presented through pandemic but excluded hygiene to boost second appointment value and beyond with upsell to more comprehensive care);
5. Existing in-house membership plan starting at $29/month;
6. Introduction to doctor and team;
7. Critical call-to-action data (map, website, phone#);
8. Highlight of differentiating features;
9. Inside pages include value-added educational content and subtle service promotion;
10. Healthy recipes appeal and extend shelf life.

Choice Dental Associates (Figs. 18 and 19)
1. Prominent branding;
2. Mother-daughter image;
3. Free consultation/second opinion (implants, Invisalign, sedation);
4. $79 new patient special that includes exam, x-rays, and cleaning (objective to drive significant new-patient flow and include cleaning at a slightly higher introductory rate to interest a younger, slightly less affluent demographic who are more concerned with initial visit convenience);
5. Emergency exams for $25;
6. Introduction to doctor and team;
7. Critical call-to-action data (map, website, phone#);
8. Highlight of differentiating features;
9. Inside pages include value-added educational content and subtle service promotion;
10. Healthy recipes appeal and extend shelf life.

In both instances, the offers were aggressive. It was understood the pandemic created a unique opportunity to introduce new patients to these two practice locations who may be looking for urgent care, not receiving communication from a current provider, who were more concerned about their health and wellness in light of COVID, disenfranchised, or looking for a change. The goal would be to quickly build the practice base to set up for continued future success.

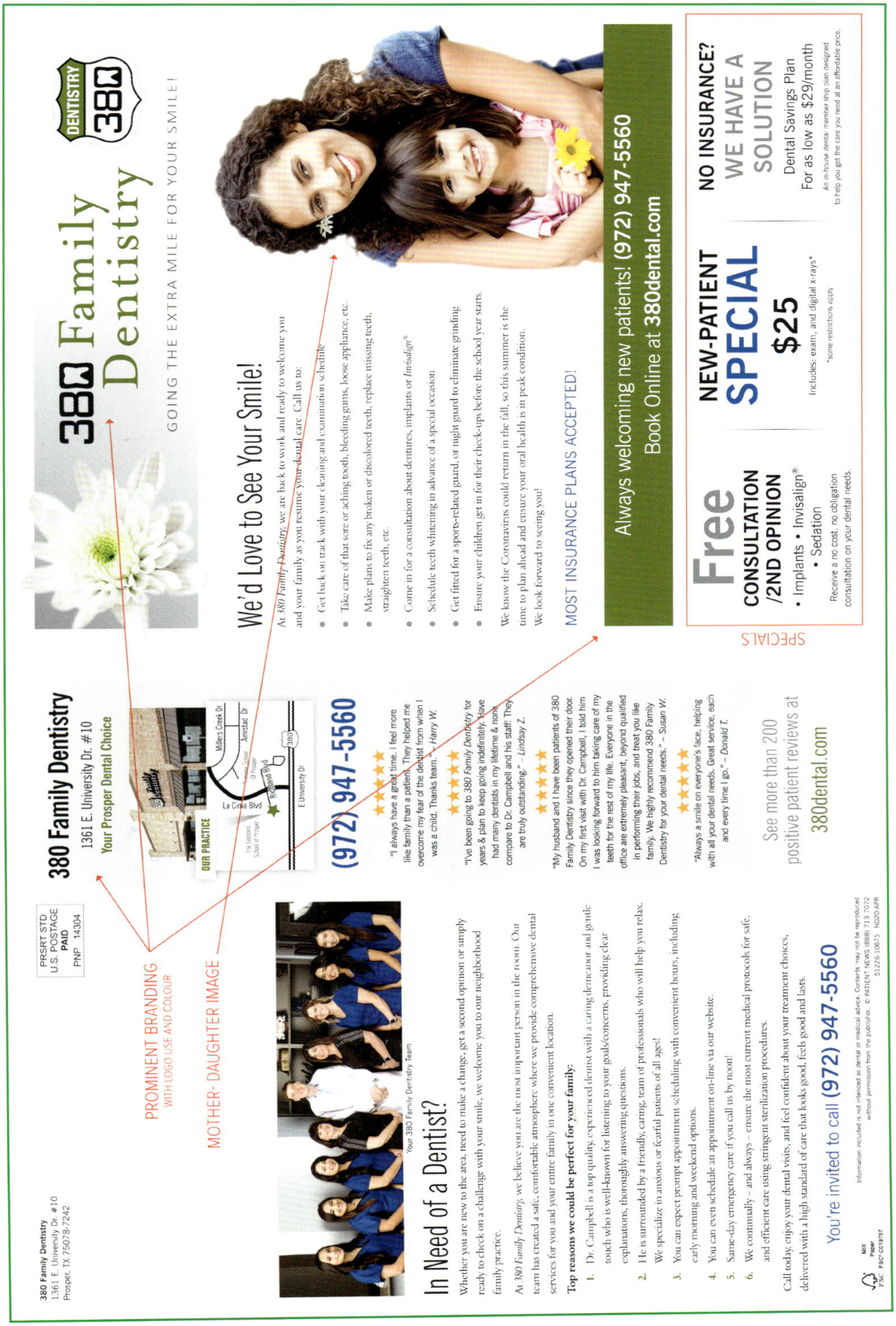

Figure 16. Example of 380 Dental's newsletter direct mail piece. Front side.

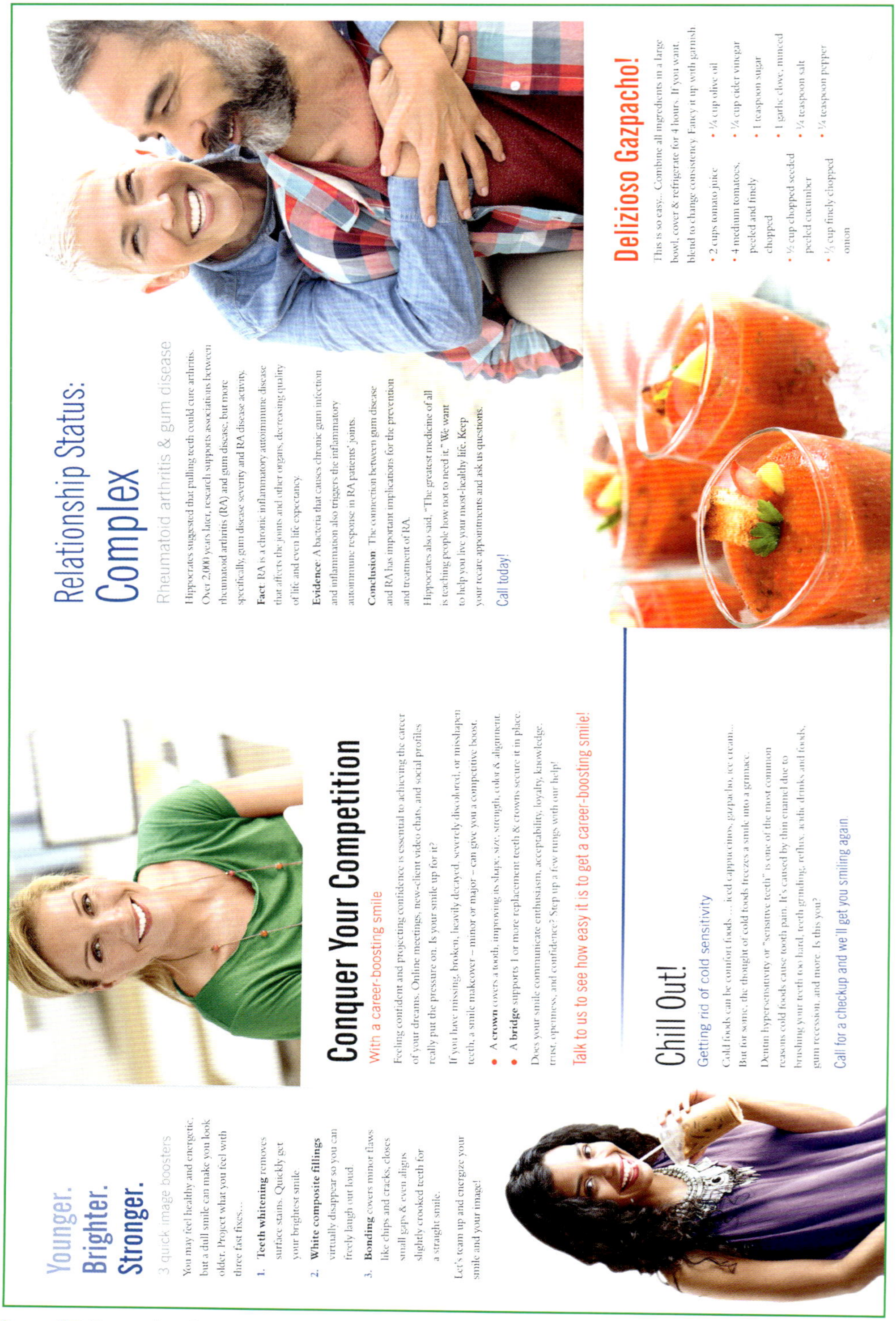

Younger.
Brighter.
Stronger.

3 quick image boosters

You may feel healthy and energetic, but a dull smile can make you look older. Project what you feel with three fast fixes...

1. **Teeth whitening** removes surface stains. Quickly get your brightest smile.
2. **White composite fillings** virtually disappear so you can freely laugh out loud.
3. **Bonding** covers minor flaws like chips and cracks, closes small gaps & even aligns slightly crooked teeth for a straight smile.

Let's team up and energize your smile and your image!

Conquer Your Competition

With a career-boosting smile

Feeling confident and projecting confidence is essential to achieving the career of your dreams. Online meetings, new-client video chats, and social profiles really put the pressure on. Is your smile up for it?

If you have missing, broken, heavily decayed, severely discolored, or misshapen teeth, a smile makeover – minor or major – can give you a competitive boost.

- A **crown** covers a tooth, improving its shape, size, strength, color & alignment.
- A **bridge** supports 1 or more replacement teeth & crowns secure it in place.

Does your smile communicate enthusiasm, acceptability, loyalty, knowledge, trust, openness, and confidence? Step up a few rungs with our help!

Talk to us to see how easy it is to get a career-boosting smile!

Chill Out!

Getting rid of cold sensitivity

Cold foods can be comfort foods ... iced cappuccinos, gazpacho, ice cream... But for some, the thought of cold foods freezes a smile into a grimace.

Dentin hypersensitivity or "sensitive teeth" is one of the most common reasons cold foods cause tooth pain. It's caused by thin enamel due to brushing your teeth too hard, teeth grinding, reflux, acidic drinks and foods, gum recession, and more. Is this you?

Call for a checkup and we'll get you smiling again.

Relationship Status:
Complex

Rheumatoid arthritis & gum disease

Hippocrates suggested that pulling teeth could cure arthritis. Over 2,000 years later, research supports associations between rheumatoid arthritis (RA) and gum disease, but more specifically, gum disease severity and RA disease activity.

Fact: RA is a chronic inflammatory autoimmune disease that affects the joints and other organs, decreasing quality of life and even life expectancy.

Evidence: A bacteria that causes chronic gum infection and inflammation also triggers the inflammatory autoimmune response in RA patients' joints.

Conclusion: The connection between gum disease and RA has important implications for the prevention and treatment of RA.

Hippocrates also said, "The greatest medicine of all is teaching people how not to need it." We want to help you live your most-healthy life. Keep your recare appointments and ask us questions.

Call today!

Delizioso Gazpacho!

This is so easy... Combine all ingredients in a large bowl, cover & refrigerate for 4 hours. If you want, blend to change consistency. Fancy it up with garnish.

- 2 cups tomato juice
- 4 medium tomatoes, peeled and finely chopped
- ½ cup chopped seeded peeled cucumber
- ⅓ cup finely chopped onion
- ¼ cup olive oil
- ¼ cup cider vinegar
- 1 teaspoon sugar
- 1 garlic clove, minced
- ¼ teaspoon salt
- ¼ teaspoon pepper

Figure 17. Example of 380 Dental's newsletter direct mail piece. Back side.

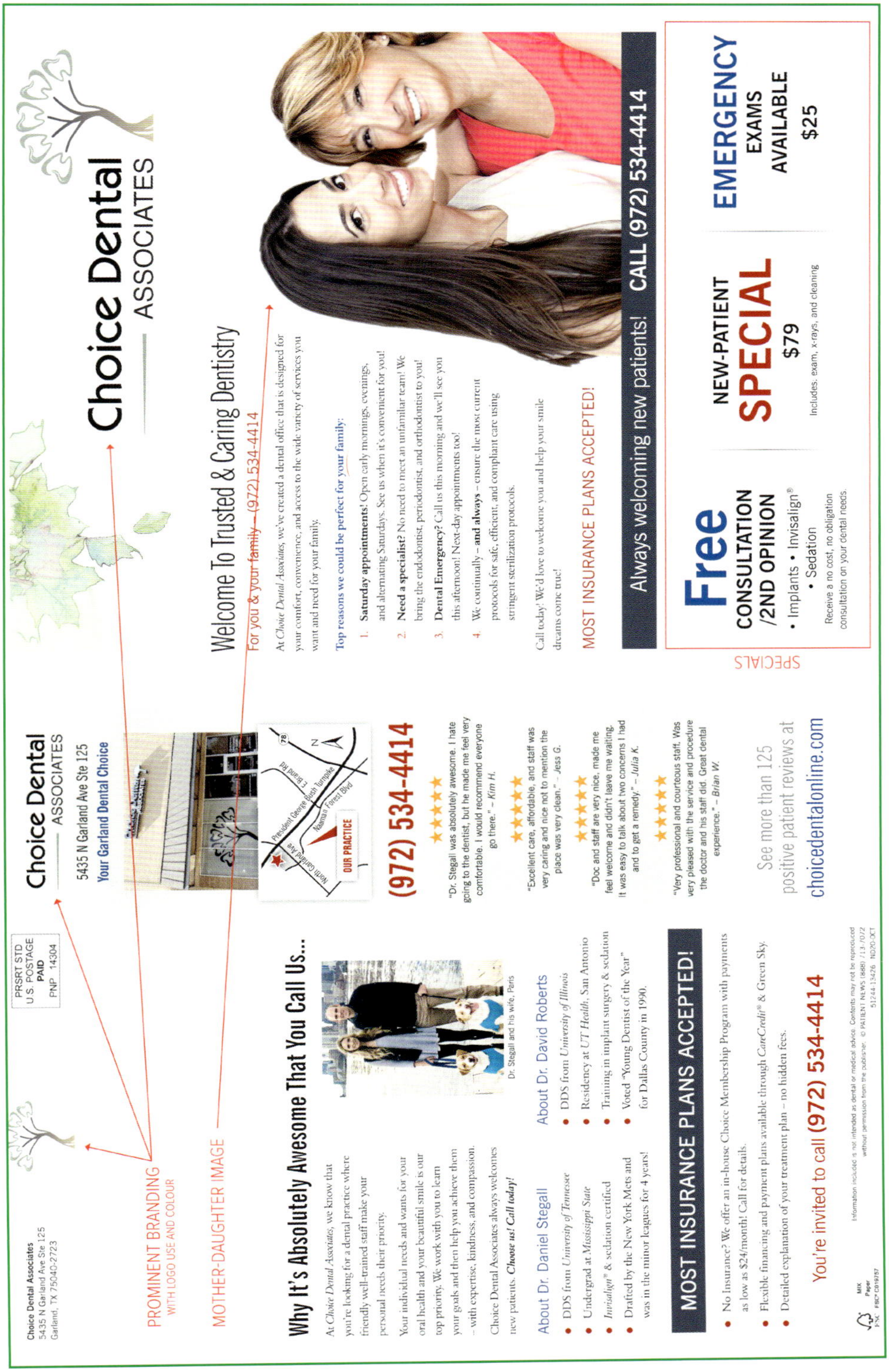

Figure 18. Example of Choice Dental's newsletter direct mail piece. Front side.

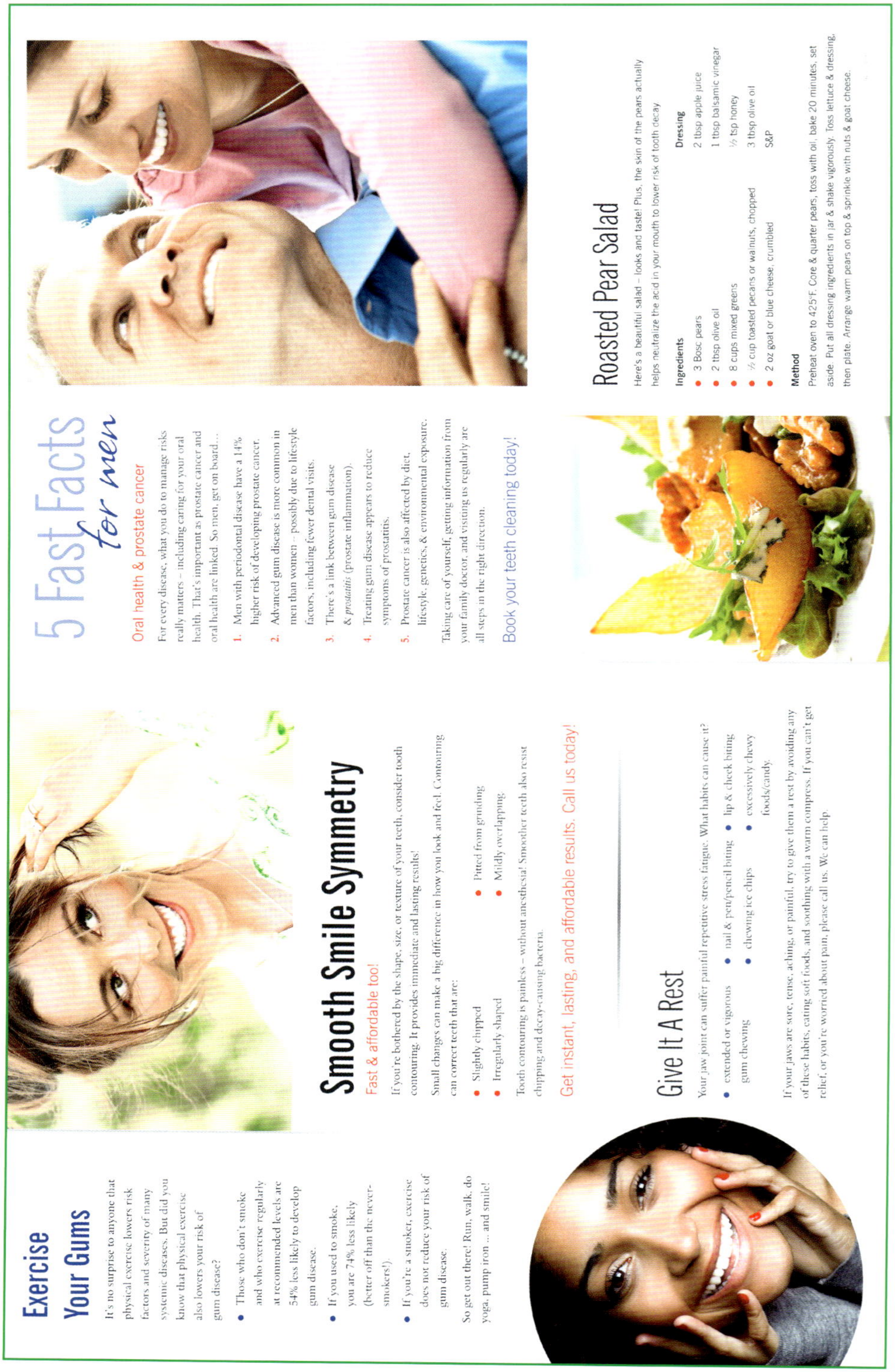
Exercise Your Gums
It's no surprise to anyone that physical exercise lowers risk factors and severity of many systemic diseases. But did you know that physical exercise also lowers your risk of gum disease?
• Those who don't smoke and who exercise regularly at recommended levels are 54% less likely to develop gum disease.
• If you used to smoke, you are 74% less likely (better off than the never-smokers!).
• If you're a smoker, exercise does not reduce your risk of gum disease.
So get out there! Run, walk, do yoga, pump iron ... and smile!
Smooth Smile Symmetry
Fast & affordable too!
If you're bothered by the shape, size, or texture of your teeth, consider tooth contouring. It provides immediate and lasting results!
Small changes can make a big difference in how you look and feel. Contouring can correct teeth that are:
• Slightly chipped
• Irregularly shaped
• Pitted from grinding
• Mildly overlapping
Tooth contouring is painless – without anesthesia! Smoother teeth also resist chipping and decay-causing bacteria.
Get instant, lasting, and affordable results. Call us today!
Give It A Rest
Your jaw joint can suffer painful repetitive stress fatigue. What habits can cause it?
• extended or vigorous gum chewing
• nail & pen/pencil biting
• chewing ice chips
• lip & cheek biting
• excessively chewy foods/candy.
If your jaws are sore, tense, aching, or painful, try to give them a rest by avoiding any of these habits, eating soft foods, and soothing with a warm compress. If you can't get relief, or you're worried about pain, please call us. We can help.
5 Fast Facts for men
Oral health & prostate cancer
For every disease, what you do to manage risks really matters – including caring for your oral health. That's important as prostate cancer and oral health are linked. So men, get on board...
1. Men with periodontal disease have a 14% higher risk of developing prostate cancer.
2. Advanced gum disease is more common in men than women – possibly due to lifestyle factors, including fewer dental visits.
3. There's a link between gum disease & prostatitis (prostate inflammation).
4. Treating gum disease appears to reduce symptoms of prostatitis.
5. Prostate cancer is also affected by diet, lifestyle, genetics, & environmental exposure.
Taking care of yourself, getting information from your family doctor, and visiting us regularly are all steps in the right direction.
Book your teeth cleaning today!
Roasted Pear Salad
Here's a beautiful salad – looks and taste! Plus, the skin of the pears actually helps neutralize the acid in your mouth to lower risk of tooth decay.
Ingredients
• 3 Bosc pears
• 2 tbsp olive oil
• 8 cups mixed greens
• ½ cup toasted pecans or walnuts, chopped
• 2 oz goat or blue cheese, crumbled
Dressing
2 tbsp apple juice
1 tbsp balsamic vinegar
½ tsp honey
3 tbsp olive oil
S&P
Method
Preheat oven to 425°F. Core & quarter pears, toss with oil, bake 20 minutes, set aside. Put all dressing ingredients in jar & shake vigorously. Toss lettuce & dressing, then plate. Arrange warm pears on top & sprinkle with nuts & goat cheese.

Figure 19. Example of Choice Dental's newsletter direct mail piece. Back side.

Results

This is where it gets interesting. Both practices were hitting it out of the park from campaign launch. While 380 Family Dentistry is continuing to mail and see significant new-patient flow, the direct mail campaign at Choice Dental Associates was halted due to different influencing factors in November 2020 resulting in a steady decline of new patients post campaign.

Here are the results as presented graphically in Practice ZEBRA:

380 Family Dentistry

New-Patient Flow by Month (pre-campaign and through ongoing campaign).

In Figure 20, you'll see the dramatic impact on overall new-patient flow during the time of the direct mail campaign, with no other change to the practice marketing effort. The newsletter, as an awareness-building and direct-response vehicle, drove new patients, existing patients, lapsing patients, and referrals to the phone, website, and the practice.

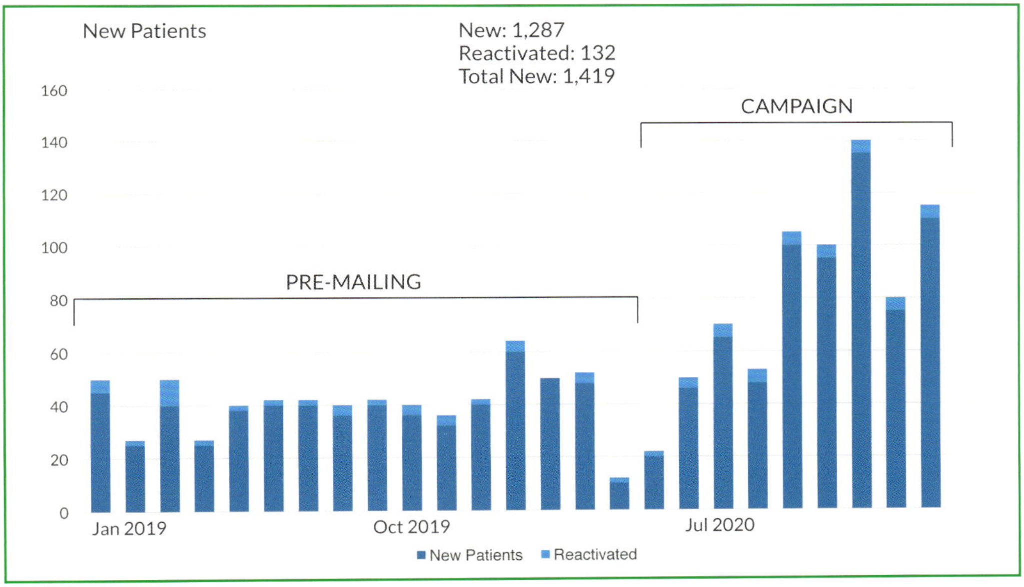

Figure 20. Data showing how new patient count rose at 380 Dental with an active newsletter campaign.

Choice Dental Associates

In Figure 21 you can see the new-patient flow by month (pre-campaign, through ongoing campaign, and through discontinuation). New patients dropped from a peak campaign volume of 76 in August 2020, to 23, 19, and 17 post campaign in the months of December 2020, and January and February 2021, respectively.

380 Family Dentistry and Choice Dental Associates comparative ROI analysis

In this detailed ROI analysis, information is presented for each location including results of annual new-patient flow pre-campaign and pre-pandemic in 2019. These are compared with both the total consolidated results for 2020 and the growth of monthly new patients

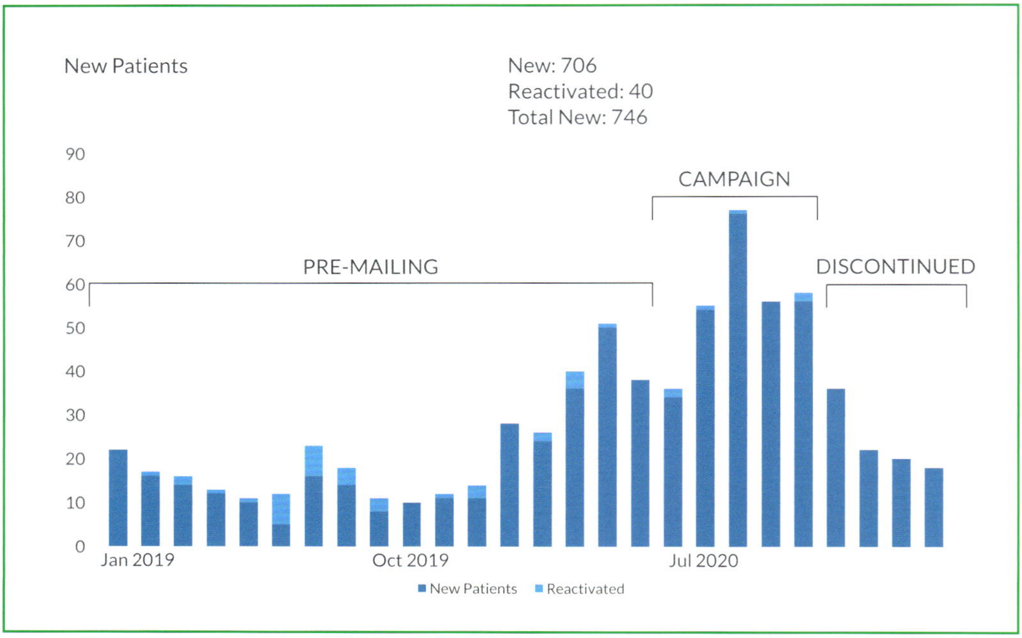

Figure 21. Data showing Choice Dental's new patient flow during and after stopping their newsletter campaign.

	380 Family Dentistry	Choice Dental Associates
2019 total new patients (pre-campaign)	488	178
2020 total new patients (with campaign)	815	531
2019 average new patients / month (pre-campaign)	36	13
2020 average new patients / month (during campaign)	79	55
Additional new patients / month	+43 (2x)	+42 (4x)
New-patient value (as reported by practice software)	$2,718	$1,063
Additional annualized revenue*	$1,402,488	$443,000
DM investment	$40,000	$22,000
Current projected new-patient revenue from campaign (*based on actual practice new-patient value*)	$366,930	$62,118
Direct mail ROI	9:1	3:1**

* Additional annualized revenue = additional new patients/mo × new-patient value × 12 months.
** While Choice Dental Associates did achieve a considerable increase in new-patient flow and a current 3:1 return on investment, they were further negatively affected by a lower average new-patient value vs 380 Family Dentistry and a less consistent campaign with shorter duration.

Figure 22. ROI analysis from both offices' newsletter campaigns.

through the specific campaign time period. In both cases the campaign results are significant with new patients doubling and even quadrupling during mailing months.

The results are then expressed in terms of overall impact on practice production and production as isolated from the campaign to date.

From this case study, you can see the benefits of working with a marketing company to help you identify your target market, to use technology and track where these patients live and work and how best to put your messages in front of them, in this case, using direct mail newsletters. When you have your market, message, medium, content, and offers in alignment and you have some way to track the actual ROI of your results, you can see how effective your marketing dollars can become. For Dr. Campbell, that meant a 9:1 ROI for his main practice and a 3:1 ROI for his satellite office. It also shows us why we need to track the actual ROI, as the average spend per patient was completely different at his two locations, despite netting around the same new patient count per month. Both newsletter campaigns were still effective but showing that more effort may be needed to boost the ROI at the satellite office.

3. <u>Postcard</u>
   People like receiving postcards, whether it's from a friend to wish them a happy birthday or to say hello from their latest vacation excursion. When we see them in the mail, they get our attention. That's why postcards have proven to be an effective format to use in direct mail marketing. They can be used to promote specific niche services you provide such as sedation dentistry or dental implants or to place incentives and other new patient specials to try to attract potential new patients to your practice. There are four main sizes available to choose from.

- **Small (4.25" by 6")**: With the least amount of real estate, this postcard is compact, making it optimal for simple, straight-to-the-point designs. It is also the *only size* within this guide recognized as a traditional "postcard" by the US Postal Service (USPS). According to the USPS, a postcard measures between 3.5" x 5" and 4.25" x 6" – *anything larger is considered a "letter."* Therefore, if your size falls into this space, you can send at first-class rates, which carry a lower cost of postage than other direct mail formats.
- **Standard (6" by 9")**: Out of the four main sizes, standard offers the most versatility and is the most commonly size selected. It is larger than standard envelopes, which allows it to stand out in the mailbox in comparison. It's also small enough to fit in all types of mailboxes, from large to small. See Figure 23 for an example.
- **Jumbo (6" by 11")**: Generally the largest utilized on the market, jumbo postcard size offers the same versatility as the standard size, with larger proportions. Given its size, you'll likely want a vertical design similar to that of a poster. This is the postcard size I utilized the most to advertise niche procedures such as dental implant edentulous arch appliances. It gives more real estate for your photos, messages, and offer while keeping you in a reasonable postage range. From a postage standpoint, staying in the letter-size rate is important. Once you exceed 6.125 by 11.5, the rate category shifts to a flat rate. That would increase the postage rate from 28.7 to 59.8 cents.
- **Extra Large (9" by 12")**: Extra-large postcards fall under the flat rate pricing outlined above, so expect extra postage costs. The biggest advantage of this size is an increased

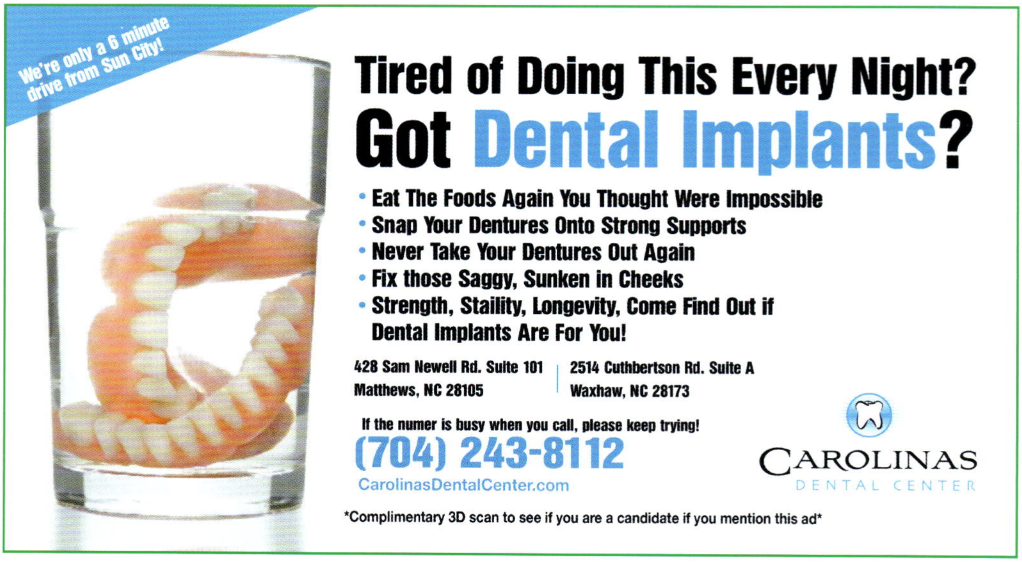

Figure 23. Example of a 6-by-9-inch postcard campaign for dental implants.

chance your target market will see it, as compared to the standard-sized letters and other postcard marketing they may receive in their mailbox. This one definitely stands out.

4. <u>*Self-Published Magazine*</u>
   The largest direct mail format you can use comes from using customized magazines. These are usually 8" by 11" in sizes with a soft, glossy cover that usually totals 8–16 front and back pages. The main focus of these magazines is to put you and your practice at the center of attention while also providing your potential new patient readers educational content about their oral health. Its size and the amount of space you have to put your marketing messages is probably the biggest advantage of this direct mail format. A secondary advantage comes from Dr. Cialdini's authority principle, which, if you remember, states that we look to credible, trustworthy authorities to lead us and tell us what to do. Because of this principle, we often look to cues that signify that someone might be an expert or someone of importance. Through time and experience we've learned that one of these cues is when people are featured on the cover of a magazine. Here are some tips to run a successful direct mail magazine campaign.

- Have a good understanding of who your target market is and what messages you want to promote to them.
- Make sure you have a professional, custom photo shoot planned to capture imagery that will engage the reader and interest him or her in booking an appointment.
- Engage copywriters who will reflect your office's strengths and benefits and elicit phone calls.
- Make sure it has an attractive, professional design.

CASE STUDY

Drs. Eric Jones and Katie Copeland are general dentists who practice in Flowery Branch, Georgia, a town with a population of approximately 8500 and with a median household income of $81,000, an amount that is approximately $20,000 higher than the median household income of all Georgia residents. Their practice does all aspects of general dentistry but has a focus on sedation, cosmetic, and implant dental services. For the last 5 years, Dr. Jones has directed a large percentage of their marketing budget toward this medium of self-publishing his own dental focused magazine (Fig. 24).

Dr. Jones's target market is those who live within a 10-mile radius, those with an average household income of $100,000 or more, those over the age of 55, and those who fit either of those criteria but also have great credit worthiness. The messages that are featured in the magazine relate back to what he considers his unique selling proposition (USP), that USP being something that makes you stand out from others, that really differentiates you because few others do the same. From him these are:

a. A promise not to judge: To Dr. Jones, many of the patients he has treated have avoided the dentist because they were embarrassed that they had let their dental condition deteriorate as much as it had. In doing so, they were afraid that when they finally saw a dentist, they would be shamed in some way for letting their condition worsen like they had. His patients were pleasantly surprised that he in fact did the opposite with them, not blaming them for their current state but instead choosing to support them in building a solution to the problems at hand moving forward.

b. A written guarantee: In Dr. Jones's experience, few dentists guarantee their work, much less put that guarantee down in writing. Dr. Jones stands by his work and guarantees it for 10 years, promising to fix any issues that occur as long as the patient is committed to coming in for hygiene two times per year.

c. An experience they won't remember: Sedation dentistry is a big part of Dr. Jones's practice, offering both oral and IV sedation. With amnesia being one of the side effects of the sedation process, patients come from miles around to get the work they need while remembering very little of their visit, guaranteeing them a great experience.

d. One location, one doc, one fee: When it comes to more complicated procedures such as "all-on-X" and other type of implant-related edentulous arch treatments, patients often are uncertain when they have to travel between multiple offices for everything from consultations, treatment planning, and then the actual surgeries and prosthodontic appointments. With each office visited comes more potential for confusion in the patient's mindset, confusion and uncertainty about what they are getting done, how much the whole thing will cost them, and more. At Dr. Jones's practice, he tries to alleviate this by offering all of the work they need, from planning to completion, in one location and performed by one dentist. He also offers these as treatment bundles with one fee, depending on the final prosthodontic restoration the patient chooses.

By targeting his list of potential new patients, an average of about 30,000 magazines go out through this medium every quarter, with a total investment in printing and postage costing approximately $7000. The content featured in the magazine showcases many before and

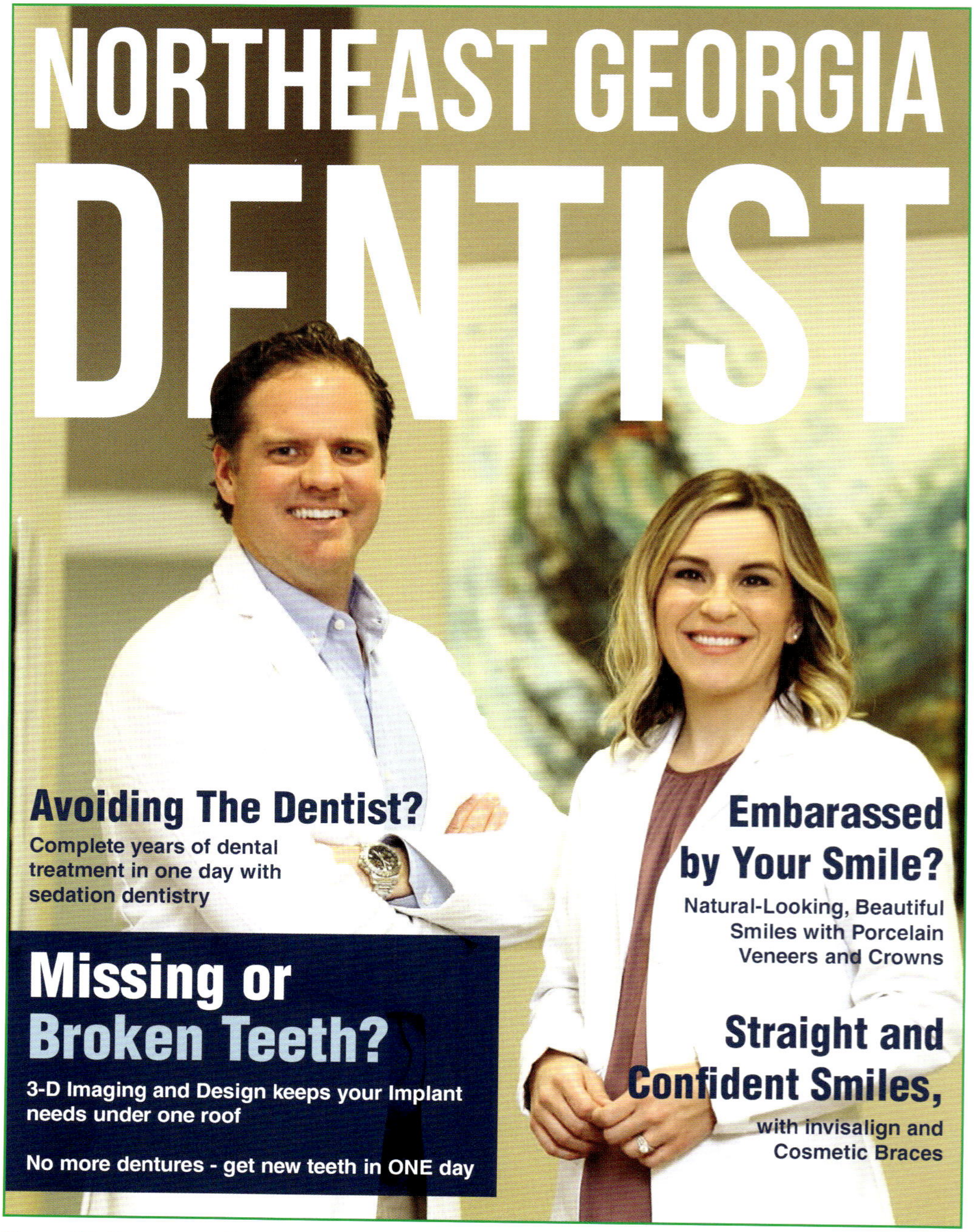

Figure 24. Example of Drs. Jones and Copeland's self-published direct mail magazine.

NEW PATIENT OPPORTUNITIES

New patient opportunities	131	
Appointments booked	114	87.02%
Appointments not booked	17	12.98%

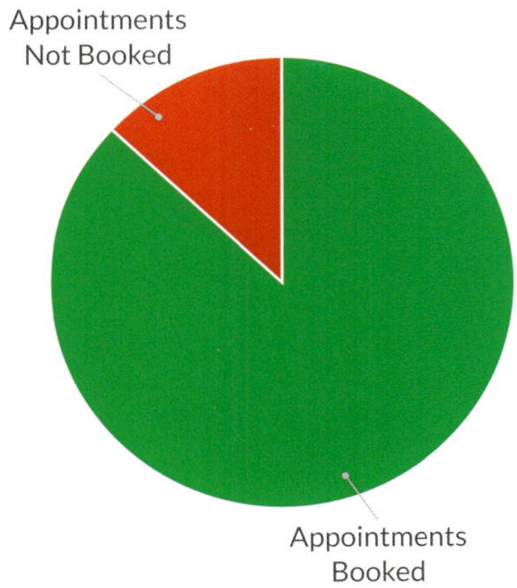

Figure 25. **Dr. Jones's call tracking data showing the number of new patients acquired from all of his marketing efforts over a four-month period as well as the team's success rate on turning those opportunities into appointments.**

after photos, along with pictures of happy, smiling patients who have undergone treatment. It also highlights stories from patients who talk about the hope that was restored in their life after having dental work done by Dr. Jones rather than just discussing the specific procedure they had performed. Each magazine ranges from 8 to 10 pages in total, printed on full color, glossy style paper, giving it the weight and feel of other magazines a potential patient might receive in the mail or have in their home.

When it comes to offers that might entice more patients to call for an appointment, he taps into Cialdini's authority principle by offering a free second opinion. You see, people look to credible, trustworthy experts for advice on what they should do. The more experts recommending something, the more likely people are to say yes. The free second opinion taps into this principle because it's another expert confirming their dental need and recommending some type of treatment.

Another offer Dr. Jones employs is a complimentary initial consultation. This offer is for patients who are early in the discovery process of what their current dental condition is. At this point, money might be a concern as they are unsure of the amount or scope of work that they will need done. By offering the complimentary consultation, it helps to remove that potential barrier in patients' minds.

With tracking and ROI, Dr. Jones incorporates unique call tracking numbers that are specific to each of his various marketing endeavors, such as his self-published magazine. Each call that comes in from this number is recorded, analyzed, and the data is ported to his monthly call tracking report. In Figure 25, you can see how many new patient opportunity calls were generated from all of Dr. Jones's marketing efforts and how many turned into actual appointments. From there, as shown in Figure 26, he can determine how many actually showed up to his office for care and how much each one spent at his office, determining whether the actual ROI makes this an investment instead of an expense.

To aid in his tracking efforts, Dr. Jones has also created a dedicated landing page, a limited website that is separate from the one he has for his main office but whose web address is heavily featured throughout the magazine. On this landing page is a different call tracking number, allowing Dr. Jones to not only see how many calls came directly from the magazine tracking number but also factor in how many people liked what they saw in the magazine and wanted to go to a website to search for more information, directing them to his dedicated landing page. From there, once their search and interest were satisfied and they were ready to make an appointment, they'd call from the landing page call tracking number they saw in front of them. Combining these two sources, Dr. Jones now has the whole truth as to how many patients showed up to his office from this direct mail medium, allowing his team to track how much they spend in the office over a period of time.

Source Name	Opportunities
Direct landing page	40
Direct mail magazine	6
Neighborhood ads	2
Brochure style flyers	26
Organic search	44
PPC Adwords campaigns	13
Total	**131**

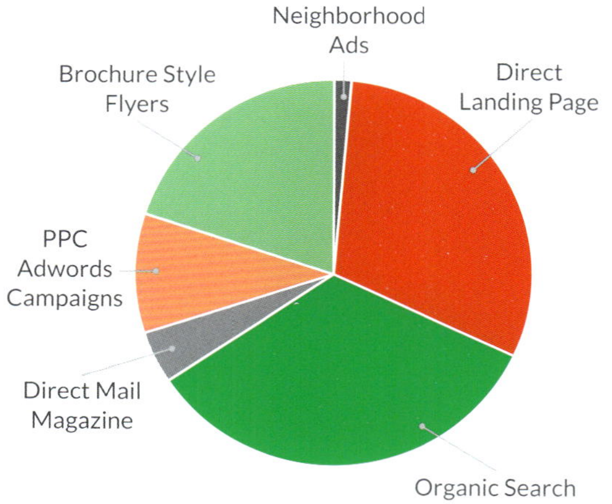

Figure 26. Call tracker ROI "Whole Truth Report," showing the number of new patient opportunities for each source.

To date, Dr. Jones invests around $28,000 per year into this medium and nets a 4:1 actual ROI of $112,000 in collections over their first six months in the practice. The longer they stay on as patients, the higher the return becomes. For Dr. Jones, this has been a very successful and predictable medium that he's been able to utilize to find more patients who are looking to do the type of dentistry he wants to do more of.

Newspaper Inserts

In advertising, an insert is a separate advertisement put in a magazine, newspaper, or other publication. In my practices, I chose to put my inserts into our local newspaper, the *Charlotte Observer*. According to a recent consumer usage report on newspaper advertising, 83 percent of adults regularly or occasionally read newspaper inserts while 70 percent reported they responded to them.

The newspaper inserts I used were usually 8.5" by 11" size, which are printed on both the front and back sides in full color on glossy paper. I targeted those who got the local paper and lived within a 10-mile radius around my practice. While you could insert your piece on any given day of the week, the two most popular times were Wednesdays and Sundays.

If your target market is younger, maybe a family demographic, then Wednesdays might give you the best chance to reach them as that was the coupon day because Wednesday is the day the majority of coupons are inserted into the newspaper and many women would sift through these, clip out their coupons of interest in preparation for their shopping that weekend. If you were after an older demographic, then Sundays proved to be the best day to insert your piece. Sunday is the day of the week that most consumers actively read newspapers and search out any inserts present. In fact, studies show that 48 percent of adults check inserts from the newspaper on this day. Sundays also allow you to reach a larger audience than during the weekday as a large percentage of people only receive the newspapers on the weekend.

Here are some additional advantages of marketing using newspaper inserts:

- **Makes you stand out**: When reading the newspaper, there is no guarantee that the ads embedded into the paper will stand out and grab a potential new patient's attention. An insert, on the other hand, is something physically separate from the paper and must be handled at some point by the person reading it. This gives you a chance for your ad to be seen. I remember once asking a patient why she choose our practice, and she said that she was opening up her newspaper and "you just fell into my lap, so I knew it was a sign that you were the place I needed to go since I'm having a dental issue." In essence, she was opening the newspaper, and our insert fell out along with the other coupons inserted. Our ad just happened to be right on top and was the first thing she saw.
- **Inserts are cost effective**: My costs averaged around 5 cents per piece, which included the printing and insertion of it into the newspaper, allowing me to put my message in front of 50,000 potential new patients for around $2500.
- **Distribution is flexible**: There doesn't tend to be any contracts associated with newspaper insert campaigns. You can drop them once a month, once a quarter, or even once a year if you desire. With a unique tracking number embedded into the ad, you can test their effectiveness over a single drop and then choose your distribution pattern from there. For my practices, I noticed that a single drop of around 50,000 pieces on a Sunday would net me 60 new patients over a three-month period with an ROI of 12:1.
- **Real staying power**: Stand-alone flyers and ads are often dumped into the trash can or recycling bin, but if you include an insert into a newspaper that people have already subscribed to, the shelf life of your campaign can be measured for a longer period of time. Because these inserts are easily removed from the paper, people have a tendency to hold onto them for a longer period of time, perhaps when dental care becomes more top of mind or pressing at a later date. I remember a sedation dentistry patient who had just completed over $10,000 of work with us. As I was escorting her in a wheelchair to her daughter's car to leave, I noticed the patient had one of our newspaper inserts folded up and sitting prominently on top of her purse. What intrigued me about this was that I had not ran a newspaper insert campaign for almost two years, choosing to focus on testing other marketing media instead, yet here was this patient with our ad from two years ago. When I asked her about the ad, she told me that she saw it in her newspaper a while ago but at that time she wasn't ready to seek out help for her dental condition. Because she loved the ad and its messages, she told me she put it away in a drawer so that when she was ready, she'd know exactly which dentist could help her.

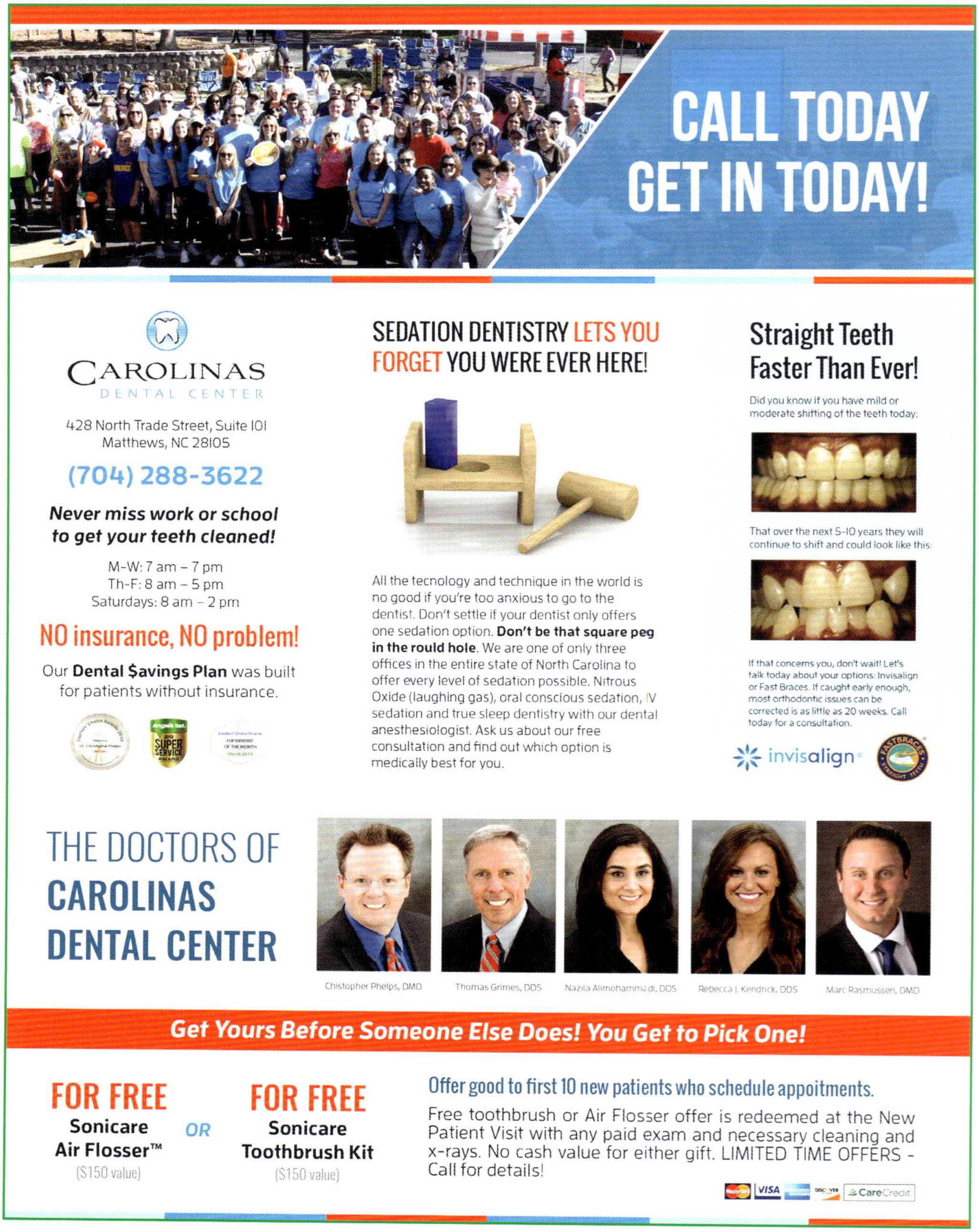

Figure 27. Example of newspaper insert advertisement. Front side.

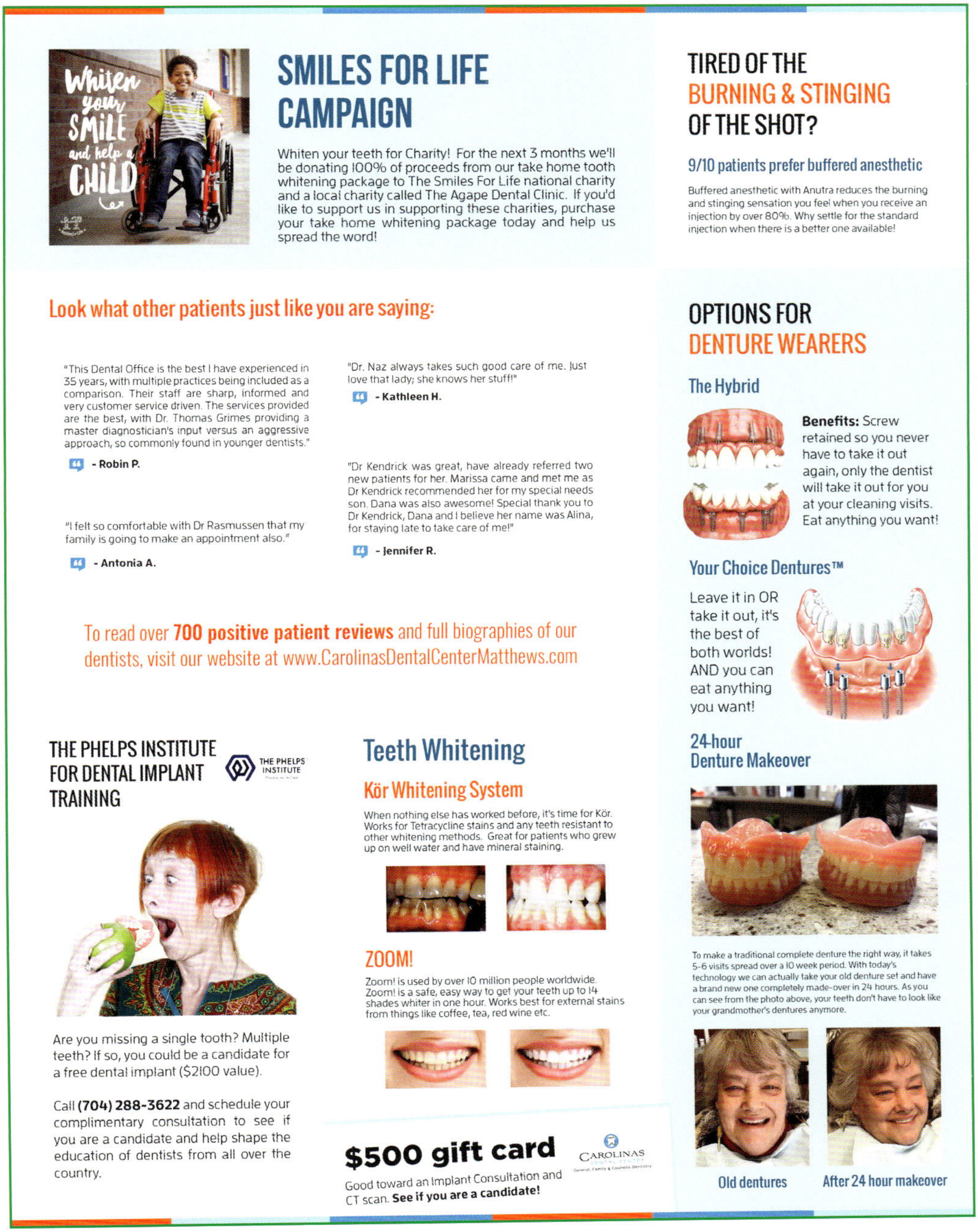

Figure 28. Example of newspaper insert advertisement. Back side.

Radio

Despite all the changes in the last decade in how Americans access music, AM/FM radio is still a cost-effective advertising medium to reach your existing and potential patients. With the widespread access people have to radio, even indirectly through shopping centers and supermarkets, radio continues to have a big presence in the advertising industry. Some advantages of radio marketing include:

- **Selective targeting**: Radio stations already target specific demographics and market segments. Therefore, by choosing which station to broadcast with, you can lock onto your potential customers and increase the frequency of delivering your message. This is why understanding your target market is key as it will aid in your selection process. AM stations tend to attract more male listeners while FM stations tend to attract more female listeners. Radio stations have also done a lot of research into where their demographic lives and works. Our job is to find a station whose demographic lines up best with where our target market lives and works as well.
- **Increased frequency**: Advertising works with frequency and reaching your audience repeatedly. Radio is the perfect medium for this, being able to expose your ad to the audience repeatedly to build awareness. Also due to the loyalty of people listening to the same station, you are able to influence the same people more often.
- **More memorable**: Compared to written advertisement, sound is more effectively stored in memory. In addition, there is the ability to instill emotion and also allows listeners to use their imagination to create their own image of the product/service.
- **Cost effective**: Radio advertising have significantly less costs compared to other types of media. Television and print ads can go up to hundreds of thousands including costs for video equipment, studio time, actors, and models. Radio ads require less resources while being able to reach the same target audience that a television spot would have resulted in.
- **Time efficiency**: Lead times with print and television ads can be very long, especially with planning, and may take up to a year for the ad to run. In contrast, producing a radio spot can take between two and three weeks. Another advantage of this is the ability to adapt and react quickly to changing market conditions. Adding a new offer or changing your main message can be done fairly quickly, making it easier to measure any change in response from potential new patients.

Another advantage of radio ads is their measurable results. With dedicated call tracking numbers, you can track results quickly and accurately. Results for radio ads can be analyzed on a daily basis, and if the message is not working to help generate calls in a week or two, a new radio spot can replace it efficiently as mentioned above. When I first started advertising using radio, I tested three different messages in my commercials, one focused on basic information about our dental practice, one on sedation dentistry, and one on how we provided "comprehensive care" or specialty services so patients didn't have to go to four or five offices to get their dental work performed. Each commercial had a different call tracking number associated with them so I could look at our call volume and see which message was producing the highest number of calls. After a few weeks I found the sedation and comprehensive care messages generated the most calls, and those patients were spending at a level that gave us the highest ROI for our investment.

Once I had established which messages provided the best results, I then was able to start experimenting with the frequency of my commercials. Most radio advertisers want you to purchase a large package of airtime as their research shows that to get the best results, your potential new patient would need hear your commercial run 3.4 times per week. The best way they recommend achieving this is by running 21 ads per week for 52 weeks. By using detailed call tracking reports from call tracker ROI, I was able to make changes to this schedule and see if it changed my results. The first thing I modified was discontinuing my commercials on the weekends. Radio listeners tend to be impulse buyers. They hear an ad, get excited about it, and want to take action right then and there. Unfortunately, our office wasn't open on the weekends, so I noticed a good number of calls coming in when we couldn't service them.

The next ads I dropped came after our office was closed during the week. Each month I made one change and then evaluated the call tracking data to see the impact. When no negative impact was seen, I made the next modification. Eventually I narrowed down my commercial runs to Mondays, Tuesdays, and Wednesdays and focused them during the times people would be driving into work and when people would be driving home from work.

Through methodical tracking I was able to reduce the costs of my radio advertising from $14,000 per month to just over $7000 per month. Regardless of its frequency, we'd average 15–20 new patients a month who came in for sedation dentistry or comprehensive care, and their average spend with us was $2500. With our collections from radio averaging $50,000/month and by taking our expenditure from $14,000 to $7000 month we were able to increase our ROI from 3.6:1 to 7:1.

Once you've identified which radio station's demographic best identifies with your target market, you've ironed out what your potential messages will be, and fleshed out a tentative schedule on when to run your ads, it's now time to decide who you'll use to record your commercial.

1. Self-Recording

As its name implies, this is when you are the one speaking in the commercial about your practice. To decide if you're the right fit, do some practice recordings at the radio studio and have some family and friends give you some honest opinions about what they hear. Do you have a voice for radio? Are you clear? Is the tone and volume of your voice loud enough to come through over other background noise the listener may hear in their car or at work?

2. Standard Radio Announcer Recording

Of the three recording options, this seems to be the most popular among businesses that use this medium. This recording is performed by someone who works at the radio station and has that proven voice for radio. Whether it's you or the standard announcer recording your commercials, you must put some thought into what will be said. Here are some things to consider when writing your commercial:

- Define what you're trying to say. Keep your messages simple and limit them to as few sentences as possible.
- Establish a connection. To be able to engage with listeners you need to understand their problems and empathize with them. How can the product or service you're promoting help the listener? How can it be translated in a way that will make the listener care?

- Data tells but stories sell. Every good ad has a story to engage with listeners, even if it's really simple. Your story needs a problem and solution, preferably one that puts the listener front and center whilst flowing naturally from beginning to end. That can be tricky, especially with a short 30-second ad but not if you keep it simple and to the point.
- Create a call to action. This could be directing them to your website to gather more info or to pick up the phone and call to schedule an appointment and perhaps tap into an offer you've mentioned.

3. Celebrity Endorsement Recording

While being the most expensive of the three recording formats, studies have shown that using celebrities in advertising does increase the message's persuasiveness, which results in consumers having a better recall and recognition for the product or brand. I found this to be true, and it was a big influence on why I chose this specific format. While there are all types of celebrities you could engage to speak about you and your practice, the ones I found to have the biggest impact in the radio industry where those people who recorded the 6–10 a.m. drive into work radio program or who recorded the 3–7 p.m. drive home from work radio program. In my town, I worked exclusively with the drive home from work hosts on the *Matt and Ramona* show. Their program aired on an FM radio station with a strong female demographic whose listeners were between the ages of 35 and 65 and mainly lived 5–7 miles from my practices. I invited Matt and Ramona to become patients of the practice and took care of any dental work they needed so that when they spoke about me and my practices, it was from their own true experiences.

While they had recorded commercials that played at the different intervals I mentioned above, one advantage of hiring them directly was that during their radio program, they would stop and do a live commercial on my behalf. While the recorded spots usually ran 30 seconds, the live spots could go for up to 2–3 minutes depending on what they wanted to say about their experience at my practices.

Utilizing their local celebrity status was also important to help me promote other marketing events I was running such as our patient appreciation party that I spoke about earlier in the book. Using radio gave us exposure to a much larger audience than we could have promoted to on our own. Having Matt and Ramona out in person to our event was a huge draw to encourage our existing patients to come out as well as enticing more potential new patients to join our party.

Another big advantage of using these radio celebrities was that when they endorsed me and my practices, even though I was a paid advertiser, it was like a direct referral. Many times I'd have patients in the chair telling me they were there because "Matt and Ramona said I should come here." These people were so popular that their listeners thought of them as good friends, friends who were referring them to us. Because of their endorsement and referral, it gave me and my practices an elevated authority status and automatically set the stage for higher case acceptance rates on these patients.

Television

According to Cengage Learning, television advertising still rules when advertisers make media purchases. Approximately 40 cents of each dollar spent on advertising across all industries is derived from TV advertising. Television advertising enables companies to reach local and national viewing markets. The largest share of TV advertising revenue is generated by businesses or organizations with nationwide advertising budgets, but small businesses such as dental practices do have an opportunity to reach potential new patients using this medium.

Standard television commercials, whether seen from a nationwide cable provider or satellite TV provider are approximately 30 seconds to 1 minute in length and can be placed over broadcast and/or cable channels. Having a clear understanding of who your target market is can help you decide whether one or both of these options are right for you to test.

1. Broadcast Reaches More People

Broadcast TV advertising uses all your local channels (ABC, NBC, FOX, etc.). Because everyone has access to broadcast (it comes free over the air), your ads will show to more people. This means you cannot target your advertising as well, but if your goal is general brand awareness, this is a good fit.

2. Cable/Satellite Targets by Interest

Cable and satellite advertising offers you all the channels you have to pay for such as MTV, HGTV, and Science Channel. TV shows that air on cable or satellite TV can attract a very specific audience—and usually has a much smaller reach than advertising on broadcast TV. For example, there is a big difference between the interests of those who watch HGTV and those who watch MTV. If you're trying to target a very specific demographic or group and have a limited budget, cable may be your best option. For my practices, I found my target market tended to spend more time watching channels such as HGTV and Food Network, so I chose to narrow my TV marketing efforts to these areas.

3. Streaming Services

Streaming TV advertising refers to running paid advertisements on streaming services such as Hulu, Amazon Prime Video, or YouTube TV. These ads typically run in either 15- or 30-second segments. One advantage is that many of these sites keep movie and TV content free to the viewer, but the consumer is forced to watch your advertisement as the price of admission. That's why there tends to be a 96 percent view rate that's shown with this option, potentially making it likely that your target market could see your messaging.

TV Advertising advantages

According to advertising researchers, the average consumer is exposed to three hundred to three thousand advertising messages each day. Newspapers, direct mail, branded clothing with shirt-slogans, flyers, and more may consciously or unconsciously increase the prospective buyer's awareness of needed or desired products and services. The best TV ads have many advantages, including viewers' improved market awareness, intrusive–not obnoxious–messaging, and positive engagement. Here are some of the advantages of TV advertising:

Multi-sensory attention

Consumer competition is fierce. TV advertising is one of the best ways to get the attention of potential buyers. Afterward, the advertiser may seek to foster awareness, the first step necessary to encourage prospective buyer action. Without TV advertising, the only medium with sight, motion, and sound properties, the advertiser is limited to "flat" media. Radio ads have only sound, and print ads and billboard ads have only sight to engage the viewer. Television is considered the dominant "mass medium." TV advertising continues to offer the greatest potential to reach the largest number of prospective retail customers.

Reach

Much like Google's reach within the local SEO and digital space, national broadcasters FOX, CBS, ABC, and NBC reach over 120 million viewing households and almost 300 million individual viewers. TV succeeds at reaching almost everyone. Ad Age says it reaches an astounding 95 percent of US consumers. Of course, not all advertisers want to reach every man, woman, and child in America. By segmenting potential viewers by age, race, and gender groups, advertisers select specific programs, channels, and networks for the best potential results.

TV Penetration

Cable TV's share of advertising spend and revenues has continued to grow over the past decade. Satellite TV has also contributed to cable penetration growth. About 75 percent of American households have cable. Cable audiences have actually grown as media researchers predicted their demise. Cable programming—or the focus on content, content, content—is a natural fit for marketers in search of the narrowest target audiences. Narrowcasting on special interest cable channels, including cooking, fitness, health, history, shopping, or home and garden, allows marketers to successfully niche market to an almost unlimited array of specialized audiences.

Always evolving

TV advertising continues to evolve, grow, and thrive. Some recent trends in TV advertising include super-abbreviated spots of 15 seconds. The spots are cheaper to make and easier for small businesses such as dental practices to purchase. Like a video ad that bursts onto a web page unannounced, the ultra-brief TV ad spot is so quick that viewers lack remote control reaction time. These TV ads are so brief, most viewers choose to watch and wait.

TV programming is actually more robust than ever, too. The popularity of websites that offer complete, high-res episodes of everyone's favorite TV shows reflects their importance to viewers. Many cable providers offer subscriber access to a wide array of TV programs to stream on smartphones, computers, and other devices. These TV shows frequently come with advertising. Free TV streaming sites also trade viewer ad views for access.

Banner logo ads and flickering or scrolling superimposed ads may appear during a national sporting event. Streaming headlines on some TV stations may seem like they're from the newsroom, but corporate advertisers and their logos are often present in these news streams.

TV advertising disadvantages

There is a short list of TV advertising disadvantages. The most frequently cited disadvantage of TV advertising by small businesses is its cost. TV campaigns are expensive. Additional disadvantages include ineffective market research and targeting, negative audience perceptions, and fleeting and difficult to recall advertising messages.

Cost

Costs of TV advertising, including commercial production and spot purchases, are substantial. According to small business author Marc Prosser, it costs between $5000 and $20,000 to make a commercial in a major US city. Large cities such as New York and Los Angeles bear higher commercial production costs.

Some TV advertising, like a $3.5 million Super Bowl commercial in 2012, is pedigreed and pricey. Small businesses benefit by working with a local TV station invested in their success. If a TV station has the necessary equipment and studio space, it may produce the advertiser's TV commercial at no cost if the business agrees to spot purchases over several months.

Inefficient targeting

Some TV ads are inefficient at reaching a target audience. If the advertiser wants to reach 100,000 homeowners in a city with an offer, it's wasteful to purchase spots on network news. Research, including ideal customer interviews and surveys, helps the advertiser make efficient media buys.

Viewers skip commercials

TV advertising may contain a fleeting or ephemeral message. Some messages are simply lost when viewers lose interest, get a snack, or change channels. To create greater viewer focus, some businesses decide on longer infomercials. Although some perennially successful infomercials such as the Bowflex Gym or ProActiv Solution Acne Treatment manage to stimulate customer awareness and sell products, others somehow cross the information line and turn viewers off.

4. Dentomercial

"Dentomercial" is a term I use to describe the dental version of an infomercial. An infomercial is a form of advertisement that is a program aimed at educating the customer about a product or a series of products via television. It is an especially long television commercial, typically between thirty minutes and one-hour long and can be featured on broadcast, cable, satellite, or streaming services. For my area, I was able to secure a private recording studio and hired a host to help me record a 30-minute spot, which we split into two formats. The first was more of a talk show style interview format where the host would interview me and ask me questions about my family, upbringing, education, hobbies, and so forth, trying to give my potential new patients opportunities to find commonalities with me in the process. The second part was geared more like a newsroom interview where the host and I were in a different area, and I got into more detail about the dental-related topic of focus, in my case being dental implants and edentulous arch treatments.

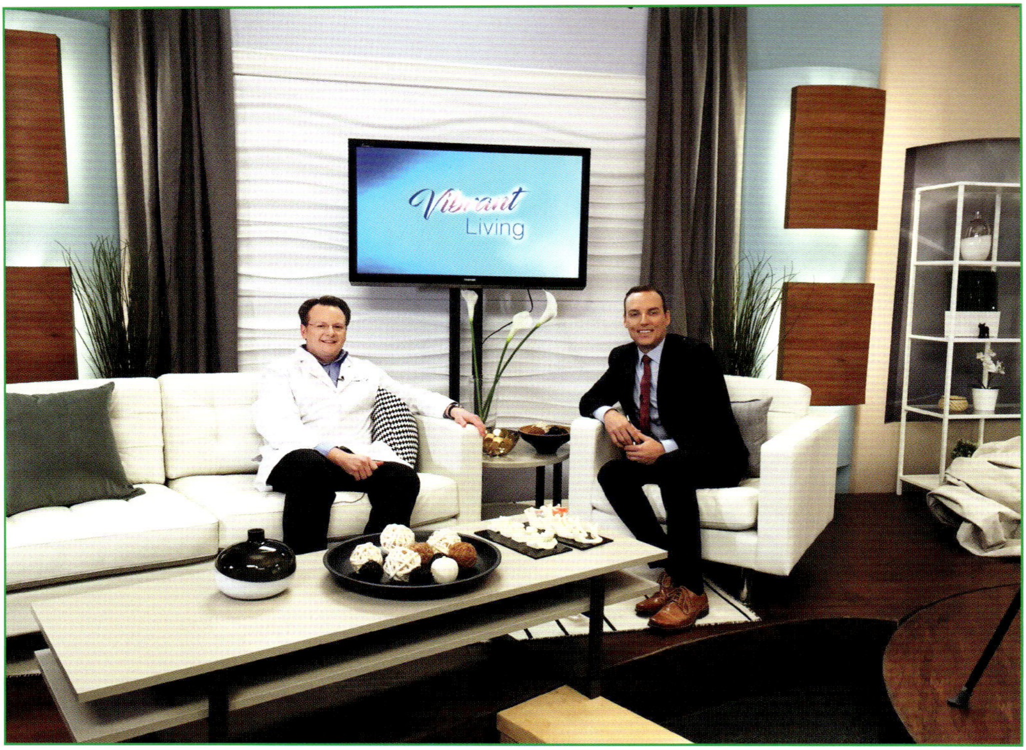

Figure 29. Picture of Dr. Phelps recording a dentomercial for his practice.

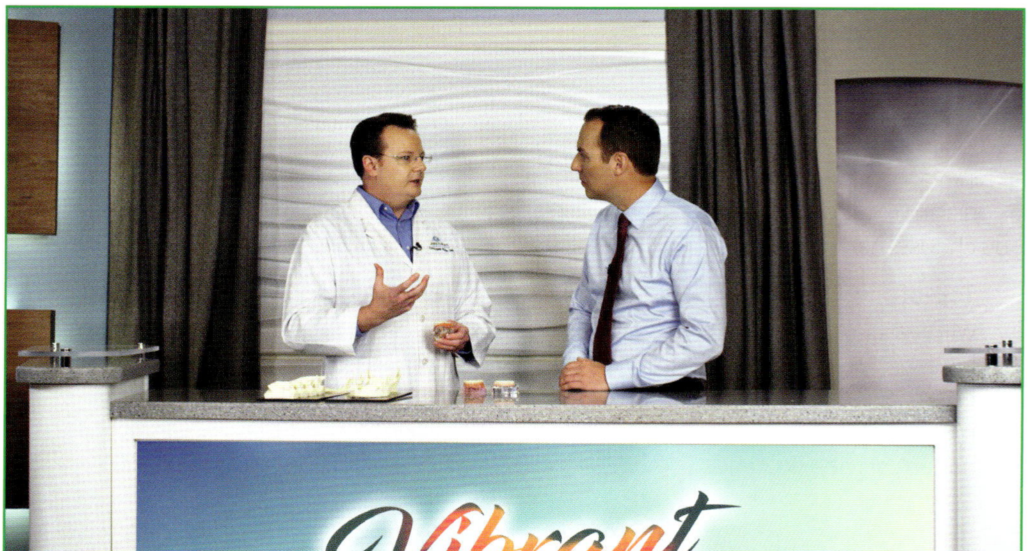

Figure 30. Dr. Phelps being interviewed during a dentomercial recording for his practice.

One of the most well-known dentomercials is called *The Wellness Hour*, hosted by Randy Alvarez. By their own account, *The Wellness Hour TV Show* has become a television and social media platform for doctors to discuss new breakthroughs in their specialty with the communities they serve. As of today's date, they have more than 1800 half-hour programs airing on broadcast, cable, satellite, and direct TV, with a reach of more than 74 million homes each week.

In this dentomercial, the dentist flies into to a private recording studio where they are interviewed as a dental expert looking to promote this area. Traditionally this has been used to promote cosmetic and implant dentistry options for patients. Once the 30-minute spot has been finalized, TV time is bought up on local public access TV as well as other cable TV stations that fits your advertising budget. One of the biggest advantages this dentomercial has over standard TV commercials goes back to those cues and trappings of authority we seek when making our decisions. We've learned that if you're on TV, you are important, and if you're being interviewed by someone on TV, you must be an important person who is an expert in the area in question. When searching for a dentist to solve their dental issue, patients are uncertain about which dentist to choose. Many will see these dentomercials and view the dentist as a leading expert in their area, influencing more to seek them and their treatment options out over others advertising the same messages in other media.

Billboards

A billboard or bulletin is a large outdoor advertising space that is meant to target and attract the attention of pedestrians and motorists in the surrounding area. It's hard to drive down a highway or major road fare these days and not see billboards up and down both sides of your path. It's been reported that the average American spends 48 minutes per day driving, giving ample time for some of them to view billboards. In one survey it was reported that 58 percent of those who looked at billboards learned about an interesting event or about a restaurant they later visited.

In today's world, they come in two forms. Static and digital. Static billboards are a solitary set of words and images that doesn't change. They tend to be the most expensive of the two options because you can't share the billboard space with anyone else. Digital billboards are essentially large computer screens that can be programmed to display messages in a range of innovative ways. They are attractive to many because multiple advertisers can use it with a constant rotation occurring, which helps offset its cost of use. Regardless of which format you choose, here are some tips for effective dental billboard marketing.

- **Top-of-mind messaging**: Billboards have the most impact when their messages line up with what you are actively looking for in that moment. You may be driving down the highway for hours and not notice one, yet as soon as you're hungry, suddenly every billboard that mentions food starts to stand out to you. The same idea should apply to your messaging with billboards. Focus on what might be top of mind for that potential new patient driving down the road that would motivate them to remember your ad and call. Maybe it's a cosmetic message or one geared toward emergency treatment. Having a tooth ache would definitely make finding a dentist top of mind. So sharing that you take emergency patients or that you can see emergency patients on the same day they call could be powerful messages that would get people's attention.

- **Make it memorable**: When possible, make it funny. Remember, people are driving past your message at a quick rate. You may have a few seconds at best of their attention. *When the ad was humorous, 56 percent of people surveyed after being exposed to billboards reported remembering key details.*
- **Keep it simple**: Provide people with precious little information. In fact, depending on who you consult, it's recommended that the billboard type be confined to no more than 10 words. Only 28 percent of billboard watchers reported remembering a long website address, and only 26 percent remembered the listed phone number. When possible, keep both of these simple. Try having a dedicated landing page, something with a very short and easy name to remember, and refer billboard watchers here. Once they go to this site, it can redirect them to your main website. Consider purchasing a number that's easy to remember as well, For instance, 444-4444 has worked extremely well for a large nationwide taxi car company.
- **It works well with others**: Consider pairing your billboard with other online marketing efforts or a direct mail campaign. The branding seen on the billboard should match the branding used in these other media. Studies show that your billboard will create a familiarity in that person's mind because they are constantly exposed to it in their daily travels. When they get something like a direct mail piece in their mailbox, automatically they will be more drawn to it than any other dental ad present because of that familiarity. When it comes time to choose a dental provider, people will typically refer back to what seemed the most familiar to them, even though they won't be able to attest to why it's the most familiar.

Magazines

Magazine advertising has long been considered one of the best ways to use print media to promote a business, a product, or even just an exciting opportunity. A magazine is more than a simple news source or bit of entertainment. It's a periodical piece of literature that many subscribers save to review more than once. This gives your advertisement the potential for repetitive exposures. Traditionally, when you think of magazine marketing, you may think of placing your ad in popular nationwide magazines such as *People*, *Entertainment Weekly*, *Elle*, or *Men's Health*.

With dental marketing, I recommend you narrow your focus down to more regional magazines. Their name may match up with your city, such as *Charlotte Magazine*, be directed toward a certain region of your city, such as *South Charlotte Living*, or they'll cater to a higher retail section of town, such as *Ballantyne Magazine*. These are usually free magazines that you'd find in grocery stores or pharmacies. Sometimes the publisher will mail a copy to everyone in a certain geographic area.

Your business doesn't have to tie directly into the topics of any one of the magazines, as long as the readers of those magazines would also be interested in your product or service. Remember, it's the audience that counts, and you can find that audience in any number of places. When selecting one of these types of magazines to advertise in, there are some factors you need to consider:

- What's the magazine's circulation? Is it within a certain radius around your practice?
- What are the demographics of the readers? Does it match up with your target market?

- How often is the magazine published?
- How is it distributed? Is it available in grocery stores or mailed out to residents in an area?
- Where will your ad be placed? On the front inside cover, back cover for best visibility, or somewhere in the middle?

There are three other important factors to consider in order to maximize your magazine marketing opportunity. The first comes from finding out what other articles or advertisements may be placed around your marketing piece. From an influence standpoint, what people are exposed to first can affect their perception when they see your ad next. This is one reason I don't like marketing on the front page of the newspaper. Sure, it's great exposure and your ad is likely to be seen, but many times the stories showcased on the front page are extremely negative. Murder, corrupt politicians, violence tend to dominate this page and can form a negative mindset in that person, who then finds your ad.

A dentist friend of mine had purchased a one-page, full-color ad in his town's most popular local magazine. I helped him with the design and messaging, and we confirmed that his target market were avid readers of this publication. I was surprised when we looked at his call tracking data and found that after the ad had run for two months, he hadn't really received a single call. Perplexed, I had him find a hard copy of the magazine and take some pictures of the pages leading up his ad, in particular the advertisement that shared space immediately to the left of his ad. Both of us were surprised to find out the ad people saw just before his ad was provocative and sexual in nature and definitely did not put people in a mindset on oral health. Before we gave up on this medium, we asked the magazine to change his ad's position so that it was next to an article instead of a racy ad. Amazingly, calls started rolling in that next month, and he ended up getting a 3:1 return for his investment.

A second thing to consider when using these regional magazines is getting the most exposure possible while reducing costs. Many times if you agree to a longer-term advertising contract, you can negotiate and decrease the price of your advertisement, sometimes leveraging their desire to get you into a longer-term contract to get you greater exposure in return. When I began advertising with *South Charlotte Weekly*, I was spending $1000 per month for a full-page, color ad that was centered in the magazine. The sales rep for the magazine advised me that if I committed to a six-month contract, I could get the cost of each ad down to $800 per month. Before I commit to a longer-term contract on any advertisement, I must test it out and track its results first. Once it's shown to provide me with a positive ROI, then I consider going to a longer term to save.

After three months, I reviewed my call tracking data and realized my ad was giving me a 4:1 ROI each month, a success to be sure, which led me to inquire about the longer-term deal. When the rep came by, he asked if I was ready to commit to the six-month agreement. Instead, I told him that I'd be willing to commit to a 12-month agreement if the magazine would consider doing a feature article about my two practices and put myself and my partner on that month's cover. After conferring with the publisher, the rep came back in agreement and in two months' time, I was on the cover of the magazine.

Our ROI for that month's issue was well over 8:1, and I had numerous friends, colleagues, and new patients who told me they saw me on that cover. I was able to leverage the cover issue by showcasing it on our social media channels: we put a link to it on our website so potential new patients who found us might be influenced by this authority cue. I also had the magazine cover and our feature article professional printed out and mounted, which we hung in our reception area to further establish our authority status when new patients were exposed to it when they arrived at our practice for the first time.

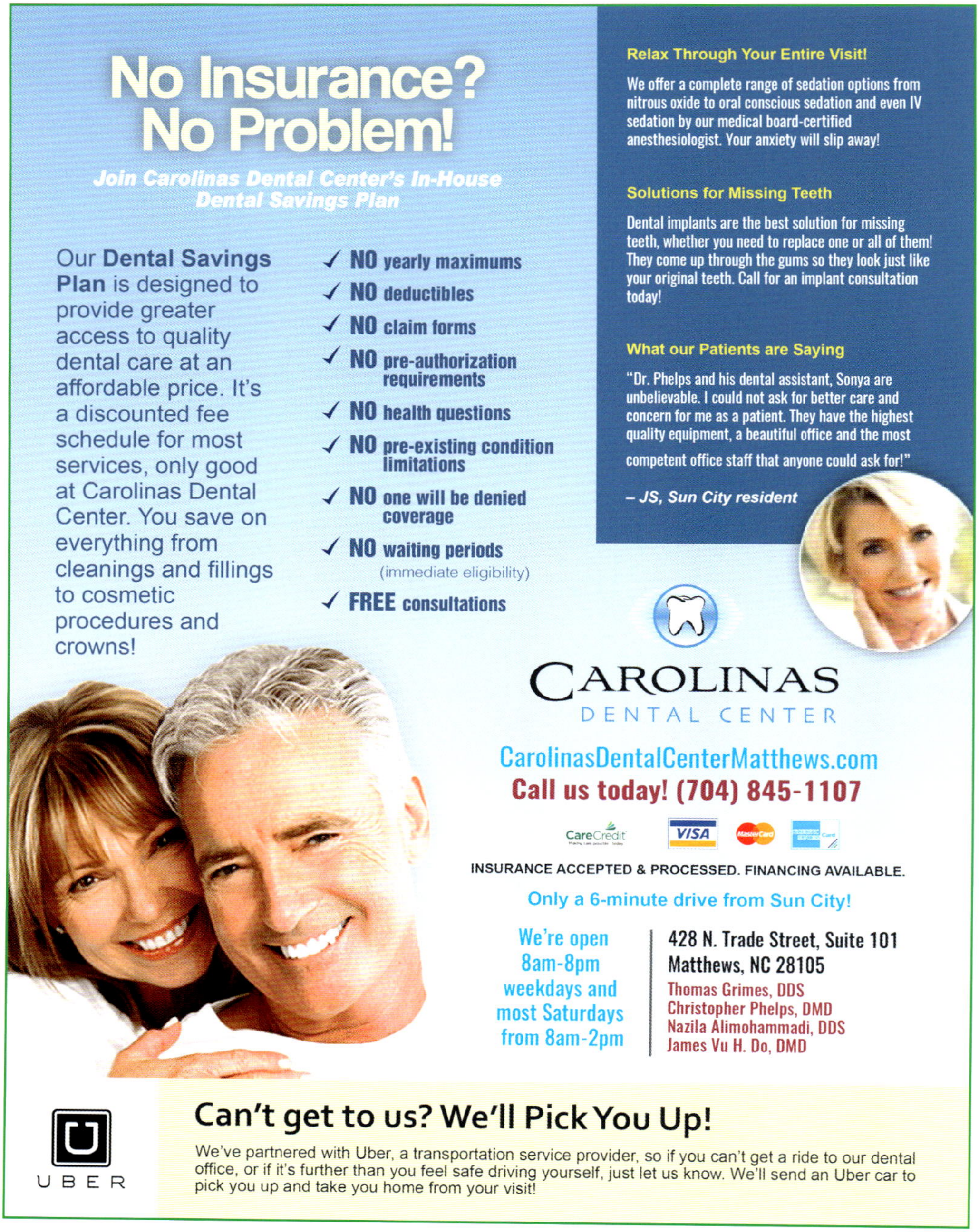

Figure 31. Example from one of Dr. Phelps's magazine advertisements.

A final thought to consider when using these regional magazines is to find ones specific to certain communities you may be targeting. Because they speak to a smaller audience, the ad rates tend to be a half to a fourth of the price of larger regional magazines, plus that audience tends to be more in line with our target market. Del Webb is a builder and developer of 55+ and older active, independent living retirement communities throughout the United States. In my book *Grow Your Dental Membership Plan* I talk about how you can find these communities and give on-site patient education seminars to promote your practice and dental membership plan. Each community offers its residents a professionally made community magazine that goes out once a month. The ad rates were reasonable but gave me lots of exposure to promote my seminars, membership plan, and practice to its residents. When you know what medium your target market is looking at to get information it should be a key indicator that this should be a place you need to test your messages.

No matter what magazine you choose to advertise in, your message will need to be strong and eye-catching. Remember, you only have a few seconds to grab the readers' attention and pull them in to read the rest of the ad. A bold graphic and an interesting headline will help you make a connection with readers right off the bat. Ultimately, the graphic and the headline must come together to pinpoint a problem and offer a solution to the reader.

B. Online External Marketing Media

Online external marketing, commonly referred to as digital marketing, comprises any marketing methods conducted through electronic devices. This includes online marketing efforts conducted on the Internet. In the process of conducting digital marketing, a business might leverage websites, search engines, blogs, social media, video, email, and similar channels to reach customers.

The best place to put your message is where you know you have a chance to get your market's attention. These days, screen time on our mobile devices is at an all-time high. Digital marketing takes advantage of this reality, allowing you to promote your dental products and services across the Internet and helps us ensure that our marketing efforts are more likely to reach customers, by targeting them where they spend most of their time.

By tapping into the various online media, practices can use digital marketing to benefit from these advantages:

- **Global reach**: Unlike traditional methods, digital marketing is not necessarily bound to a specific geographic area. The Internet is available to customers across the globe. This allows businesses to market and sell to customers who live in a different state or country, removing many traditional barriers to entry.
- **Low cost of entry**: To achieve the global reach of digital marketing through traditional channels, there would be a serious price tag attached. On the other hand, certain aspects of digital marketing can be achieved with a small investment of time and resources. For example, even small or startup businesses can create a website, manage social media, and publish blogs without breaking the bank.
- **Measurable ROI**: In order to maximize profits, practices must carefully evaluate ROI. Digital marketing provides real-time visibility into the effectiveness of each campaign,

enabling practices to make well-informed decisions about what's working and not working from their efforts.

- **Improved targeting**: Digital marketing allows practices to target very specific demographics of potential patients. By engaging potential new patients in a particular geography, industry, or social channel, your practice will have a much better chance of reaching your target market.
- **Dynamic adaptability**: Digital marketing strategies are extremely malleable and flexible, enabling practices to adjust course when needed. Unlike long-term, traditional marketing campaigns, practices can adjust their digital efforts on the fly, enabling quick pivots when necessary to realize commercial opportunity. For example, let's say a reality TV show has suddenly popularized a certain dental product and potential new patients are actively seeking that product. With a digital ad, you could modify your copy and offer instantly to let people searching know they can find this item with you. With print media, it could take several weeks before that same message could be released, missing out on valuable momentum created in those first moments.
- **Immediate connection**: People have a search problem today. Too many activities, to-do items on their list that need to be satisfied, and so forth. Because of our constant distractions, when a problem presents itself, our brains want an answer to the question at hand as soon as possible. Thus the search begins with people conducting online research and evaluating reviews. By creating a dominant online presence, we can be assured to come up early in their search to make that immediate connection to their problem at hand.
- **Relationship building**: The rise of social media has turned it into a dominant communications platform for many customer demographics. Furthermore, customers increasingly want to interact with businesses on their terms and on their preferred platform. As a result, businesses that engage in effective social media marketing practices can build longtime and loyal relationships with current and prospective customers.

"Digital" or "online marketing" are broad terms that encompass many different channels for promoting the interests of your practice to prospective new patients. That being said, there are several common methods for conducting digital marketing, including:

- **Search engine optimization (SEO)**: SEO is the practice of improving ranking within major search engines to increase online traffic.
- **Local search marketing (LSM)**: Sometimes known as local SEO, it is a form of search engine optimization that helps your practice rank highly when potential new patients are searching for a dentist but they are physically near your practice.
- **Search engine marketing (SEM)**: SEM leverages paid online advertising to increase website visibility within search engines. SEM is often used in conjunction with SEO. This includes pay-per-click and Google Ads services.
- **Pay-per-click (PPC)**: PPC is an online method for advertising where a practice only pays for its ads when a person clicks on them.
- **Google Ads**: A form of PPC specific to Google's search engine.
- **Social media marketing (SMM)**: SMM uses using social media channels such as Facebook or Instagram to promote your practice's products or services. The use of social media influencers, often referred to as influencer marketing, is prevalent in SMM.

- **Content marketing**: Content marketing refers to the publishing and distribution of text, video, or audio materials to customers online. Posting content in social media communities such as Nextdoor, creating your own blog site, posting videos, and having your own podcasts are common ways for practices to engage in content marketing.

Search engine optimization (SEO)

Search engine optimization is the process of improving the quality and quantity of viewers, called "traffic," to a website or a web page following terms they enter into a search engine such as Google, YouTube, or Bing. SEO targets unpaid, often referred to as "organic," traffic rather than direct traffic or paid traffic. Direct traffic means a person who comes to your website by directly typing in your web address instead of doing a search and then finding your website after a series of clicks. Paid, or "inorganic," traffic are viewers that come to your website after clicking a paid or sponsored link, commonly referred to as pay per click.

When a potential new patient enters their search criteria into their preferred search engine, such as Google, several hundred pages of website links populate, each one ranked in a specific order. Prior to populating this list, the search engine companies have sent out programs called "crawlers," whose job is to go out, search the content posted on every website, and bring back that information to build an index. When you put your terms of interest into the search engine, a computer algorithm tries to match up your search criteria with information in its index and bring you the most relevant sites that match. It's been reported that Google has over 200 known variables it uses in its algorithm to populate its search rankings. That's all in the SE (search engine) part of SEO.

The O part of SEO is the optimization. This comes from matching up the actual content you have on your website to as many of those algorithmic variables as possible. The more variables that line up, the more likely your website will organically rank in a higher position than others like it. In the battle of paid/inorganic ranking vs organic/unpaid rankings, many prefer the organic route since studies show a potential customer is 8.5 times more likely to click a link to your website from this route versus the paid rankings. Remember these tips to optimize your SEO efforts:

- **Remove anything that slows your website load time**. Few will wait patiently for a website that takes 4–5 minutes to load. In this world of cellular, cable, and fiber Internet speeds, people expect websites to load quickly. A popular study showed that 40 percent of people abandoned a website when it took more than three seconds to load, 80 percent of which did not return to view the site again.
- **Create links to other websites with relevant content**. YouTube is a great example. Create your own YouTube channel for your practice, where you can host different video content, short clips of you and/or your team discussing different services or procedures you offer or posting patient video testimonials. Linking those videos from another credible source to your website, your website automatically gets you higher organic search rankings than those websites that don't do this.
- **Before you can optimize, you have to be ready to track**. Your website should have Google Analytics, Google Search Console, or some other private web analytics software to help you track the number of people coming to your website as well as what they

spend their time viewing. Tools like Crazy Egg show you specifically where and what they clicked on for your site and where they navigated to after leaving you.

- **Your website needs to be responsive, not static**. A responsive website means that people can view your website in its entirety, regardless of what device they are using. Whether it's a desktop computer or your smart phone, your website should automatically adapt to what it's viewed on.
- **Google reviews**. While positive patient reviews are important to improve your search on any search engine platform, acquiring positive Google reviews is paramount. Google is the preferred search engine for over 70 percent of the marketplace. While they have over 200 variables for their search algorithm, the quantity and frequency of your Google reviews has been shown to help you rank higher than those who don't get reviews posted often or have a significant quantity. Most experts agree that you need to have at least 40 Google reviews to start making an impact on your SEO organic rankings.

Local search marketing (LSM)

Some marketers call it local SEO, but I think of local search as a more integrated approach to marketing your practice to prospective new patients who are actively searching in your immediate geographic area. Local search marketing is all about putting your practice on the map in local searches when customers are searching for terms such as "Dentist near me." It's been reported that 72 percent of consumers who perform a local search visit that store if it's within 5 miles of their current location. Here are some items to consider when attempting to maximize your local search efforts.

- **Create or claim your business listing**. If your practice is new, you'll need to create new business profiles on Google My Business, Bing Places for Business, Yahoo, Yelp, and Facebook. If you've been around for a while, a business profile has most likely already been created for you. You'll need to check these sites and claim/verify your page and then correct and/or complete any missing information on them.
- **Provide accurate, consistent NAPU**. NAPU stands for name, address, phone number, and URL, or website address. Search engines, such as Google and Bing, don't just take the information you give them as the only truth. They use information from four main sources, Infogroup, Acxiom, Localeze, and Factual. To make things even more complicated, those four sources get their information from hundreds of online business directories. That means 100s of potential business listings for your practice could be out there. If your information is different or inconsistent across those directories, that will confuse the search engine, and it won't know where or when to list your business in search results. The more consistent your information is across all of these directories, the more the search engine will trust your business and the higher it will rank you as a result.
- **Choose the right categories**. While having consistent information across all of your business listings is important, don't forget to add appropriate categories to your business as well. The more specific, the better. General dentistry is probably too broad a category. Instead, consider putting categories of dentistry that you would like your practice to be known for. Cosmetic dentistry, sedation dentistry, implant dentistry are just some examples of how you could categorize your practice in your business listing. A word of caution, remember "less is better." According to Google's current guidelines, you should use as few categories as possible so pick the ones that might really speak to your target market.

Search engine marketing (SEM)

Search engine marketing is the practice of marketing a business using paid advertisements. These links usually appear at the very top of search engine results and are signified by having the word "Sponsored" or "AD" in front of them. Keywords are critical to this pay-to-play form of digital marketing. Advertisers bid on keywords that users of services such as Google and Bing might enter when looking for certain products or services, which gives the advertiser the opportunity for their ads to appear above organic/unpaid results for those search queries.

These ads, often known by the term "pay-per-click" (PPC), come in a variety of formats. Its foundation is built on an auction/bidding system. To start, you select a target keyword that you want to display for, and then you decide how much you're willing to pay every time someone clicks on that ad. If you win the auction for any given keyword, you ad will show up at the top of the search results when someone uses your keyword in their search. Where in traditional print media you're paying for the advertisement space and hoping patients will respond, the biggest advantage of PPC ads is that it only costs you when someone clicks on your advertisement link. This makes it a very cost-effective medium to add to your overall attraction plan. A different form of PPC is Google Ads. Google Ads is Google's proprietary service that offers PPC services for its search engine and that of its many partner websites.

For any SEM marketing strategy, it is advisable to use both Google Ads and PPC services available on other search engines such as Bing. It's unlikely that a potential new patient would run the same search for a dentist on both Google and Bing, so by focusing on only one area, your message may not be seen by a significant number of people. Because these keywords work on an auction/bidding system, if there is more competition for a word or phrase, then it will drive up its cost of use. Since Google runs the majority of worldwide searches, it would be easy to surmise that they have the highest competition among advertisers who were bidding. By running your campaign on sites like Bing, you may find the competition for those keywords to be less, which may help your marketing budget go a lot further.

Because of its focus on keywords, SEM's greatest strength is that it offers your practice the opportunity to put your message in front of motivated customers who are ready to buy at the precise moment they're ready to make a purchase. You're targeting the most popular keywords they are searching for, and by showing up at the top of their search results, you put yourself in a prime position for your message to be seen.

Social media marketing (SMM)

Social media marketing is the action of creating content to promote your practice on various social media platforms such as Facebook, Instagram, and Twitter. It's about meeting your target market where they are and as they socially interact with each other and your brand. While there are newly emerging opportunities to place paid advertisements on social media channels, SMM first started with publishing. Businesses were sharing their content on social media to generate traffic to their websites and, hopefully, sales. But social media has matured far beyond being just a place to broadcast content.

Nowadays, businesses use social media in a myriad of different ways. For example, a business that is concerned about what people are saying about its brand would monitor social media conversations and respond to relevant mentions (social media listening and engagement). A business that wants to understand how it's performing on social media would analyze its reach, engagement, and sales on social media with an analytics tool (social media analytics). A business that wants to reach a specific set of audience at scale would run highly targeted social media ads (social media advertising). In dentistry, we need to have some focus in all three of these areas.

Here are some of the most popular social media sites today. Facebook, Instagram, Twitter, LinkedIn, Pinterest, YouTube, and Snapchat. There are also smaller and up-and-coming platforms, such as Tumblr, Tik Tok, and Anchor, plus social messaging platforms, such as Messenger, WhatsApp, WeChat, and Nextdoor. With all of these possible media to engage, where does one start? Ideally it would be best to target just a few of these platforms instead of investing time and money to reach them all. To decide which ones are best for you, go back to your target market and decide which of these companies might be engaging with our target market the most.

Popular Examples

- **Facebook**: 1.7 billion daily active users worldwide. In North America, 68 percent of people engage with this platform daily. Currently the majority of its users are reported to be of generation X and millennials. Generation X is defined as those born between 1965 and 1980, while Millennials are those born between 1981 and 1996. Current recommendations are to use this platform to improve your brand awareness and for paid advertisements to support direct phone calls to your office or to promote lead generation marketing attempts.
- **LinkedIn**: 675 million active monthly users. Main user demographic is the baby boomers, born between 1946 and 1964, followed by generation X and then millennials. Current recommendations are to use this platform to promote your practice to other businesses and business owners, such as to promote a dental membership plan and show how they can provide this to their employees as a cost-effective employee health benefit.
- **YouTube**: Over 2 billion logged in monthly users worldwide. Main user demographic are millennials followed by generation X. Current recommendations are to use this platform to increase brand awareness, provide entertaining perspectives on dentistry and the dental experience, and to host how-to or patient education videos on services you wish to promote. Linking these videos to your website also increases your SEO efforts as described earlier.
- **Instagram**: One billion monthly active users, the majority of which are millennials. Current recommendations are to use this platform to post natural-looking media, fun behind-the-scenes images from your practice/team, and for paid advertisement spots.

Social media metrics

To track these platforms, we need data related to the success of your posts, your impact on your audience using these platforms. These metrics may include data about your level of engagement, likes, follows, shares, and all other interactions on each platform.

Here are 10 of the most important metrics for you to track:

- **Engagement**: This includes clicks, comments, likes, and replies on your social media posts. There are also platform-specific types of engagement such as "saved" posts on Instagram and "pinned" posts on Pinterest.
- **Reach**: The number of people who have seen any content associated with your page or profile is your reach.
- **Followers**: This is the number of people you have on your profile who have clicked your "Follow" button and see your content in their feeds regularly.
- **Impressions**: This is the number of times a post from your profile or page is seen, whether or not your audience members click on it. This is often what happens when someone is scrolling through their newsfeed, but not clicking on anything.
- **Video views**: On Facebook, Snapchat, Instagram, or any other social channel with video capabilities, this is the number of views each gets.
- **Profile visits**: The number of people who have opened your social media page is your number of profile visits.
- **Mentions**: This is the number of times your profile has been mentioned by audience members in their posts.
- **Tags**: This is when your audience adds the name of your company's profile or your hashtag to another post.
- **Reposts**: This is when a member of your audience posts a piece of your content on their profile.
- **Shares**: These are the posts your followers and audience take from your profile and share with their network.

You can influence all of these metrics, increase your social following, and improve overall engagement on your profile by using these seven pillars of marketing we're discussing.

Content Marketing

Forbes magazine defines content marketing as the technique of creating and distributing valuable, relevant, and consistent content to attract and acquire a clearly defined audience – with the objective of driving profitable customer action. The key word here is "valuable." It's what distinguishes this definition from one that could describe almost any form of advertising or marketing. You can tell if a piece of content is the sort that could be part of a content marketing campaign if people seek it out, if people want to consume it, rather than avoiding it.

Perhaps more important than understanding what content marketing is is understanding why content marketing is important to your practice. To do that, we need to understand the four steps of the buying cycle:

- **Awareness**. Prior to awareness a customer may have a need, but they are not aware there is a solution.

- **Research**. Once a customer is aware there is a solution, they will perform research to educate themselves. For example, a car buyer will try to find out what different types of cars exist and which one will fit their needs.
- **Consideration**. At this point the customer starts comparing different products from different vendors to make sure they're getting a high-quality product at a fair price.
- **Buy**. Finally, the customer makes their decision and moves forward with the transaction.

Traditional advertising and marketing is great when it comes to the last two steps. Content marketing helps you reach the potential new patient in the first two stages of their buying process, raising awareness of solutions and educating them about a product or service that they may have never considered before, which you happen to provide. The key is finding the right place to put your content.

From a behavioral science standpoint, people enjoy community. They enjoy conversing with one another, sharing pictures/stories about their lives, and learning about the events happening with others in their community. Now that technology has made these conversations happen more quickly and on a larger scale, we've seen the rise of the social media powerhouses described above. One community-based social media company that has gained the most traction recently is called Nextdoor.

Founded in 2010, this San Francisco–based company has grown to over 30 million users nationwide, bringing over 236,000 neighborhoods in the US together to share information. During the COVID-19 pandemic of 2020, usage of the app by its members reportedly increased over 80 percent, quickly becoming the go-to place to find out relevant information about what's going on in your community. For the last couple of years, I have found this website to be a great area to engage potential new patients via content marketing.

Why? Because content marketing is all about sharing valuable information, information people seek out and want to share. From a dental standpoint, the information people are actively searching for on Nextdoor is unbiased answers to the dental problems and questions they have. If you live relatively close to your practice, you or your team can register and instantly gain access to their direct communities as well as the different neighborhood communities they are adjacent to. Once a day I would have my team search through the different community forums and look for questions people were asking related to dentistry or a dental problem they had.

Once my team found these opportunities, I would log in and attempt to give them an unbiased opinion on the topic of interest. I wasn't diagnosing by any means and made that point clear in all of my posts, but many times the questions had fairly straightforward answers or at least I could provide them with a differential diagnosis of possible things they would need to rule out with a dental professional. While my profile had my "Dr." title in it, I did not mention my dental practice at all in those conversations. Over time, I noticed two distinct things occurring. At first, you wouldn't find too many additional comments from those exposed to my answers. As time went on, perhaps after I had established some history on the site of providing unbiased answers, more and more people felt safe to post additional follow-up questions to the original one. Eventually, others in the community would start to tag my name when someone posted a dental-based question in a different community forum or thread, alerting me to the opportunity to answer.

Ultimately, I noticed that my efforts to provide more awareness of the solutions to the dental problems in question and educating people on their options had become a marketing funnel to my practice. By giving those unbiased answers, the community started to look to me as the dental authority in the area. A credible, knowledgeable professional willing to help them. For many, when it came down to solving their problem in question or if a new dental issue developed, it influenced those patients to seek me out for their care. While maybe not providing my practices a huge quantity of new patients, the numbers were still significant, and I found them to be of high quality and accepting of the treatment recommendations I gave them.

2. MARKET, MESSAGE, MEDIUM: THE SEQUENCE MATTERS

A. Where Do Most People Start in This Sequence?

When I meet with dentists following any marketing talk I've given, I usually get asked a similar question when it comes to media. Does direct mail work? Should I do radio ads? Do I need to be spending any money with Google Ads? In essence all of these questions tell me that dentists tend to start their marketing efforts by focusing on what medium they should use, when instead they're starting at the end of the sequence, not at the beginning. "Does direct mail work?" they ask to which I reply, "Sometimes yes, sometimes no." Truthfully it depends on whether or not you've taken the time to address the first two areas in the sequence.

- Who is your target market? The person you're really trying to attract with direct mail or in any marketing medium.
- What are your unique, differentiating messages (collectively defined as your headline, content, offer, and influence principles) that will cause them to take notice of your advertisement and motivate them to want to respond?

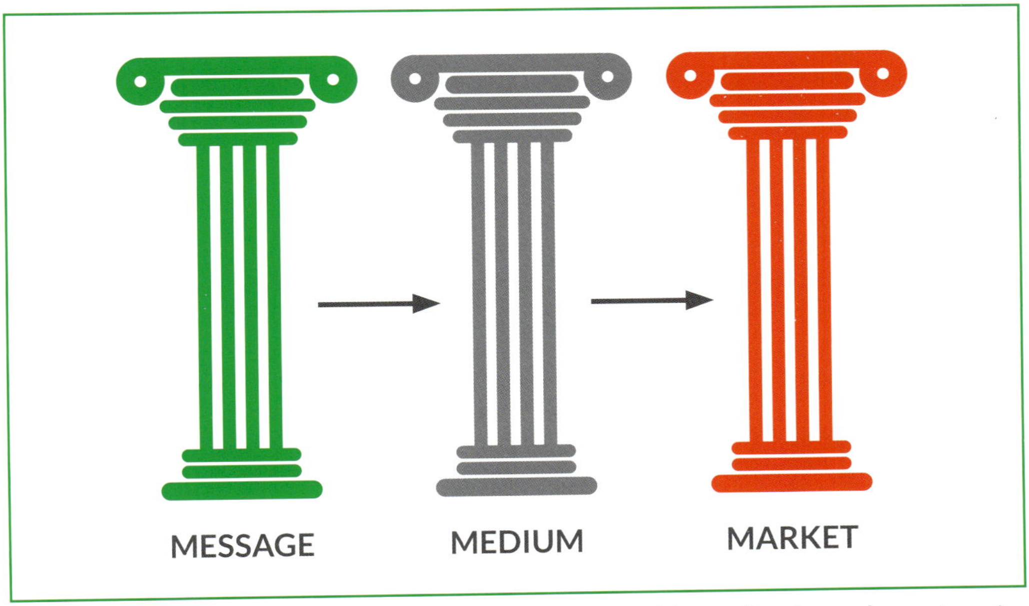

Figure 32. Showcasing how your message needs to be in the right medium to reach your target market.

B. What Happens When You Get the Sequence Right?

One day I was talking with a patient who I'd considered my target market, someone I had recently placed two dental implants and restored with his final crowns. This patient was an active, independent living retiree, someone who came to see us because of the dental membership plan we offered, who still valued being in great oral health, and who didn't want missing teeth. After I delivered his crowns, I decided to do a short interview with him to ask some questions that could give me insights into how to find others just like him.

"Bill, why did you decide to have these implants and crowns completed at our office?" I asked. He responded by telling me that he had some consultations at other offices but liked that we could offer both the implant and final restorative work in one location and that with our dental membership plan discount, he ended up saving around 10 percent compared to the other offices he had consultations with. So now my target market is giving me some insights into key messages I could use in future marketing to grab their attention and stand out: Avoid having to travel to multiple offices to get the work completed and a mindset of saving or getting a discount off a service they intended to do somewhere. The second question I asked him was geared more toward learning about his hobbies and interests. Then I asked him where he is getting his information from. He mentioned the Internet, newspaper, magazines, and Facebook. I also attempted to interject some humor into the question as well.

"Bill, you said you're retired these days. Is that correct? What do you do now that you're retired? Just sitting around the house being a couch potato?" Bill responded, "Well, Doc, I start out every morning the same. I get out of bed. I go to the front door and grab the newspaper. I open it up to the obituary section and look to see if I'm in there! If not, then I continue on my day...."

Now Bill and I both had a good laugh after his comment, and I wished him well as he left the office. Later that day I started to relay this story to one of my associate dentists when it hit me. What medium did my target market just tell me he looks at every day? The newspaper. But not just the newspaper or the ads you may see scattered throughout. No, he told me he reads the obituary section of the newspaper every day. Even though it was said in jest, when your target market speaks, you need to listen. Over the next two weeks I decided to see if any of my other implant patients did a similar action as Bill. Most were in my hygiene chairs and I'd ask them, "This may sound like a weird question, but do you ever read the obituary section of the newspaper?" Each of the next three patients confirmed that they did in fact read that section every day. When I asked one of my female patients why she read that section every day, she told me, "Well, I guess I read it to see if any of my friends are dead."

Not long after this confirmation, my wife and I were on an airplane and about to take off for a vacation. The man sitting next to me looked like he might fit my target market profile of an active, independent living retiree. He wife was traveling with him but sitting in the seat across from our aisle. As we're about to take off, I notice he had the newspaper open to the obituary section and to my surprise, he leaned over the aisle to his wife and said, "Honey, look at this. Ted just passed away. Can you believe it?" Yet another example that my target market looks at this section of the newspaper fairly often.

C. Putting It All Together

100:1 ROI

Putting the pieces together, I knew who my target market was. From the questions I asked patients who had already said yes to treatment, I discovered some differentiating messages I could use to attract more like them to my office. Thanks to the joke my patient made about the obituary section, I now had a good idea of a strategic medium I could use, a place I could put my messages where my target market might have a chance to see and respond to.

I called the advertising department our local newspaper to inquire about what marketing opportunities they had available. Unfortunately, none of the options included the obituary section of the newspaper. Not wanting to let this opportunity be wasted, I asked the representative if it would be possible to put an ad in this section of the paper. I believe I was the first to ever ask this question based on the confusion the representative had with my request and the fact that he had to check with two different supervisors to see if it was possible. Eventually he came back on the phone with me and told me that in fact I could advertise in this section with certain restrictions.

- I had to run the advertisement for a minimum of seven days;
- I could not use any pictures outside of our practice logo;
- The total dimensions had to be no more than two by three inches.

At a cost of $1200, I committed to running this small ad for the next seven days. Since we didn't have a lot of space to use, we were limited in what could be said, so I settled on: "Patients Needed for Dental Implants. Significant cost savings if you're a candidate. Email Shelley at Shelley@carolinasdentalcenter.com for more information.

The result? The office received over 134 emails from interested patients that week. Many potential new patients went to Google and used Shelley's email to find our website for more information. In an upcoming section we'll discuss call tracking in more detail, but from our tracking process, we discovered that over 20 patients called from our website tracking number, once they had seen the advertisement in the obituary section. Over the next three months, the office collected over $120,000 in implant-related fees from that $1200 investment. A 100:1 ROI.

Never stop asking questions to understand your target market

Over the next year I ran this advertisement once every four months. Each time it delivered an astounding ROI and became one of my go-to media to attract larger implant cases. In my initial discussions and conversations with the patients who said yes to those larger dental hybrid cases, I began to notice another pattern emerging. Of those who said yes to treatment, the vast majority had first been to a popular nationwide dental implant center, one that specializes in dental hybrids and treating edentulous arches. This was a group it was rumored would spend over $100,000 a month in marketing their practice in that area and who typically had a 20 percent case acceptance rate.

At that time, one arch of treatment at the center nearest to my practice would cost the patient around $30,000. My fee at that time for a similar dental hybrid appliance happened to be $22,500. What I discovered from my target market was that not only did they look at the obituary section of the newspaper for information, but many of these larger edentulous arch cases had first been to this implant center for education and consultation. While they liked what they heard about the treatment and the options, they were still unsure about the price and whether to move forward with this group, hence them coming to me for a second opinion.

We mentioned earlier how these patients had a focus on saving or getting a discount off the treatment they planned to get somewhere. In contrast to the $30,000 price, my price for the same procedure was 25 percent less. With this discovery, I decided to refine my message in the obituary ad, to dial in and narrow the focus of my messaging to attract my new target market: someone who had been to this popular implant center, someone who liked the options on what they heard but just didn't like the price. So the next iteration of the ad became: "Patients needed for dental implants. If you've been to a popular implant center for consultation, we can save you a minimum of 25%. Call or email Shelley to see if you are a candidate as our appointments are limited." Then we provided the office number and Shelley's email.

By narrowing the focus of who the ad was speaking to, this version decreased the quantity of new patients who responded but significantly increased the quality, netting me one or two edentulous arch implant cases per month with a consistent 100:1 ROI over its lifetime of use. To this day, when I want to do more implant and full arch hybrids cases, I turn to this ad to generate potential new patient opportunities.

Could we refine this even more?

Over time, asking questions and listening to my patients, I realized the scope of who my target market was had changed. I wanted to attract a very specific type of patient now, one who had been to this popular implant center but wasn't satisfied with their visit. I had also learned some unique messaging that had consistently attracted these patients to my practice when they had left this implant center undecided. I asked myself, what was the best way to get my message in front of my target market, ideally, in front of them when finding a solution for their loose-fitting dentures was at the top of their mindset. Then one day I was in my car and at a stop light and was surprised with what pulled up next to me.

It was a billboard on wheels. I had seen these vehicles all over town, promoting various other types of businesses, but it never occurred to me that there could be an opportunity to use this medium to strategically get my message in front of my target market when it mattered the most, as they were leaving this popular implant center and had decided to not move forward with treatment there. Given this was estimated to be 80 percent of those who came in for consultations, there was a considerable opportunity here. Imagine a patient walking out of this center, liking what they heard but deciding not to move forward there and they see my billboard drive past them stating: "Like what you heard but didn't like the price? We can save you 25% or more. Email or call us for more info. While I contacted the company responsible for these billboards and validated that it would be legal to have this mobile billboard drive around the parking lot and area where this popular implant center was situated, other circumstances kept me from testing this medium out. One day I do plan to return to it, but I bring it up to illustrate the point. When your market speaks, you should listen. When they tell you opportune places to strategically put your messages in front of them, you set the stage to grab their focus on and attention. On top of this, finding out why they say yes to treatment, what attracted them to your office, and other questions such as these are important to defining who they are. They are also critical to helping you to continue to refine who they are and give you ideas on what creative media, like the billboard on the back of the truck, you can strategically tap into to get your unique message to your target audience.

When the sequence is wrong, your quantity of potential new patients suffers

Now let's look at the reverse situation. See Figure 33. You may understand who your target market is, meaning you know who you want more of in your practice. For example, people who need simple or more complex implants and restorations, sedation dentistry, or sleep apnea or clear aligner therapy. You may have some messages or headlines that could stand out to them. But if you haven't taken the time to really talk with your target market and research where they are getting their information from, you could be putting your efforts into a medium that they are not even using. They won't see your message and have zero chance to respond. This leads to a low or negative ROI and your marketing becomes a wasted expense.

You may understand who your target market is. You may have taken the time to talk with them in great detail, to learn what media such as radio, TV, or Internet they are using to find information. Yet if you're marketing messages that don't stand out and grab their attention, the result is the same. Your potential new patient doesn't see your advertisement. This leads to a low or negative ROI, and your marketing becomes a wasted expense. See Figure 34.

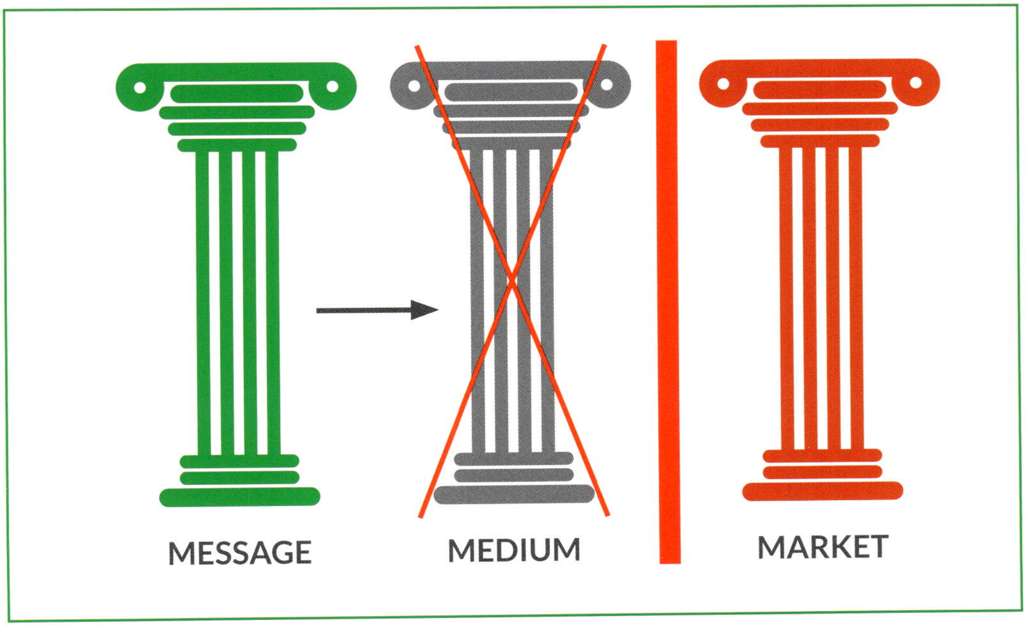

Figure 33. **Despite having the right message, one your target market would respond to if exposed to it, if you choose the wrong medium, then your message will never reach and influence your target market.**

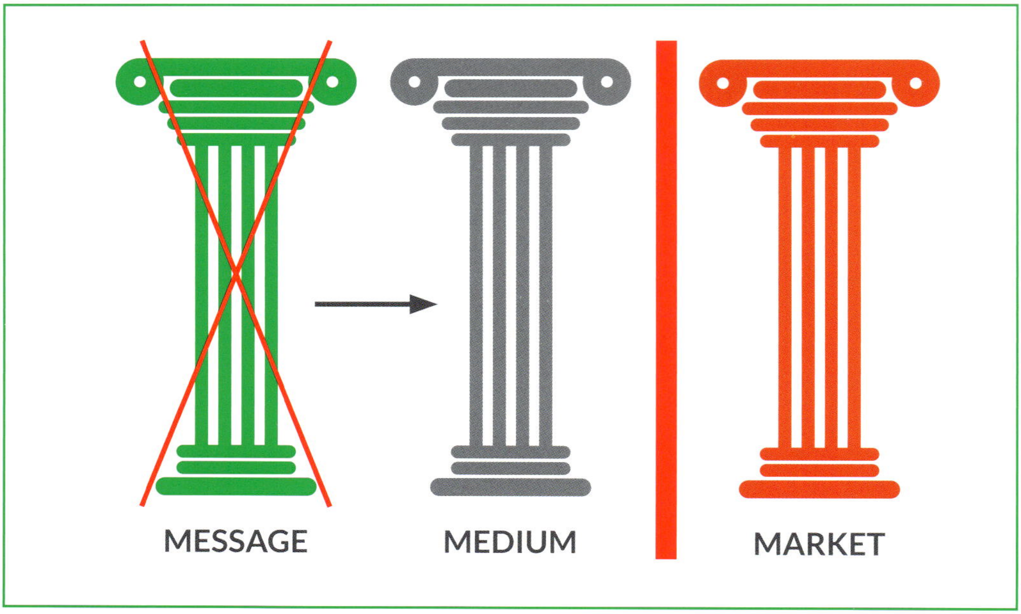

Figure 34. When you pick the right medium but your message doesn't stand out or resonate with your target market, you have little chance to grab their attention and influence them toward your direction.

In this section we've covered many of the most popular marketing media available to us to promote our dental practices. Each involves different levels of time and financial commitment, but all have the potential to help you reach your new patient attraction goals. The idea is not for one source to help you reach your goals but instead to find some balance over numerous areas that fit your time and monetary budget. Remember, you won't necessarily find one thing that consistently attracts 100 new patients per month, but you should be able to find four or five that let you reach that total. Focus on really defining who your target market is and identifying what unique messages will attract their attention. Between these two it should give you some insights into what media you can strategically test and analyze for the best results.

CASE STUDY

Dr. Nate Jeal is a practicing general dentist in Winnipeg, Canada. Like myself, Dr. Jeal has spent a lot of time learning how to become a better marketer and has used those skills to help promote the growth of multiple practices in his town. During the COVID-19 pandemic of 2020, Dr. Jeal decided to take on a bold marketing endeavor. His plan was to have an "Invisalign Day," one day out of the whole year where he would offer patients an opportunity to start Invisalign treatments at a reduced cost.

Dr. Jeal's target market was people who were unhappy about their current tooth positions, possibly those who had orthodontic therapy as kids but have since had orthodontic relapse as a result of not wearing their retainers, and were ready to make a change. His message to them was simple. If they wanted to make that change, then they had only one day this year they could do it and receive a significant discount. While his treatment fee was normally around $6000 Canadian dollars, he was offering those who started treatment on this day a rate of $5000 dollars. In addition, he paired this with a contest, offering a free Invisalign treatment to one lucky person, one chosen at random from those who started treatment that day.

To promote this event, he tapped into two different media. Six months earlier, he began posting content to the practice's Instagram page. Content related to the Invisalign treatment process, existing patient stories of success, their before and after photos, and details about the "one day only" event and contest ahead. Due to prior efforts, the practice had over 7000 followers who were exposed to these messages. One week before the Saturday event, he spent around $400 on paid Instagram ads that would air each day, leading up to the big day. In addition, he reached out to a local radio station whose demographic fit that of his target market, paying for them to promote his event and free Invisalign contest to their listeners, even having them onsite the day of the event to broadcast live and to encourage those listening to come down and attend.

All in all, Dr. Jeal scheduled 22 consultations for Invisalign that day. Each one had placed a credit card on file to hold their appointment time. Of those, 20 of the 22 moved forward and paid $5000 that day to start their Invisalign treatment. One of the 22 was the winner of the contest and received their treatment for free. When you factor in the cost of the Instagram ads leading up to the event, the radio ads and onsite broadcast performed, and the cost of performing the free Invisalign treatment on the lucky winner, Dr. Jeal had invested around $5000 for this event, collecting $100,000 and netting a 20:1 ROI for that investment. That's not counting the hygiene revenue those 21 people would bring to the practice moving forward or the restorative treatment many of them had to complete first, before they could actually begin their ortho treatment.

That's the power that can occur when you really understand your target market, when you have messages you know will capture their attention and appeal to them and when you choose the right medium to get those messages out to them. A $100,000+ collections day. Despite it being the height of the COVID-19 pandemic, without any viral vaccine readily available and despite a massive rise in the number of people who had lost their jobs and went on unemployment or state-supported benefits.

Chapter 6
Internal Marketing

The act of internal marketing means you are sending advertising messages to your existing patient base. Of all the media, this one is ideal as it involves very little of your time directly and doesn't tend have a large expense. It can be leveraged in two ways.

- Marketing specific procedures and contests to your existing patient base to increase revenue from scheduled treatment;
- Influencing your existing patient base to recruit new patients to the practice.

MARKETING SPECIFIC PROCEDURES TO YOUR EXISTING PATIENT BASE

When it comes to marketing specific procedures and contests to your existing patient base, I recommend you focus your efforts in two areas. Limited time and limited day promotions. Previously in this book we've talked about Dr. Cialdini's principle of scarcity. This principle states that when resources are dwindling or about to disappear, it motivates us to want those resources more, increasing the time, effort, energy, and money we are willing to put in to get them. This principle motivates us to take action because it taps into a primal need for resources, situations where if this resource truly ran out, it could mean life or death. Let's say that the oxygen was running out in the room you are sitting in now. I think everyone reading this would prefer to know that the oxygen is running out well before it actually runs out. Having that information beforehand will motivate you to go out and find more oxygen. Because of this principle it's fair to say that many times we don't want something until we find out we can't have it.

Let's look at the Black Friday phenomenon as an example. In the United States, Thanksgiving is a day our country sets aside to rest and connect with our families. It's a day of peace and fellowship, to love your fellow man, yet the very next day you may find yourself in the early morning hours about to fight someone over a deeply discounted TV. Why do our mindsets suddenly change in less than 24 hours? It goes back to scarcity of the things we want and desire around us. Our motivation to attain these scarce resources is elevated even more if there is competition at play. Thus, if we are aware that others are interested and making attempts at gaining resources that we are interested in, and those resources are about to run out, then our motivation to get them first rises to new levels. The Black Friday phenomenon affects us because of the scarcity of time to get the discounted items of interest. It's the only day of the year in fact that you tend to see those levels of savings, and retailers count on the effect this principle has on us to drive customers their way, for many, into the black and making a profit for the first time all year. So how can we apply this scarcity principle and competition to our dental marketing efforts?

1. Limited Time: End-of-the-Year Seasonal Promotions

Use it or lose it dental insurance promotion

On January 1, most dental insurance plans start a new calendar year. With this reset comes a fixed amount of money patients can use toward any dental treatment needed that year. On average, this amount is around $1000. If that patient has not used up any or all of that benefit, then potentially it could be lost when the policy resets the next January 1. Unused benefit amounts are not transferable to the next year. That makes this $1000 benefit a potential scarce resource because if the patient doesn't use it, they lose it to the next year.

One November, I decided to run a report from my practice management software geared toward my target market. This report was targeted in two ways, first to patients who had outstanding dental treatment that had not been scheduled, and second, to those who still had some of their annual dental insurance benefit that had not been utilized. I knew that my message or headline would focus on the scarcity of what they were about to lose, which was their $1000 in unused dental insurance benefit for the year. To get this message out, I decided to run a 6-by-10-inch postcard direct mail campaign (see Figure 35). From the report generated on those who had unscheduled treatment but still had insurance benefit to utilize, I exported those names and addresses and sent them to our direct mail company to send our postcard to. A unique call tracking number was placed on the card for each of

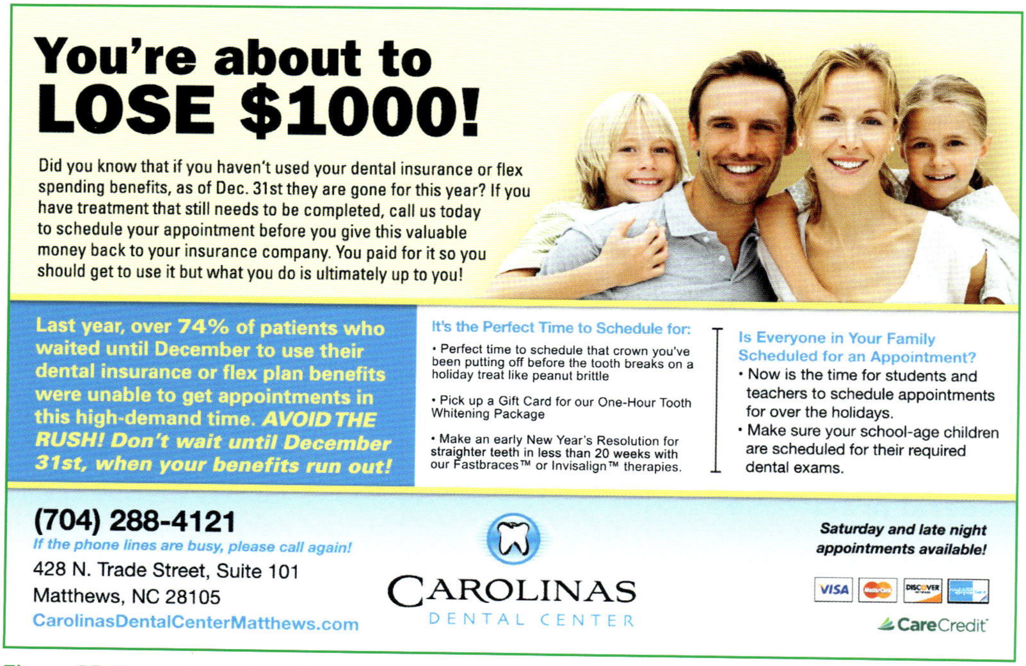
You're about to
LOSE $1000!
Did you know that if you haven't used your dental insurance or flex spending benefits, as of Dec. 31st they are gone for this year? If you have treatment that still needs to be completed, call us today to schedule your appointment before you give this valuable money back to your insurance company. You paid for it so you should get to use it but what you do is ultimately up to you!
Last year, over 74% of patients who waited until December to use their dental insurance or flex plan benefits were unable to get appointments in this high-demand time. AVOID THE RUSH! Don't wait until December 31st, when your benefits run out!
It's the Perfect Time to Schedule for:
• Perfect time to schedule that crown you've been putting off before the tooth breaks on a holiday treat like peanut brittle
• Pick up a Gift Card for our One-Hour Tooth Whitening Package
• Make an early New Year's Resolution for straighter teeth in less than 20 weeks with our Fastbraces™ or Invisalign™ therapies.
Is Everyone in Your Family Scheduled for an Appointment?
• Now is the time for students and teachers to schedule appointments for over the holidays.
• Make sure your school-age children are scheduled for their required dental exams.
(704) 288-4121
If the phone lines are busy, please call again!
428 N. Trade Street, Suite 101
Matthews, NC 28105
CarolinasDentalCenterMatthews.com
CAROLINAS
DENTAL CENTER
Saturday and late night appointments available!
VISA
DISCOVER
CareCredit

Figure 35. Example use it or lose it end-of-year promotion.

my two offices so we could evaluate who responded to the advertisement and track what each person spent for this campaign. The postcards were slated to hit patient mailboxes on December 1. In total, approximately $3500 was spent on this campaign. From the call tracking data we found that 25–35 patients had called and scheduled to come in and get some dental work completed before the year end. All in all, over $35,000 in revenue was collected at each of the two offices that month causing record collection months at both offices, giving our campaign a 20:1 ROI for our efforts.

2. Limited Time: Beginning of the Year Promotions

Once the end-of-the-year scarcity effect has concluded, I then turn my marketing efforts to the new year, new mindset that occurs in January and February, a mindset to motivate more existing and new patients to move forward with treatment they may need. Studies show that the beginning of the year brings a change mindset to people. It is a time to move forward with things that were on hold, a time to do something different or stop procrastinating on things, a time of New Year's resolutions. Because this mindset is universal to most out there, we can tailor our marketing and messaging to tap into it. In January and February, I like to run a "New Year, New You!" promotion, a special that offers people a chance to purchase a $100 gift card to our office for only $80. At most, people can purchase up to 5 gifts cards, totaling $500 in treatment for $400. We run this promotion internally to our existing patient base as well as externally in any advertisements we have in play. The goal here is threefold:

- To offer people some savings on doing something they know they need to do anyway and to help motivate people who've been procrastinating on visiting the dentist to move our direction.
- To attract more patients with newly reset dental insurance benefits and those who do not have dental insurance. The majority of those who respond tend to be those who don't carry any type of dental insurance plan.
- To motivate more treatment being scheduled per patient. Studies show that people who have a gift card tend to spend more money per trip than those who don't have a gift card. Think of this as if you were out a restaurant and had a gift card. Normally you might skip the appetizer, dessert, or bottle of wine, but if you have a gift card, suddenly you might want to splurge. This makes your overall bill and ensuing tip you'll give higher, spending more money overall than you would have without having that gift card. In our world, we'll see this as patients agreeing to move forward with both crowns you have treatment planned, instead of one crown today and the other down the road. Maybe they do the two fillings with the crown instead of just one or the other.

Influencing Your Existing Patient Base to Recruit New Patients to the Practice

General practice referrals

A great way to increase new patients is by influencing your existing patient base to refer their friends, family, and coworkers to your practice. Getting our best and favorite patients to send others like them to your practice should be the goal of every dental office. Another benefit to attracting new patients through referrals is that doesn't typically cost you a lot of money, so it's not really hurting your marketing budget. To maximize the chances that an existing patient will feel comfortable referring someone to our practice, I developed an "influence-based, ask-for-the-referral" system, which utilizes five out of six of Cialdini's principles of persuasion.

Reciprocity: $5 gift cards to places people enjoy

As mentioned earlier about the reciprocity principle, when someone has received a gift that they value, an obligation is created inside of them to reciprocate, to give back in kind to what was given to them. These gifts can be intangible things such as doing someone a favor, taking a task off their plate, showing them respect, or giving them attention. These gifts can also be more tangible things such as gift cards. Studies show that a $5 gift card has more influence to getting someone to say yes to your request than offering them a $50 reward to comply.

To tap into this power that giving gifts can create, we need to make sure we find gifts that are unexpected and have some significance to that individual. If the person knows that you'll be giving them something, that expectation isn't really perceived as a gift. It's perceived as an entitlement. Something they are owed. If that gift has no significance to that person, there is no real influence power here either. You've probably heard dental consultants out there who recommend you give your new patients some type of gift, a stainless steel coffee mug for instance, something designed to keep your coffee hot all day. Now picture that I'm a new patient in your practice and that you've just given me this gift. There is only one problem. I don't like or drink coffee.

So what have you really given me? Something I don't appreciate or find value in. Something that's now become an inconvenience as I now have to figure out what to do with this "gift" you've given me. Maybe I can re-gift it to someone else who might enjoy it. Regardless, without any meaning to me, it holds no influence power. So we need to find a way to give a choice of gifts that people will find unexpected but also really value, keeping in mind that a $5 gift card has more influence power than a $50 reward or incentive. As an added bonus, when they pick one of your gift card options, they've now chosen the gift that has the most meaning to them. To figure out what kind of gift cards to offer, you should survey your patients and see what they are spending their money on. Where are they shopping for their goods and services? The most common ones my patients brought up were Amazon, iTunes, Target, and Starbucks.

Next, we need to decide who will be receiving these gift cards, who will be asking for a referral, and when will we be asking. Here's the who, what, when, where, and how:

- **WHO RECEIVES**: Existing patients who had been with the practice for at least one year, something that implied that they liked us, had a good relationship with us, and have enjoyed their experiences with us thus far.
- **WHO RECEIVES**: I also looked for patients who had no dental treatment to be scheduled. Had there been dental treatment planned, asking to schedule this treatment would have been our priority over asking for a referral.
- **WHO GIVES**: The person who has the best relationship is typically the best person to ask them for the referral. Sometimes this is the doctor, but oftentimes it's the person who had spent the most time with that person to date. Usually that meant my hygienist or dental assistant would be the one giving the choice of gift cards and then asking for the referral.
- **WHAT'S GIVEN**: $5 gift cards to popular places people tend to spend their money in. This includes things like gas stations, restaurants, and high-end in-person or online retail stores.

- **WHEN**: Typically the longer the time between when a gift is given to when a request is made, the less influence you have. As such, we chose to give the existing patient a choice of gift card options at the end of their treatment that day, just before it's time to make their next appointment.
- **WHERE**: Usually in the hygienist chair after they have finish their cleaning or in the doctor's chair if they had just completed the last item on their treatment plan.
- **HOW MANY**: Studies show that the more choices a person has to choose from, the less likely they are to choose anything. Too many choices overwhelm people and makes it difficult for them to decide. For our purposes here, I like to limit the number you present to patients from two to no more than four gift card options.
- **WHAT'S NEXT**: We've now identified an existing patient who has no treatment planned, one that has had positive experiences with us in the past and ideally a great experience today. As you start to sit the patient up at the end of their visit, the hygienist or assistant working with them would say, "Mrs. Jones, Dr. Phelps and I just wanted to thank you for coming in today and for being our patient. We know you have a choice in that matter and that you chose us for your care means a lot to us. As a small thank-you from us both, here's a couple of gift cards. Why don't you pick one?" Once the person picks one of your gift card selections, you know they've chosen the one that has some meaning to them; you should receive a genuine "thank you" from that patient. Once heard, you respond by making your request. "My pleasure. Now we need to get you set up for your next appointment, but before we do that, I have a question for you. Do you know of anyone who is looking for a good dentist or dental office?"

Consistency – Get more commitments to influence more referrals

When people make a real commitment to something, there is a lot of internal and external pressure on them to stay consistent and do what they said they would do. When you think of people who are inconsistent in their actions, who don't do what they say they would do, what names or labels have we created for those people? Flaky, wishy-washy, liars. It's because of this that there is an external influence on us to be consistent and avoid being labeled as this type of person. The internal influence comes from us not wanting to view ourselves and our actions as falling in line with these negative terms as well.

While getting commitments is crucial, it's important to note that there are specific type of commitments we need to focus our efforts into attaining:

Voluntary commitments

This type of commitment revolves around giving people a choice. When people have a choice in the matter, they don't feel pressured or backed into a corner. By asking patients if they know of anyone who could use a good dentist, we're giving them a choice to recommend someone or not. It's up to them.

Active commitments

This type of commitment comes in three forms: verbal, written, and effort involved. For verbal, people tend to live up to what they've told someone they will do. For our purposes, the best way to get active verbal commitments is to ask questions. We're going to ask, "Do you know of anyone who needs a good dentist or dental office?"

After the patient says that they do, you'll follow this by asking, "Great. What's their name?" While sitting in your dental chair, most people's mindset is on themselves and their oral health care. In that moment they are not likely to be specifically thinking of someone who they could refer to you. By asking them who they'd recommend and giving them some time to think, most people will give you a name in a fairly short amount of time. Usually they'll respond with, "Oh, my husband needs to come in" or "I need to get my kids in." Sometimes they'll think of a friend or coworker. Regardless, they almost always come up with a name. By giving you that name, they're now even more committed to referring that specific person. We're also going to let them know that you're asking for a specific name because you have a gift bag to give this potential referral and that you'd like to write their name on this gift.

Once we've got them committed to referring and now referring a specific person to the practice, we need to ask one more important active commitment question. Something that's going to require that they put some effort into their commitment to us. "Thank you for referring (whomever they said). Would you help me out by taking this gift bag and pass this on to them on our behalf? When you give this to them, please let them know that we look forward to meeting them."

What's in the Gift Bags?

What we see first, can change our perception of what we see or experience next, typically putting more emphasis, good or bad, on that second item. As stated earlier, this is known to behavioral scientists as the contrast effect. For our purposes, you'll want a combination of expected vs unexpected items to achieve the desired result. The first thing I want the potential new patient to see when opening this gift bag are the expected items one might get from a dental office. A toothbrush, floss, and toothpaste, for instance. When exposed to these expected items first, the contrast effect should heighten their reaction when they see the unexpected gift items we've placed inside the bag for them.

For the unexpected gift items, you'll want to use different gift cards. the first being one of the $5 gift card options you offered your existing patient before you made your request for a referral. Since our existing patient knows this potential new patient the best, I like to ask our existing patient to pick out one of the $5 gift card options and put it in the gift bag for the person they'll be referring. By getting your existing patient involved with picking out a gift card for this person, we're adding more influence power to set the stage for this person to show up in our office.

The second gift card I like to include is a gift card to your own office. Gift cards have more influence than gift certificates and even more influence than coupons. To create a gift card for your office, you can look to online sites by doing an Internet search for custom gift cards to help. Pricing on these range from 25 to 30 cents per card you have printed up, and you can customize their design any way that you wish. For my offices, I offered a card that entitled the bearer to save $200 off $500 in treatment or $500 off $1000 more in treatment.

Now an initial concern one may have is that $500 off will be too much of a discount to offer a lot of people, especially if they are using this to get a single crown. The good news for us is that this rarely occurs thanks to the psychology of gift cards. People who have a gift card tend to spend more money with that business than people without a gift card. In my practices, I saw this to be true. The majority of those who used this gift card tended to use it toward larger treatment plans that they needed, agreeing to getting three or four crowns done instead of just one. Plus, these gift cards were only going out to potential referred new patients. We didn't offer these in our marketing efforts to attract new patients using other media.

In an earlier section, we talked about how the principle of scarcity can be a powerful motivator for people to take action. One way we can increase this influence is by limiting the amount of time people have to take advantage of your offer or gift. On the gift card to our practice, we make sure to put and highlight that this gift expires 30 days from receipt. In our internal tracking efforts, we make note of the potential new patient's name and what date the gift bag is estimated to be delivered to that person. This way we can honor the expiration after 30 days seen on the gift card. Because the scarcity principle motivates action, the good news for us is that those who are really interested in using your gift card will not wait 30 days. They'll move today.

Public commitments

This type revolves around the patient making a commitment in front of more than one person. The more people that know about the commitment you've made, the more influence there is on you to follow through with what you've said you would do. In this context, it would be ideal to have at least two people present in the dental operatory when the existing patient is committing to referring someone to the practice and have agreed to pass on the new patient gift bag. If we can't have two people in the operatory when the request and commitments were made, then we need to share this commitment to others on our team. "Thank you for agreeing to refer (whomever they said) and agreeing to pass on the gift bag to them. I'll let Dr. Phelps and the other team members know you're going to do this for us. I know he'll be thankful as well. The team will be excited when (whomever they said) gives us a call to schedule."

Reminder of the commitment made

While the consistency principle states that when real commitments are made, people tend to follow through with them, I think many of us have experienced times where this turned out to not be the case. People sometimes don't follow through with what they've said they'd do. They don't give us a Google review or refer someone like they said they would. Why is this? Are they all flakes? Wishy-washy? Are they all liars? No. Studies show that the majority of times when people don't follow through with their commitments, it's not that they intended to do this. Instead, it's more likely that while they meant to do it, it got overshadowed by other things going on in their life. It dropped on that person's to-do list. In their mind they still mean to do it, but because it's not a priority, it drops off their radar of things that need to get done. One influence technique that helps counteract this tendency is to find ways to remind people of the commitments that they have made. That simple reminder is enough to bring their commitment back to their top-of-mind thinking and gives you a greater shot for them to follow through with the commitment they've made. The potential new patient gift bags that our existing patient has agreed to pass on our behalf serve this purpose as a commitment reminder. Most people will take that gift bag home and feature it somewhere prominently. They'll put it on their kitchen counter or by the front door to remind themselves that they need to pass this on. Every day that passes and they see this gift bag waiting to be passed on will put more influence on them to make arrangements to do so.

Raving fans while building trust

Once the patient leaves your office and makes arrangements to pass on the potential new patient gift bag, Cialdini's principles of liking and authority will take center stage. The principle of liking states that people prefer to say yes and do business with those that they like. But it's also about things they may share in common, that connect them, such as shared interests, hobbies, or families. When your existing patient goes to pass on the gift bag, they are going to tell this potential new patient everything that they like about you, your office, and your team. They'll also point out everything that this person may have in common with you and potentially like about you. In essence, you've now turned a patient who probably hasn't said many things to anyone about your practice into a raving fan.

In addition to speaking about all of the liking and connections this person may have with you, they are also going to give their testimonial about you. They will tell that person about their past experiences, things like how you didn't hurt them when they had their dental work done, how they didn't feel the shot or injection, or how nice and friendly everyone at your office is. Cialdini's authority principle states that people look to credible, trustworthy authorities to tell us what we should do, mostly as a shortcut measure since we don't have time to learn how to be an expert in everything. By giving their testimonial, sharing their experiences with your office, they are speaking to why they trust you as their dental authority and reaffirming why this person will too.

They'll be excited when they hand this person the gift bag and recount how they had a hand in picking out a special gift card just for them. When the potential new patient opens the bag, discovers the expected items like the toothbrush but then discover the unexpected items like the gift cards, a mindset shift typically occurs from the reciprocity in action. They'll start to think, "Wow, I've never had a dentist give me a gift before I've even met them. Maybe (the person who referred them) is right? Maybe they do things differently there. Since I do need a dental home, I'll make an appointment there and see it for myself."

How do we track this?

Using Excel, Google Sheets, or some equivalent spreadsheet, the team tracks the following variables:

- What team member gave the gift card and asked for the referral?
- Date this occurred.
- What gift card was chosen by the patient?
- What gift card did the patient choose for the potential referred patient?
- What is the name of the potential referred patient?
- Date they scheduled and came into our office?

Other logistical concerns

- Presentation of the $5 gift card choices. When you're offering a choice of gift cards, you don't allow your team members to be fumbling around the operatory, trying to find and present these to your existing patient. Instead, you should have some way to prominently display them to your patients. Perhaps a nice collage of pictures of the gift cards? Maybe it could take on more of a menu of choice look? Ideally this should be readily available to grab in the moment and clearly show the patients the options they have to choose from.

- Gift cards are stored centrally and tracked. A mistake many have made in the name of convenience is keeping a certain number of the gift card options in the operatory itself. It's not a fun day when a team member discovers that $100 worth of gift cards has suddenly disappeared. Was it a patient going through drawers when the team member wasn't present? Was it the cleaning crew who discovered it one night and decided these cards wouldn't be missed? Was it your team member who took them for personal use? Regardless of the answer, these are questions you never want to be in a position to have to ask as it puts you and the team member in an uncomfortable position. Instead, the gift cards should be kept in a lock box and stored in a central location. There should be two people in charge of this box for verification purposes. A sign out sheet should be used so the doctor knows what gift card has been given out, who signed it out, and who verified it. Once the patient has seen their menu of gift card options and made their selection, it's easy for the team member to come up and grab the gift card selected. Once they return and physically hand the gift card to that existing patient, they can continue the sequence as laid out above and ask for the referral.
- Document that a gift was given in the patient chart. For reciprocity to have influence, gifts have to be given unexpectedly to someone. If they come to expect it, then it turns into an entitlement, something we owe them. It's important to document that we've given this patient a gift and asked for a referral. This way we don't make a mistake of repeating this process when they are back in the office six months later and train our patients to expect this gift choice each time they come in. My recommendation to keep this unexpected is to run this cycle once every two years. In the dental space where this process will most likely come out of hygiene, that means waiting three or four cleaning visits before repeating this process.
- Note any patterns. In addition to giving unexpected gifts, the ultimate goal with reciprocity is to give gifts that people really value and appreciate. We can accomplish this by offering them a choice of gift card. What does it tell us if out of 100 gift cards given out, 50 percent of the people chose gift card A, 50 percent chose gift card B, but no one chose gift cards C or D? It tells us that no one really valued those companies, that service, restaurant, and so forth. It means we should switch these cards out for other ones people might value more. The more options we have that people might value, the greater the chance a gift card selection will occur and we can influence them to refer.
- Should we fear a no? Asking for a referral is one of the most inexpensive yet effective marketing media you can use to grow your practice, but oftentimes it's the one thing few practices are actually implementing. One answer is an aspect of all human behavior. People don't like rejection. They don't like for others to tell them no. So to avoid hearing no, we tend to avoid requests that might generate them, ultimately missing out on a great opportunity to attract more new patients without having to spend more money in other marketing media.

Let's look at this fear from a behavioral science standpoint. If people fear rejection from others, that means that people really don't like hearing no from others. If people really don't like hearing no, that means they typically don't like telling people no. With the principle of reciprocity, there is another aspect that might aid us in our cause to combat this fear of rejection. Instead of being afraid of hearing no after our request is made, what if we changed our mindset and were just prepared for the no? Studies show that people like to offer a concession when people have first offered a concession to them.

As mentioned previously, a concession is an alternative option or plan to the one first presented. If a request is made and is rejected, and then the person who made the request asks for something else in that moment or offers an alternative option, they are now more likely to get a yes. If a second no is given and another request or backup option is given, they are even more likely to get a yes to this request. So if a fear of rejection is what's holding us back from asking for more referrals, we can now be confident that we shouldn't be afraid of a no; we should just be ready for it, ready to ask for something else if no is heard.

Team member: Do you know of anyone who could use a good dentist or dental home?

Patient: No, I'm sorry. I don't.

Team member: That's okay. If you think of anyone, please let us know. In the meantime, you mentioned you had a great visit with us today, right?

Patient: Yes, I did. You guys are great!

Team member: Thank you; we love hearing that from our patients. Would you mind helping me out then? Would you be willing to give us a 5-star Google review and let others out there know about your experience with us? That would really help us out a lot.

Patient: Of course. I'm happy to do that for you guys.

Utilizing five of Cialdini's six principles of persuasion, you can influence more of your existing patients to refer new patients to your practice. The costs of this system are minimal: $5 gift cards for the existing patient and potential new patient and the costs of the gift bag, toothbrush, toothpaste, and floss. The results are powerful. For offices who've run this system like outlined above, around 68 percent of the potential new patient names attained ended up becoming new patients in their practice. In many cases this doubled or tripled their new patient count from existing referral sources, providing a high ROI in return.

Dental specialty practice referrals

Dental specialty practices are no strangers to this idea of using referrals to help them achieve their new patient goals. In fact, historically this medium has been almost 100 percent of their marketing efforts. Dental specialists spend a lot of time building relationships with area general dentists, taking them out to lunch, getting to know more about that potential referring dentists practice and team, educating them about their specialty practice and how they can work together on future cases.

While there isn't typically a huge marketing investment spent, there is a large cost to the time involved to build and continually maintain these referral relationships. Through my call tracker ROI system, I have had the fortune to be able to study these referral relationships from specialty offices across the US and Canada and have identified two main areas of lost opportunity that are preventing these type of practices from getting more new patients, one that affects the amount of new patient calls coming in and one that affects the actual number of new patients that make an appointment.

Increase in the amount of new patient calls

When interviewing my specialty dental colleagues, I asked them to categorize the general dentists who are actively referring patients to their practice. For most, they broke them up into three categories: best, okay, and absent referral sources. Their best referral sources were the ones who were actively referring 10 or more patients per month to their practice. Okay referral sources generated 2–9 new patients per month. Absent referral sources generated 0–1 patient per month. One aspect of how they accounted for these categories was by the number of patients who showed up to their office and were now sitting in their chairs. As customary, the specialty dentist would send their referring dentist a letter that summarized what was discussed and/or any treatment performed at that initial consultation visit. This made it easy to calculate how many patients each dentist in their area referred.

Using my call tracker ROI system, I was able to review the potential new patient phone calls of orthodontic, oral surgery, endo, and periodontal offices across the US and Canada. Because this was a tracking system, I was able to distinguish what general dental offices had referred these new patients to the practice. I was then able to correlate each of these calls back to the best, okay, and absent referral categories the dental specialists had placed these referring general dentists in. In my analysis of these phone calls, a definitive pattern emerged for each category.

Those offices who were considered to be the "best" referrals had tapped into Dr. Robert Cialdini's principles of liking, authority, and consistency. It was obvious that the referring dentist liked the person they were referring to. They had relayed stories and commonalities they had with them to their patients, connections such as family, hobbies, interests that the patient may have had in common with them too. They had done an excellent job of endorsing the specialty dentist as an authority to their patient by presenting their credentials, training, and expertise to them, relaying why they trusted this specialty dentist with their patient's care, taking barriers to scheduling off that patient's plate. Instead of giving the patient a referral slip with the office's number on it and then putting it back on the patient to call them and make an appointment, offices in this category chose to make that call on their patients' behalf, helping them make an appointment while they were still in their office, giving the patient one less thing to do later, which they could have possibly forgotten.

In the okay and absent referral categories, it was clear from the conversations overheard that these offices had not done a good job or invested any time to create liking, promote authority, and create more consistency in their patients to ensure they called that specialty office. Therefore, if you want to increase the number of new patient calls from referral sources, you must invest time on the following:

- Spend time with your current and potential referring dentists.
- Don't forget about spending time with their teams as in many offices it's the team that ends up helping the patient decide which specialty office they'll go to.
- Find liking connections with the dentist and team members. Share with them all of the things you feel comfortable with others knowing about you: your hobbies, interests, favorite sports teams, etc. Anything they or their patients might find in common with you.
- Educate them on your credentials, training, and expertise. Convince them you are an authority in this arena.
- Share patient testimonials and positive Google reviews from patients they've referred to you or that you've received from other patients.
- Identify barriers potential patients may have to scheduling, and train your referring dentist's team on how to remove those barriers and get more commitments to scheduling with your office today.

Increase the amount of new patients who make appointments

A few years back, I ran into a local oral surgeon at an annual dental society meeting, someone I hadn't really spoken to for a couple of years. Before this, the surgeon had routinely taken me out for lunches and sent annual Christmas and birthday gifts to our office. Yet as time went on, we lost touch. He stopped reaching out to schedule those lunches. Truthfully, I didn't give it much thought as my own schedule had become pretty hectic from practicing dentistry, running multiple offices, and starting up new companies such as Call Tracker ROI, Golden Goose Scheduling, and Dental Membership Direct. Yet I found it interesting when I ran back into him at this dental society meeting and he asked me why I stopped referring to him. You see, in my mind I had not stopped referring to him, so his question kind of caught me off guard. In fact, I was sure that in the week leading up to this meeting I had referred one or two patients his way.

From his point of view he had stopped seeing patients I referred in his chair, which caused me to go from a best referral source to an absent one. Because of this he decreased any time he might have invested with me over lunch, dinner, or birthdays, instead probably putting those energies into his other best referral sources or potential new referral sources. From my point of view, I had noticed a decrease in the time he invested with me, but I had not let that affect the referrals I attempted to send his way. So what was the disconnect here?

The answer was found on those new patient telephone calls coming into his office. From our Call Tracker ROI data, I know that the average general dental office does not answer around 32 percent of their incoming new patient calls. To make matters worse, when the office does answer the phone, the team only makes that patient an appointment about 34 percent of the time. We'll cover the why on this in more detail and what to do about it in a later section. For specialty offices, you might assume that their answer rate and new patient scheduling conversion rates would be higher than in general practice. A referred patient has been influenced by the liking, authority, and consistency principles we mentioned above, which should translate into more appointments scheduled vs a non-referred patient, who has no real connection or trust established with you yet.

The Call Tracker ROI data we amassed show this not to be true for most specialty practices. Like the general dentist's results, the average specialty practice only converts around 34 percent of their new patient calls into actual appointments, even in endodontic practices, where the patient being in pain is a high motivation factor influencing them to schedule. Compound this with a significant number of new patient calls going unanswered, and you can see why the surgeon and I had that disconnect. After some more research and tracking his office's new patient calls, it was discovered that he had a team member that was sabotaging his results. Dentists like myself had tried to send referrals his way, but the phone calls either weren't getting answered or the patient left the call without making an appointment, usually avoiding care by a specialist altogether or leading them to research a different office and make an appointment there.

In other offices we tracked, there wasn't a team member putting up a barrier for that new patient to schedule. Instead, it really went back to a lack of training on how to handle the barriers new patients may bring up when they are attempting to schedule, how to make it more convenient for that new patient to schedule with them, how to handle patients' uncertainty about whether this is the right office for them. Can they trust this office to take care of them and treat them well? These uncertainty issues had already been satisfied by the actions of those who were their best referring offices but were sorely missing in the okay and absent referral offices.

To increase the number of new patients who make appointments from referral sources you must:

1. Have data on all of your potential new patient calls from referral sources;
2. Identify any deficiencies in your ability to answer new patient calls;
3. Identify any challenges your team members have with scheduling new patient calls;
4. Track their conversion percentages by referral source so you can identify patterns from your best, okay, and absent referral cites;
5. Provide training for those answering the telephone, which helps them overcome barriers patients may bring up while scheduling and that help them avoid putting up barriers that could be preventing more patients from scheduling.

Let's look at an influence-based system I created that ties all of these points together and should help increase referrals to any specialty practice, one that uses tracking, reciprocity, and accountability.

Tracking

1. Utilize a call tracking company like Call Tracker ROI and acquire 10 unique tracking numbers. You will assign one unique number to your website. When a new patient calls this number, that call will be recorded for analysis and will be set up to automatically forward to your main office line.
2. Pick 9 general dental offices to work with. Three offices should be from your best referral source group, three should come from the okay referral source group, and three

should come from your absent referral source group, maybe people who used to send you a significant number of patients in the past but now it seems that they do not. Assign one unique tracking number to each of these 9 offices. Each of these numbers, when dialed, should automatically forward to your main office line.

3. Create new referral pads. You will need to invest in a new series of referral pads, 9 unique ones. Each referral pad will have a different call tracking number shown as the number to call to reach your office. Why 9 different referral pads? Because anything worth doing is worth testing and investing in.

Reciprocity

- Give a gift of value to each referral source. Earlier we talked about how giving gifts of value will influence those to give back to you or say yes to a request you may ask them, in this case, to send you more referrals. To do this, I want you to focus your gift efforts on the referring dentist as well as their team members, since both can play a hand in influencing a referred patient your direction. One of the gifts I've found that both groups really value is having their car washed.
- Hire a mobile car wash group to go out to wash and detail the cars of your referring dentist and team members. Average cost for this runs about $20 per car washed.
- Have one of your key team members go to that referring office on the day the cars are being washed. Let them know this gift is on behalf of the specialist dentist and then swap out any old referral pads they may have with one of your new unique call tracking number referral pads. Make a note of which office received which call tracking number.
- Let the office and their team know that you appreciate them and would love to help treat their patients if they have any specialty needs that arise in the future.

If the general dentist and their team really appreciate the gift you've given, it should generate more referrals calls out of all three categories you're testing, from the best group referring even more to seeing the absent group send something, if they hadn't sent anything before.

Accountability

At the Phelps Institute, we provide our clients with a telephone training presentation and video to help your team increase their phone conversions. This is done by giving them strategies to overcome the barriers that patients may create when attempting to schedule as well as how to avoid creating barriers on their end that might push a potential new patient away. Once a month I recommend that you review the reports from your call tracking numbers. Look at those calls that didn't end with an appointment scheduled and look at the reasons why this occurred. Review these calls with your team members monthly and attempt to reinforce the telephone training strategies that they have learned. By giving them better telephone communication skills and having monthly accountability meetings, you will see their new patient scheduling conversion rates increase significantly, translating into more new patients now sitting in your chairs.

By having this tracking data, you'll also get a more accurate assessment of which dental offices are really attempting to refer patients to your practice. This may lead to you reclassifying these into your higher categories of referral sources. For those that are attempting to refer patients your way, spend time with them to continue to develop that relationship. Speak with those dentists and team members from your best referral offices and find out what they are doing to endorse you as an authority. What barriers to scheduling are they eliminating on your behalf? Share this information with the offices who are attempting to refer patients to you, and you will bear the fruit of this investment.

As stated earlier, I usually recommend starting this system with 9 offices: three from your absent, three from your okay, and three from your best referral categories. You should have a unique tracking number assigned to each of these 9 offices so you can track what potential new patients are coming from what sources. A 10th number will go on your website. When calls originate from this source, it's important for your team to ask, "How did you hear about us?" to that potential new patient as they may have been referred by one of the offices you're tracking but did not call you using the unique call tracking referral slip they were given from that office. Using reciprocity should motivate more referrals from all three categories while sharing best practices from your best referral sources should initiate more referrals from your other two categories as well. Ultimately this should result in more new patient opportunities being generated.

Utilizing your data from your call tracking program, you'll know exactly how many potential new patients you had, which office they truly came from, and what your team was able to do with those opportunities. Get your team the tools they need to be more successful on the telephone. Meet with them monthly to praise any successes or progress made from the previous month. Review their data with them in areas where improvement can be made. Use the data from your tracking reports to make smarter decisions. Sometimes the reasons you didn't schedule an appointment could not be helped by the team at all. For example, you may find that the team is unable to answer a significant number of new patient calls. You may be down a team member so you have less people to handle the volume of calls coming in. Maybe patients are calling when everyone in the office is out to lunch? Regardless, there is usually a pattern and a solution to help. Consider outsourcing your new patient opportunity calls to dedicated dental scheduling services. I created Golden Goose Scheduling for this very reason. Whether my team is acting as backup for our client offices or handling the bulk of their potential new patient calls, our offices know that we are an extension of their team and that they will see more new patients showing up in their office.

Using this referral system, you will be able to increase the number of potential new patient calls generated. Being data and training driven, you'll help your team schedule more of those opportunity calls that come in. By utilizing a well-trained third-party scheduling service your capacity to answer and schedule more new patient calls will significantly increase. Added all together, this should translate into more new patients in your chairs that generate a great return for your investment.

Patient appreciation party

From the outset of this book, I've referred back to an old adage in dental marketing is that there isn't typically one thing you can do that will net you over a 100 new patients. With most of the media I've tested over the years I have found this statement to be true. But I have found one exception to this rule. Something that consistently netted me over 100 new patients when implemented. It's called a patient appreciation party. This idea of having a party to celebrate my existing patients came to me one day when I was studying Cialdini's principle

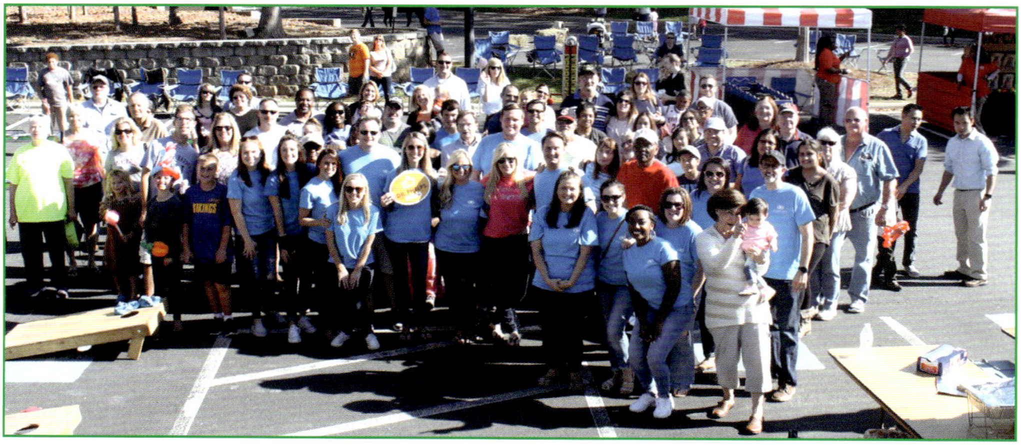

Figure 36. **Picture from patient appreciation party.**

of reciprocity. My initial goals for this party were simple. If I celebrate and give to my existing patients, then they would most likely reciprocate and give back to our office in kind, hopefully in the way of increasing case acceptance and getting more treatment scheduled or through increased referrals.

Where would we have this party?

Each of my offices measured around 3500 sq. ft. of space with 8 dental chairs inside. They were in commercial buildings that had ample parking with empty lots adjoining them. This gave me options. If we had a small number of patients attend, we could host everyone inside our office. If the attendance numbers grew, we could host the event both inside and outside of our office. I checked with our buildings condominium association as well as the other business owners in our development to get everyone's approval for the event I had planned. I invited all of the businesses in our complex to participate and asked them to invite their client base to this event in an attempt to cross-promote and possibly attract some of them to become our patients as well. In exchange, we'd be offering them exposure to my patients for their business as a reciprocity exchange for them doing the same with their clients. If logistically it didn't make sense to hold this event at our office, then I would have looked at renting a larger venue and would have hosted it there. Fortunately, I had the permission from those businesses around me and ample outside space to accommodate several hundred people if it was a success.

What would I give those that attended?

By throwing an event specifically for them, I was showing them admiration, showing them that myself and my team really appreciated that they had chosen us for their dental care. But we needed more. Food is always an easy gift to give, so I wanted to provide a free meal to those who might attend this event. Lastly, I wanted to give them a chance to win something that they really might value. Large flat screen TVs, nice stereo headphones, Apple laptops, iPads, a grilling and tailgating package, and a four-day cruise were just some of the prizes I purchased and raffled off at these events. The more expensive the gifts I purchased to give away, the higher the attendance appeared to be for that event.

When would we have this appreciation party?

Between my two offices, I held these events twice per year, once per office, each time rotating the date of the event, testing different seasons and its effect on the number who attended. During the summer months, we had great attendance with 400+ people showing, but the heat and humidity we had in Charlotte, North Carolina, almost made it unbearable. We avoided the heat during the winter months but noticed that we couldn't predict how cold our area would be on the day of the party. Some years it was more moderate in temperature and made for a great event. Other years it was so cold outside that it made the event have lower attendance and engagement by those who did attend. Eventually I settled on dates around August, September, and October. Our weather temperatures were consistently moderate. Not too hot, not too cold from year to year. Plus, we didn't have to worry about rain ruining our event like we did during the spring season. During this time, we were consistently able to get 250–300+ people to attend.

What was my goal for this party?

Initially, my goal was to use this as a goodwill gesture and as a thank-you to my existing patients. Because my practices were fee for service, patients had a litany of choices around them who were in network with their dental insurance plan but chose our practice in spite of this. I genuinely was thankful to them for this and wanted to give back to them.

At the same time, my practices needed more new patients, so I wanted to use this event as a new patient attraction vehicle. What better way to achieve this goal than by influencing my existing patients to refer more new patients to our practice? Plus, I was able to attract new patients by promoting this event in some other marketing media such as newspaper inserts and our celebrity endorsement radio ads that were currently airing.

Lastly, I wanted to use the principle of scarcity and the idea of a limited-time promotion to collect enough revenue the day of the event that would more than cover the total costs for throwing the event. It was at these events that I ran an annual discount special off Invisalign orthodontic treatment. I limited the special to this one day a year and targeted existing patients who had already received a treatment plan for aligner or bracket and wire therapy but had not moved forward with treatment. I also mentioned the special in my other external marketing ads to attract potential new patients who were seeking this therapy and whose mindset was focused on getting a deal.

How would you organize an event like this?

- Hire an event planner.
- Get the team involved and assigned certain roles.
- Finalize the prize list that you'll be raffling off during the event.
- Create engagement activities for your guests to enjoy throughout the event.
- Map out a plan for how people can win prizes and let them know the schedule of when the prize winners will be announced.
- Promote, promote, promote!
- Record, record, record!

Given the scope of this endeavor and my lack of experience hosting an event of this potential size, I hired an event planner to aid me. An event planner, also known as a meeting planner, is someone who can coordinate all aspects of a professional meeting or event. From choosing a meeting location to hiring food truck vendors, negotiating with party event vendors for tables, chairs, arranging for petting zoos, and so forth, this person was instrumental in the early years for making this event possible. As time went on and our experience with these events increased, I was able to delegate the event planner's responsibilities to my team.

Once the event planner was hired, it's time to sit down with your team and get them committed to participating. The first questions that usually come up from them are typically:

- When are you going to have this event?
- How long will it last?
- Will they be paid for participating?

As mentioned earlier, I recommend you hold this event during the fall months. September and October tend to be well received temperature wise in all parts of the country. You'll want to hold this event on a Saturday as that will give you an opportunity to have the greatest number of people attend. Since lunch will be served, I like to start the event at noon and have it last around three hours in total. Many of those who'll attend this event are families with children of various ages. A lot of the engagement activities we use are tailored to younger children and pre-teens. That means that you don't want to have the event too early in the morning as then you'll be competing with the various sporting events their children may be into. Typically, the bulk of those games are held in the morning for kids in this age range, so we want to hold our event during a time when they'd be free to participate. These events are also popular with our older patient base, those of retirement age who enjoy bringing their kids and young grandchildren out as a fun family activity as well.

For larger crowds, anything shorter doesn't really give people a lot of time to participate in everything you may have to engage them, and anything longer and they tend to lose their focus. It's doubtful you'll have all of your participants stay the full length of time as many will attend early for lunch, try to win some prizes, and then take off as others arrive for a later lunch/snack and finish the event out. If you are anticipating less than 100 people, you may consider shortening the total time for the event down to 1.5 to 2 hours.

Staff participation in these events is critical. Many times it's our team members who have the best relationships with our patients, so people will come to these events to see them just as much as they may be coming to see you. To reduce any barrier that may keep a team member from attending and participating in this event, I decided early on that I would pay them to attend. As you'll see from the list of engagement activities that are being held, our team members will be working very hard and will be very busy both leading up to and during these events.

Giveaways are essential. It's the idea of winning a big prize that motivates people to attend, especially the first time you throw this event as people won't know what to expect or know why they should attend. Attracting them with the right giveaway could be just the motivation they need to show up. I tend to get gifts from four main categories:

- Popular technology items such as flat-screen TVs, iPads, Apple watches, and such.
- Items related to popular activities they may enjoy such as tickets for great seats to a professional football or basketball game or a four-day Bahamas cruise.

- Items related to treatment or services at our office such as a certificate for Zoom Whitening or one of our Dental Savings Plans, a membership plan that would provide someone without dental insurance all of their preventative care needed for the year.
- Items donated from other businesses who were participating at our events. This included things such as $5 to $10 gift cards to area restaurants, free or discounted membership to local tennis and racquet clubs, and gift certificates that could be used at our supporting businesses.

Creating engagement activities is important. Some will come and go in a short amount of time but many will choose to stay for the whole event. That means you have to keep them occupied, so I tried to have activities for adults, activities for kids, and things both could enjoy together.

For the kids activities we included things such as:

- Cotton candy and popcorn machines;
- Mini tennis;
- Mini golf;
- Air brush painting station;
- Bean bag toss;
- Bounce houses;
- Petting zoo;
- Pony rides;
- Halloween costume contest.

For the adult activities, we included things such as:

- **Match the mouth**: This was a series of before and after cosmetic dentistry photos that had been jumbled up. Those who matched up all of the before and after photos to the correct mouth would be entered into a raffle to win one of the technology prizes mentioned above.
- **Live music**: At every event, I hired a professional musician to come out and play music throughout the duration of our event. I was then able to use the audio equipment they had set up to make periodic announcements to the crowd and announce who won the various prizes we gave away.
- **More giveaways**: Every adult who attended received a little branded gift from us for attending. Each year it was something different, but I tried to put our branding around things they might use such as a portable wine and beverage glass or a foldable chair.

Activities adults and kids might enjoy

Behavioral science researchers have long realized that when people are tasked with scavenger hunts, more people become engaged in completing the quest and report having an improved overall experience. Add in the potential reward of winning a prize for fully completing the assigned tasks, and you'll see even more engagement from both adults and kids alike. For our events, I decided to create a type of scavenger hunt that encouraged people to attend all of the engagement activities we had laid out for them. At each station they'd receive a stamp by one of my team members or someone who was manning that area. Once all stations were visited and the map was complete, they could turn their map in to be entered to win an adult prize or a kid prize. On average, I found that 30–40 percent of those who attended the event got a stamp from every station and were entered into the drawing.

Now it's time to finalize your plan for the raffle tickets. Things that must be decided:

- How you'll handle feeding the crowd, but keep an accurate count so your food vendors don't overcharge you.
- Prize raffle ticket assignment and additional opportunities. How do your patients get raffle tickets? How can they get more tickets if they want a better chance to win? Where do they put these raffle tickets if they want to win specific prizes? How can we use the raffle tickets to satisfy our goals of using this as a new patient attraction event as well as influencing more people to sign up and pay for adult orthodontic therapy?
- Schedule of giveaways.

Feeding the crowd

Mobile food trucks offer an easy solution to feeding a large crowd. Having a variety of these vendors present also gives the crowd choices and should help keep your overall food expenses down. For my events, the most popular food trucks were typically a hot dog, a barbeque truck, and some company with a vegetarian offering. When people first arrived at the event, we asked them to sign in and register. At registration, each person was given a white raffle ticket for every person in their party. With each food vendor, I had a prearranged deal in place with them. For example, if a person turned in one white ticket at the hot dog truck, that one ticket would get them two hot dogs and a bag of potato chips. At the barbeque vendor, that one ticket would get them a barbeque sandwich and a bag of chips. At the vegetarian place it might get them a salad. For drinks, I had my team set up a drink station where we provided water and a few soft drink varieties people could choose from.

With each food package, I had also arranged a fixed price that I would pay the food truck vendor after the event was completed. At the barbeque place, for instance, for every white ticket the food vendor turned back into us, we pay them $4 per ticket, so 100 white tickets meant we wrote them a check for $400. All in all, this was a great way to simplify tracking how much food was actually consumed by our participants, and it allowed us to give the crowd more food choices than we might have been able to had we have a group cater the event for us with one fixed menu.

Awarding the prizes

One of the first things you'll want to consider is how you'll award the prizes. There are two main options to choose from. You can accept all raffle tickets at once. Store them all in the same bin if you will, and then draw a unique ticket for each of the prizes you give away. The benefit to this approach is that a greater number of attendees are likely to stay for the entire duration of your event as their name will still be in the running to win your grand prize drawing you conclude the day with. The downside to this approach is that if everyone stays the entire duration, when you reach crowds of 200+, you could find yourself with a traffic situation. On the front end it can make for a parking nightmare as most commercial real estate developments weren't designed to have that many people on-site at any one given time. At the end of the event, when everyone is ready to leave, the traffic jam that is usually created can be a source of great frustration, taking away from the amazing experience they just had with you and your team.

The second option would be to create separate ticket storing bins for each of the prizes you intend to give away. Then draw the winner from that prize's specific bin. The benefit to this approach is that it should raise the level of engagement from those attending the event. Especially if you give them opportunities to complete more activities to win additional tickets and thus increase their chances of winning the prize they want the most. The downside of this approach is that once you've had the drawing for a specific prize, many may decide to leave now that their chance of winning is over.

Having tried both ways, my recommendation is to have separate ticket bins for each of the prizes you wish to give away. This allowed for more available parking throughout the event as people left early once their prize bin was announced, which aided in parking for those who arrived fashionably late. I also noticed a significant increase in people's desire to get more tickets to win a specific prize and thus was able to leverage that motivation to get more things for our practice, things such as more Google reviews, video testimonials, treatment paid for, and money raised.

Once you have chosen how you'll want to award the prizes, you'll then need to come up with a schedule on when you want to give away each prize. Ideally you'll want to start with smaller items such as gift cards to area businesses and then work your way up to whatever grand prize you've purchased for the event, such as a large flat-screen TV or a four-day Caribbean cruise.

Raffle ticket assignment

When people start to arrive for the event, we funnel them over to a registration or check-in area just inside our office doors. At this station, you'll need to have access to your schedule, and your goal is to discover whether they are an existing patient or a potential new patient to the practice.

If they are an existing patient:

- Thank them for coming. Make sure we have them scheduled for a future appointment such as a cleaning. If we don't have them scheduled, then attempt to do so.
- Give them their welcome gift bag, promotional gift like the branded travel wine glass I mentioned previously, scavenger hunt sheets, and schedule of prize drawings (shown below). Go over the rules of the scavenger hunt and the prize they could win.
- Give them one food ticket per person in their party and explain the food options present.
- Give them one raffle ticket, review the prize list available, and explain how they can be entered to win any of those prizes.
- Explain the different options available for them to win more raffle tickets to increase their chance of winning a specific prize.

If they are a potential new patient:

- Thank them for attending. If not obvious, ask how they found out about this event and make a note of it for internal tracking purposes. This helps us identify if they were referred to the party by an existing patient or if any of our external promotional efforts attracted them our way.
- Give them their welcome gift bag, promotional gift like the branded travel wine glass I mentioned previously, scavenger hunt sheets, and schedule of prize drawings (shown below). Go over the rules of the scavenger hunt and the prize they could win.
- Give them one food ticket per person in their party and explain the food options present.
- Give them one raffle ticket and review the prize list available and explain how they can be entered to win any of those prizes.
- Explain the different options available for them to win more raffle tickets to increase their chance of winning a specific prize.
- Offer to give them a tour of your office before they start with the events festivities.
- Most importantly, ask them if they'd like to make an appointment for an initial cleaning or consultation with the dentist.

Raffle ticket additional opportunities

By attending the event, each person received one raffle ticket, which they could put toward any one prize of their choosing. Adding additional opportunities to gain more tickets is a great way to motivate people to be more engaged at your event and help you attain resources you can use in future marketing efforts. Here are some examples of ways I gave patients additional raffle ticket opportunities.

- **Prepay for treatment**: For anyone who responded to our orthodontic treatment promotion by prepaying for their Invisalign treatment at this event, we awarded them 15 extra raffle tickets. For anyone interested in starting, we took them into the office and completed an on-the-spot consultation with one of our doctors to see if they were a candidate. From here, they could have a digital scan or impression so we could begin their treatment.
- **Attract more new patients**: For every potential new patient that an existing patient brought to this event, we would give them an additional 10 raffle tickets to put toward a prize of their choosing. They could put all 10 toward one prize or split it up among several prices, their choice. This could be a spouse or other family member who had not been to the practice yet or someone outside of their family.
- **Video testimonial**: At each of these parties I hired a videographer to document and record the day's events. For any person that would sit down with our videographer and spent a few minutes to give us a video testimonial about their experience from that day and as being one of our patients, we awarded them an extra 5 raffle tickets.
- **Google reviews**: For anyone who would give us a 5-star Google review, we'd give them 5 extra raffle tickets. All they had to do was show one of my team members the review and we'd award them the extra tickets. If a patient had already given us a 5-star review in the past, all they had to do was show this to a team member, and we'd thank them by giving them the extra tickets as well.

- **Match my mouth**: For those who participated in the "Match My Mouth" contest I mentioned earlier, we'd award them an extra two raffle tickets. By turning people's focus toward the cosmetic dentistry we had performed on other patients, I knew this would influence more interest in what we might be able to do for their mouth. Using a service called Lumismile, we took a photo of those who participated and emailed them a new photo of their smile with some type of cosmetic enhancement. So they could see their potential new smile on themselves. Whiter teeth, straighter teeth, or what they'd look like with veneers or cosmetic crowns.
- **Scavenger hunt completion**: Anyone who visited and gotten a stamp from all of the booths on our scavenger hunt received two extra raffle tickets. Plus, their completed sheet was their entry for an additional adult and child prize.
- **Social media station**: Like us, follow us, or leave us a review on Facebook or Instagram, and we'd give them two additional raffle tickets.
- **Fund raising**: Additional raffle tickets were also available for purchase: $1 per ticket, 12 for $10, 25 for $20. Each year I selected a different team member and asked them to choose a charity to raise money for. All proceeds from the sale of additional raffle tickets went to the charity my team member selected that year.

Raffle ticket results

My goal for this event was to create an opportunity to give back and thank my patient base for choosing our practice. I also wanted to use this party as a new patient attraction vehicle and collect enough money from patients who prepaid for treatment that day to help offset my hard costs for hosting this event. The results?

- **Prepaid treatment**: The costs to run an event on this scale would typically be $12,000–$15,000. That's compensation for my team's participation, the food, renting the engagement activities, and purchasing the prize giveaways. During these events we would offer a discount off Invisalign or other orthodontic services, the only day of the year we offered this discount. The average fee most people paid that day ranged from $4700 for treatment that would last seven-plus months down to $2700 for treatment that lasted six months or less. We never had an event where less than 10 people prepaid for one of these two options. Treatment fees collected that day would range from $27,000 to a record $64,000 at one event.
- **Attract more new patients**: "There isn't one thing in dental marketing you can do that will net you over 100 new patients." Consider that old adage broken because our average number of new patients who scheduled appointments at these events was 116, over 90 percent of those coming from existing patients who had invited someone new to the practice to come with them. I remember one existing patient in particular who was so excited for the chance to win the 55-inch plasma TV that he brought 10 of his friends to the party and put all 100 of his extra raffle tickets in that bin to win. I'm so glad he won, but even if he hadn't, for that kind of effort, it would have been my pleasure to buy him one.
- **Video testimonials**: These are probably the hardest to attain as people don't typically like being on camera or being filmed. So you have a resistance barrier right off the bat. Despite that, we were able to get 6–8 great video testimonials from each event, videos we were then able to post on our website and on all of our social media channels.

- **Google reviews**: We'd average an additional 30+ reviews each time we held this event.
- "**Smile simulation**": Out of those who received the Lumismile projection of what their new smile could look like, over 35 percent came back at a later date for a cosmetic consultation, most of which moved forward with some type of cosmetic dentistry treatment and many of whom were people I might not have had a cosmetic consultation with before showing them what they were missing out on by not having this new smile.
- **Scavenger hunt**: 30–40 percent of the attendees completed the scavenger hunt activities. For my neighboring businesses who participated, it brought them great exposure and new clients to grow from. As time went on and I collected success stories these businesses had attracting new clients, I was then able to start charging businesses a sponsorship fee to participate. Usually $500 but with 10 or more vendors present, it became yet another way to offset my hard costs for hosting this event.
- **Fundraising**: Our team's goal was to raise $1000 from these events that could be donated to a charity of one of my team members choosing, a donation made in their name and the practice's name. We did not have one event where we did not surpass that goal.

Promote, promote, promote

Once you've finalized the logistics for your party and your team understands their role, your efforts now have to move toward promotion of this event (Fig. 37). If no one knows your event is taking place, then you shouldn't be surprised by a poor showing. At a minimum, I'd recommend three full months of promotion. Ideally, I'd like to see your promotion efforts start six months before your first event. Promotional efforts can come from either internal or external efforts or some combination of the two.

Internal Efforts: Six Months before Your Event

Informational flyers (Fig. 37) should be designed and printed for distribution at the office. Flyers are 8 by 10 inches, full color with 70-pound glossy paper. In the past, I've printed them in bulk with a local printer, but now there are so many online printers available that are competing that you should research and find who'll give you the best price.

Your flyer should include the most important information about your event:

- Date and time;
- Activities available;
- Entertainment you'll be providing;
- Prizes you'll be giving away;
- How to increase their chances of winning;
- That patients new to the practice are welcome to attend;
- Any one-day specials or treatment promotions you are offering;
- Include logos of any businesses who've paid to sponsor your event;
- RSVP recommended but not required.

One flyer should be given to each patient who had an appointment that day in your practice, those from the hygiene side and the dentist's chair. If we do this consistently for six months, then you can be assured that the large majority of your active patient base now knows about your party. If you and your team make special mention and personally invite them to the party, then that will increase the chances of more attending.

Internal efforts: three months or less before your event

Email reminders should start going out around three months before the date of your party. One reminder three months out, one reminder two months before, and then one email per week during the three weeks before the party. For the week just before the event, I send an email reminder 3–4 days earlier and the last one the day before the event. In these emails we

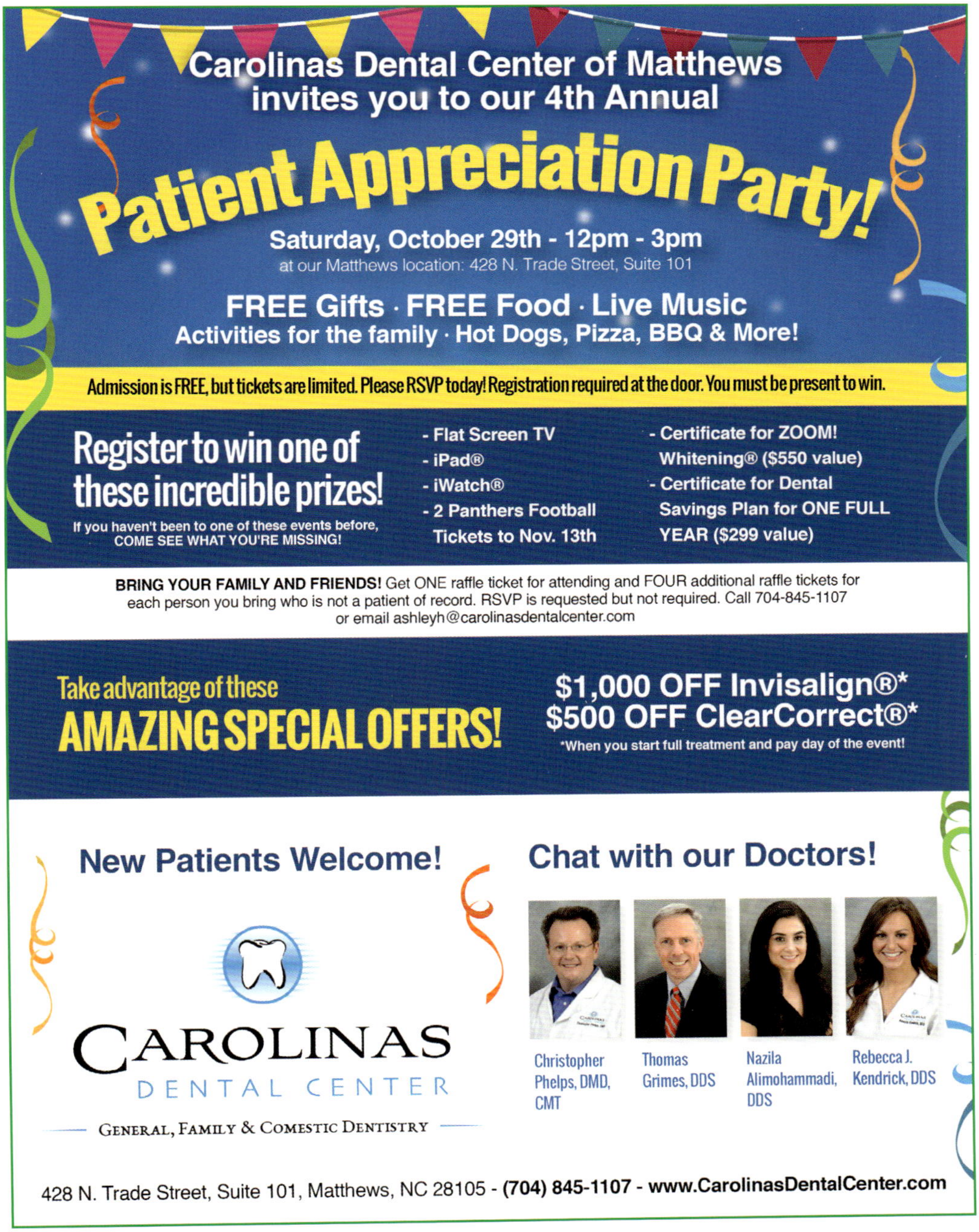
Carolinas Dental Center of Matthews
invites you to our 4th Annual
Patient Appreciation Party!
Saturday, October 29th - 12pm - 3pm
at our Matthews location: 428 N. Trade Street, Suite 101
FREE Gifts · FREE Food · Live Music
Activities for the family · Hot Dogs, Pizza, BBQ & More!
Admission is FREE, but tickets are limited. Please RSVP today! Registration required at the door. You must be present to win.
Register to win one of these incredible prizes!
If you haven't been to one of these events before, COME SEE WHAT YOU'RE MISSING!
- Flat Screen TV
- iPad®
- iWatch®
- 2 Panthers Football Tickets to Nov. 13th
- Certificate for ZOOM! Whitening® ($550 value)
- Certificate for Dental Savings Plan for ONE FULL YEAR ($299 value)
BRING YOUR FAMILY AND FRIENDS! Get ONE raffle ticket for attending and FOUR additional raffle tickets for each person you bring who is not a patient of record. RSVP is requested but not required. Call 704-845-1107 or email ashleyh@carolinasdentalcenter.com
Take advantage of these AMAZING SPECIAL OFFERS!
$1,000 OFF Invisalign®*
$500 OFF ClearCorrect®*
*When you start full treatment and pay day of the event!
New Patients Welcome!
CAROLINAS
DENTAL CENTER
GENERAL, FAMILY & COMESTIC DENTISTRY
Chat with our Doctors!
Christopher Phelps, DMD, CMT
Thomas Grimes, DDS
Nazila Alimohammadi, DDS
Rebecca J. Kendrick, DDS
428 N. Trade Street, Suite 101, Matthews, NC 28105 - (704) 845-1107 - www.CarolinasDentalCenter.com

Figure 37. Example of promotional flyer for patient appreciation party.

embed the info flyer we created and most likely gave them at their last appointment as well as make a request to RSVP for the event. It's great to have an idea of how many will attend to aid in your logistical planning. Do you have enough raffle tickets, for instance? Will there be enough people to support all of your food vendors to make the event worth their while? Do you have enough gift bags to hand out to people who attend? Asking people to RSVP will help you answer these questions and make for a more successful event.

At the same time our goal is to have as many people show up as possible. The last thing we want is to exclude anyone who might decide at the last minute to attend but wouldn't because they didn't RSVP. So I found that using the phrase "RSVP recommended but not required" helped my team on the planning side but also left the door open for more to attend. By planning for 20 percent more than the number of RSVPs we gathered, we successfully accommodated all who actually attended.

External efforts: three months or less before your event

While referrals from existing patients will be the main source of new patients that attend your patient appreciation party, I would not discount trying to use some external marketing to attract them as well. To promote this party, I mainly focused on celebrity endorsement radio ads and newspaper inserts. The radio ads were already underway, so I would just update the station with information about our party event. I would invite the radio station to have a booth at our event to promote their channel and the talk show hosts that we did paid sponsorships with. Three months leading up to the event, I'd have the talk show team discuss our party once a week during their live show. About one month before the party, I'd have them air recorded commercials that promote our party and invited their listeners to attend. These were at varying times throughout the day with the heaviest number airing the day before our event. For the newspaper inserts, I'd drop those once a month for the three months leading up to the event, with the third drop being in newspapers the day before the event.

Record, record, record

At each party I had two specific people I had hired. To me, these were two of the most important jobs for this event. One was a videographer and the other a photographer. My goal for the photographer was to engage with the crowd, document our event, take photos of me with the prize winners, and offer to take a nice professional photo of them and their family. We'd then email those patients the photo taken so they could have a copy for their own personal use. The videographer's job was to do something similar: document the event, show the people enjoying the activities we had provided for them, and assist us in capturing any video testimonials people wanted to give us to attain more raffle tickets.

Once you've attained these photos and video, it will provide you with marketing material you can use for months and years to come. Photos would be posted on our social media account for about three months following our event and then three months leading up to the next event. A page was dedicated to these parties on our website to show potential new patients what we were about and how we support the patients who support us. In the photos, we'd gather as many people together as we could to take large group shots (Fig. 36). Leveraging the principle of social proof, I'd include those group photos in my advertisements and promotions for the next year's event to show others just how many people came out, participated, and enjoyed last year's event, to plant a seed so that maybe this year they might want to attend as well. We'd send out an email to all of our patients with a photo montage of the event, thanking those for attending but also to use the scarcity principle to show my patients who did not attend what they missed out.

With the video footage, I would post each of those video patient testimonials to our website to influence and decrease potential new patients' uncertainty about what office they should choose, why people trust us, and why they should too. I had the videographer create a video montage of the event as well, which I used on our website, social media channels, and to introduce a crowd of potential new patients to our practice before I spoke to them at one of my grassroots educational seminars we'll discuss shortly.

Of all the marketing media I'll discuss in this book, the patient appreciation party is by far my favorite. It's a win for everyone involved: our existing patients, potential new patients, local businesses, and more. Yes, it takes time and effort to plan and organize these events. It takes a commitment by the whole team to participate and play a role, and it is an investment of money. From the results I hope you'll see that it's one of the best ROIs in marketing that I've invested in. Now I've found that one thing that can get me over 100 new patients. The only downside is that it can only happen once a year.

Google business reviews

Behavioral science studies show that when people are uncertain or when they have questions or doubts about a decision that needs to be made, oftentimes they look to Dr. Cialdini's principle of social proof and the behavior of others to show them what they should do or decide. We've seen businesses such as Amazon, TripAdvisor, and Facebook tap into the power of the masses to influence decisions and behavior. From a dental perspective, all of our marketing efforts are influenced by what others have said about us in the form of Google business reviews. A January 2020 report by *Search Engine Journal* looked at different studies about Google business reviews and their influence on our business. Some of the key takeaways of significance were:

- 82 percent of shoppers actually seek out negative reviews as an initial measure to decide trust. It turns out having some negative reviews actually increases the credibility of the positive ones you have.
- 91 percent of consumers between the ages of 18 and 34 trust online reviews as much or more than personal recommendations from a friend.
- The more reviews the better. On average, a business needs to have at least 40 reviews before that consumer believes their average star rating, an increase from an average of 34 reported in a 2017 study.
- Reviews increase revenue. A *Harvard Business Review* study showed that for every one star increase a business attains in their average rating, this translated into a 5–9 percent increase in revenue for that business.
- When it comes to expensive purchases, one study showed that when reviews were displayed along with information about that product or service, the conversion rate of those interested in attaining those products or services increased over 340 percent.

This is important if we're marketing higher-priced services like orthodontic care, cosmetic veneers, and full mouth rehabs or dental implant restorations for the edentulous arch patient.

- Google has over 200 variables it uses to assign a rank to your business profile compared to others in your category, yet most experts agree that the one variable that's weighted the most in Google's algorithm is having more Google reviews. Those with the most Google reviews in an area tend to show up higher in search rankings than those dental practices who don't have as many reviews.

Add these all up and you can see just how important these reviews are and why I consider them a marketing medium in their own right. So how do we get these reviews and how can we influence more people to leave them for our office? The main ways we have available to use today are to physically ask the patient to leave us a review or we can use an automated medium to ask them on our behalf.

Automated means

There are many companies such as Podium, Birdeye, and SolutionReach that offer your practice an automated ability to ask patients for reviews. These are programs tied into your practice's management system and set up to trigger after certain occurrences, usually immediately after the patient has visited your office for a cleaning or visit with the dentist. You can also set up the program to send out build requests to your patient base via email or text. This is usually set up as a quarterly run so as to not inundate your patient base with requests.

The monthly costs for these programs are manageable, and I've found offices have great success using them to generate more reviews. While the actual ROI for a review can be hard to calculate, I think after you factor in the importance of these reviews outlined above, you'll see any monthly fee to have this technology is easily covered.

Direct means

Outside of automated means, we're left with more direct means of acquiring these reviews. This comes from directly asking the patient if they'd like to leave a review. This request is usually made in person and while the patient is still in your dental chair. Below I'll outline a system I've developed to influence more patients to leave 5-star Google reviews for your practice.

Reciprocity

It all starts with a great patient experience. Asking someone for a review who's been waiting to be seated well past their appointed time is never a good idea. Instead, I like to search out people that we have good relationships with:

- Existing patients with no treatment planned or to be scheduled is ideal.
- Someone who has just completed the last step or visit of their treatment plan and are happy with their results.
- Someone who goes out of their way to compliment us about their experience at the practice. Positive comments such as "I can't believe we're done already" or "Wow, Doc, that shot didn't hurt at all!" When people relay these types of comments, whether you

realized it or not, you've given them a gift that they valued, an intangible gift that they bring up because they are looking for a way to reciprocate or return the favor. If you have given someone this type of gift, your work is done and you can move on to asking them if they would leave you a 5-star Google review. When the patient states, "Wow, Doc, that shot didn't hurt at all, you guys are great!" then you or your team member would respond by saying, "Thank you, we love hearing that. Would you mind helping us by leaving a 5-star Google review? That would really help us out by letting others know about your experience."

If an intangible gift has not been given, you can initiate reciprocity much the same way I described in my influence-based referral system previously in this book, by thanking the patient for coming in and offering them a choice of $5 gift cards.

"Mrs. Jones, Dr. Phelps and I just wanted to thank you for coming in today and for being our patient. We know you have a choice in the matter and that you chose us for your care, which means a lot to us. As a small thank-you from us both, here's a couple of gift cards. Why don't you pick one?" Once the person picks one of your gift card selections, you know they've chosen the one that has some meaning to them; you should receive a genuine "thank you" from that patient. Once heard, you respond by making your request. "You're welcome. Before you go, would you mind helping us by leaving a 5-star Google review?" Because we've tapped into the power of reciprocity, the likelihood of getting a yes to our review request is high. So what now?

It's at this point I see most practices bungling an opportunity. Yes, we've gotten a simple commitment from this person to leave a review, but we've left too many things to chance, too many distractions that could get in this patient's way of actually leaving that review. Even if we attempt to send them a text or email with a link to do the review, there is still a chance that review never manifests. So what steps can we take to influence more people from this point on to leave that review for us?

Ask them to do the review while still in the chair

It's always best to strike while the influence iron is hottest. If a patient has committed to giving us a review, then we should have no fear in asking them to pull out their phone and go ahead and leave that review before they leave the office. They may have a few minutes before the dentist comes in and does their exam or maybe the front desk is backed up, so it will be a few minutes anyway before you could check them out. Regardless, asking them in that moment is the opportune time to get it done. The key you have to remember is that the patient will need to be disconnected from your office's Wi-Fi *before* they leave their review. I can't stress the importance of that enough. If they leave a review for your office while they are on your Wi-Fi's network, Google will recognize the IP address the review was posted from as coming from your office. Google will then assume your business is posting fraudulent reviews and will penalize you for it. I've seen offices make this mistake who had 50 or more of their reviews instantly removed from their profile as punishment. Even though every one of them was a legitimate review given by a patient. When the patient is off your Wi-Fi network, then the IP address for the review will show as coming from their cellular data plan and not be seen as coming from your office.

Don't be afraid of a no

What if they are unable to do the review at the chair? It's completely possible that when you ask the patient to do that review in the moment, they will be unable to for one reason or another and may decline this request. Remember the other aspect of reciprocity where after someone says no to our request, if we immediately follow with a different request, we're likely to get a yes.

Team: I'm glad you enjoyed your visit with us today. Would you mind doing a Google review for us to share that experience?

Patient: Sure, I'd be happy to do that.

Team: Great. Would you like to do that now while we're waiting for a chance to check you out?

Patient: "Oh, I don't think I have time for that now, I have another appointment to get to.

Team: Okay, that's understandable. Do you think you can do that review later today for us?

Patient: Consider it done.

Team: Awesome, thank you. I'll let the doctor and the other team members know and to keep a look out for that review.

Get more commitments for them to do the review

Cialdini's consistency principle states that when people make a real commitment, there is a lot of influence on them to follow through and do what they said they would do. The more commitments we get from a person, the greater the chance they will follow through with the commitment made. So far, we've gotten two commitments. One was to do the review for us, and now the second is for them to do that review later today. We've also added more of a public commitment nature to our request by letting the patient know that the dentist and team will be told of the review to come and be on the lookout for it.

Another type of commitment we can leverage here is that of a voluntary choice. Presenting patients with a "this or that" option scenario. Each time they make a choice, they are now more committed to the choice they've made. While the automated platforms we use can make it easy for patients to leave reviews, at the same time they can give us false hope that this patient will use that specific format to leave the review. An example would be my 74-year-old mother. If you sent a text link to her smartphone and expect that she will be able to use this and do an online review, then I refer you to my childhood and the 1000 times I had to explain to her how to use the VCR remote control. So using her smartphone would not be the best format to make this request. On the other hand, she has gotten pretty good at using a desktop computer to navigate her way through the online world. Now if you emailed her a link or shortcut to help her post a Google review, you'd have a much better chance of seeing that review come to light.

So after a patient has told us that they are unable to do that review while they are here in the office but have agreed to do the review later in the day, we now have an opportune time to ask one more commitment question and increase our chances that the review actually gets posted. Ask them what type of device they prefer to use when they do post this review.

Patient: Oh, I don't think I have time for that now, I have another appointment to get to.

***Team*: Okay, that's understandable. Do you think you can do that review later today for us?**

Patient: Consider it done.

***Team*: Awesome, thank you. I'll let the doctor and the other team members know and to keep a look out for that review. Before you go, let me ask you this. When you go to do the review, do you think you'll post it using your smartphone/table or will you use a desktop/laptop computer?**

Patient: Oh, I'll probably use my smart phone or Oh, I'll use my computer when I'm back at work.

***Team*: Okay, great. I'll send you a text with a link that will make it easier to post the review, or if they prefer the desktop/laptop computer route you might say: Okay, great. I'll send you an email with a link that will make it easier to post the review.**

Remind them of the commitment they've made

When people make real commitments, they tend to follow through with them. That much has been established, but can you think of a time when people didn't follow through? A commitment made didn't translate into them following through. Was it because they are liars and really didn't intend to follow through with the commitment they made? Fortunately, behavioral science studies show us that for most people, it's not because they intended to be deceitful. In fact, they really did intend to follow through, but life got in the way. A distraction appeared that stole their focus on the commitment they made. In their mind, this item is still on their to-do list, albeit pushed way down on the priority scale. If you're lucky, it might rise back up in the ranks at a later date, but most of the time, it's so far down that it's never to be seen or heard from again. A simple influence trick we can use to overcome this potential barrier is to remind that person of the commitment they've made. This could be a follow-up text or email to them a couple of days after a commitment was given but no action was taken on their part. It could be a cute sticker or postcard inserted in their hygiene bag that thanks them for their 5-star review but ultimately is designed to remind them of the commitment they've made.

One of my personal favorite commitment reminders is for patients who might be technology challenged like my mother. If she is attempting to do a review for you and the slightest issue comes up while attempting it that confuses her, then that review is not going to happen. To help these patients, I asked two team members for help. One member I asked them to give our office a 5-star Google review using their smartphone while the other I asked to give us a review using a laptop or desktop computer. I then asked them to write down each step they had to take and take a screenshot picture of each step in the process. I then had our local printer create two little pamphlets with step-by-step instructions and with pictures on how to leave us a review, one using the smartphone or tablet route and the other via a desktop or laptop computer. Now we had a great reminder that could go home with patients and potentially diffuse any technology issues that the patient may have had in their attempt to leave us a review. The better we get at reminding people of the commitments they have made, the more compliance and in this case Google reviews we can expect to see.

Chapter 7
Grassroots and Other Marketing

1. GRASSROOTS MARKETING: GETTING IN FRONT OF YOUR TARGET MARKET

In the previous section we talked about how the goal of internal marketing is to transmit your message to your existing patients with the hopes of motivating them to move forward with treatment or to refer more patients to your practice. Before that we discussed the goal of external marketing: to launch your message to a large group of people and attempt to reel in some new patient opportunities. Both of these forms tend to sit on opposite sides of the spectrum when it comes to time and money. Internal marketing doesn't cost a lot of money, but it does tend to involve a lot more of your time. External marketing is the opposite, usually costing less, if any, of your time but does require more of a financial investment. Grassroots marketing is a medium I've found that sits in the middle of this time-and-money spectrum and balances the two.

Grassroots marketing, sometimes known as guerilla marketing, starts with you getting yourself and your messages directly in front of your target market. Then, instead of launching a message you hope will appeal to many people, you target your efforts to a small group and hope that they will spread your message to a much larger audience. The 2014 ALS ice bucket challenge is a prime example, a small idea that grew into a national campaign.

The concept was simple. You would take a video pouring a bucket of ice water on yourself and then use social media to challenge someone else to do the same. If you participated, you were then supposed to donate money to the ALS Association. What started out as a few devoted people trying to raise awareness and funds for this deadly disease then went viral around the world. This grassroots campaign became so successful that an independent research organization reported that donations from the 2014 ALS Ice Bucket Challenge enabled The ALS Association to increase its annual funding for research around the world by 187 percent. Having a good friend in dental school who had lost his mother to ALS, I was influenced to participate and donate to this cause as well.

Much like the Ice Bucket Challenge, your grassroots marketing content should:

- Inspire your target audience to talk about and share it with others;
- Focus on solutions to your target audience's problems; and
- Motivate people to take action.

In dentistry there are four main areas I believe we can use grassroots marketing efforts to help us attract new patients:

- Social media community forums;
- In-office patient educational seminars;
- Off-site patient educational seminars; and
- On-site patient educational seminars.

A. Social Media Community Forums: Be the Dental Authority

Cialdini's principle of social proof states that many times we look to the behavior of what others are interested in or talking about to let us know what we should be discussing as well. You've seen the power of social proof build companies such as Trip Advisor, Amazon, and Facebook, all of which are fueled by the evidence of what others are interested in or have experience with. Social proof influences us because of its primordial roots. Think of fish swimming out in the ocean. Evolution and experience has taught them that it's not safe to swim out there all alone. Dangerous things can occur, so they've adapted and learned this idea of safety in numbers. They flock together in what we call a school, knowing that it will be harder for a predator to single any one of them out from the crowd.

Despite man's evolution and development of this idea that we all want to be unique individuals, the fact remains that we still want to be unique individuals who are part of a crowd, a community. Hence, we see Facebook's popularity at an all-time high because they allow us to flock together into large and smaller communities to share information and opinions. Have you noticed how many public and private dental Facebook groups exist? I know I'm a member of over 200 of these types of groups. The good news for us is that our patients have flocked to these types of communities as well. But before we can engage them here, we have to nail down a strategy to use these platforms to present us as the dental authority.

Why an authority? In Dr. Cialdini's book, he talks about this authority principle and how we look to credible, trustworthy experts for advice to tell us what to do because we don't have time to become an expert in everything. This principle isn't about telling others you are the expert as that can come off as bragging or make others think you are too arrogant. It's not about being in authority over someone, like a boss telling their employee to do something. No, this principle is about your actions alerting people that you are a true expert on the matter. Once they start routinely coming to you for advice or counsel, so they will in person when a real need develops.

Let's now look at how we can tie this altogether. Our target market are people who are actively engaged in different social media communities. Our message to put in front of them will not be one of sales. It won't be about promoting our office or services at all. Instead, it will solely focus on education. Giving unbiased expert opinions on any dental questions that arise in these community chat forums. The media we'll use will be any of the community groups you can find on Facebook. This could include your neighborhood's Facebook page and other neighborhoods around your practice. It could also include your town or cities main page. Look for website or blog sites people are searching for dental answers. One website I've had success with is www.findatopdoc.com. Lastly, check out any up-and-coming companies or services people are using to communicate in mass, such as Nextdoor.

Once you have your media identified, your goal is simple. Either you or someone on your team should scroll through these sites once a day. At most you'll spend 20–30 minutes. See if there are any conversations occurring on these sites that relate to dentistry. Most have a search tab where you can input certain key words related to dentistry to help hasten your search. Once you find the dental questions people are asking, take some time to give thoughtful, educational answers. Avoid any attempts at promoting yourself or inviting anyone to come to your practice. People will read this as a sales attempt, and it will completely diminish any influence power you'd have gained. People will know you're a dentist because it will be shown in your profile name. With Google at the ready, it won't be hard for people to find you if they do decide to become your patient.

When you educate people instead of trying to sell them, those are the efforts that will present you as a dental authority. The more questions you answer, the more your exposure to the masses increases and the more authority you'll attain. You will automatically become the trusted expert in their mind because many have constantly turned to you for dental answers. Once that trust has been established, when it's time for them to seek out a dentist for their own care, they are now more likely than ever to become your new patient.

B. Patient Education Seminars

Patient education seminars are events put on by health care professionals to educate patients and potential patients. While not new to the medical profession (plastic surgeons and weight loss specialists have been using this medium for years), they are growing in popularity in dentistry. They can be used to promote a new treatment or service you are providing to existing patients or to attract potential new patients.

Tips to make any type of patient seminar a success:

- **Educate, don't sell**: Be their authority. You never ask the crowd directly to buy anything at one of your events. That's not to say that you won't do a little promotion about your practice. I spend about 10 percent of my time on the promotional aspect, discussing who we are and why we're different than other area offices. Usually that 10 percent is handled right at the beginning of my presentation. From there it moves to the educational piece, leaving people feeling like they were educated from my events, not sold to. Just remember to refrain from asking them to purchase anything, such as a dental membership plan, at that event.
- **Ease fears about scary procedures**: Make sure the crowd knows this is a safe place where all of their dental questions can be answered, a place where you're acknowledging people's fears about different dental procedures but demystifying those services in the process.
- **Limit the time**: To be respectful of people's time and attention spans, these events should be limited to two hours if there is a meal and dessert provided and around 50 minutes if no meal is provided.
- **Make it convenient**: Be cognizant of what activities could be competing with your event. Try to schedule them on a weeknight. Doing one on a weekend means you'll be in competition with other activities your potential patients have, causing them to choose that over your seminar. If you're not providing a meal, then don't do your event during your target market's normal dinner time. Otherwise the only thing that they'll focus

their attention on is the dinner they are going to eat. Since most of my target market was retired and usually ate dinner around 5 p.m., I held my events just after dinner, at 6 p.m., typically on a Tuesday or Thursday evening.

- **Everyone loves to be a winner**: This was one of the lessons I learned from the patient appreciation parties I mentioned earlier. People truly enjoy contests and they love to win things. Make sure you create opportunities at your events to let them do so. At each event I like to raffle off three prizes: a $500 gift card to our practice that can be used on any dental service they choose, a dental membership plan that covers all of their preventative needs for the year, and usually a nice Sonicare electric toothbrush package. In addition, each attendee receives a goodie bag that has our branded toothbrush, floss, toothpaste, and pen. It contains a flyer with information about our practice including our address, website, and telephone number. It includes a brochure outlining the details of our dental membership plan and includes an application in case they want to fill it out that night or choose to bring it in with them for an appointment. Lastly, I include some of the more popular or relevant gift cards from area business who are members of my business-to-business gift card program I'll define in more detail in the coming sections.
- **You need some type of hook to attract them**: Free goodie bags and gifts like the $500 gift card, free dental membership plan, and Sonicare might be enough of a hook to attract potential patients to your event, but I'd like you to have as many as possible. Think about what other items you could provide people that might incentivize them to come out. Appetizers or a meal? Drinks? Dessert? In my book *Grow Your Dental Membership Plan*, I talk about the two I've had the most success with. Offering high-end wine from Napa Valley or making my event an ice cream social. The answer ultimately goes back to who your target market really is and what they might enjoy.
- **Be ready if they do want to take action**: While I never directly ask the attendees to make appointments or to purchase things like my dental membership plans at the event, that does not mean I will tell them no if they bring it up to us. Make sure your team is ready to accept any completed membership plan applications if they've decided it's for them. Have the capability to have your schedule in front of you so that you can make people an appointment if they come up and ask you for one at the event.

Using these tips, I have found all of the different seminar formats available to us to be cost effective in both time and money. They have also proven to be some of my most effective ways to attract general dentistry patients as well as patients who need higher-priced services such as cosmetic dentistry, sleep apnea, sedation dentistry, and dental implant options for the edentulous arch. There are three main types of seminar events you can utilize: in office, off-site, and on-site. Each has their respective advantages and disadvantages.

1. In-Office Patient Education Seminars

In-office events are seminars that you host inside your practice location. These can be used to promote new treatments and services to existing patients, to attract potential new patients interested in those procedures, or a combination of the two. For this event, there are many logistic issues to consider.

Disadvantages

- **Logistics**: Audiovisual capabilities, seating capacity, esthetics. Do you have the space to host an event at your office? Is there enough comfortable seating for those who'd attend? Seating that can sustain them for a 30–40-minute talk plus time for questions at the end? Have you updated your décor lately? Will the area you host this event make a good first impression for someone who has never been to your practice before? These are all questions that could create challenges for you to host one of these events at your office.
- **Limited quantity attending**: Despite your best marketing and promotional efforts, having these events in your office can be a barrier that really limits the number of people who'll come out to your event. In fact, of the three formats we'll discuss, this one usually has the least number attending. If you can consistently attract 6–10 people for this event, then I would count that as a success. Since these events tend to be more intimate, plan accordingly.

Advantages

- **Only the most committed attend**. Using any of these marketing media will help put the word out there about your practice, but it doesn't necessarily bring in patients that are pre-committed to doing this treatment. On the other hand, those who come out to your office for a seminar, who've committed the time and effort of attending, are patients that are highly engaged and more likely to move forward with whatever treatment or service you are discussing. Thus you can expect higher case acceptance rates overall on these patients than on the other formats I'll discuss.
- **You can introduce yourself in a non-scary way**. Fear and uncertainty about what their experience might be is definitely a deterrent that keeps many away from our dental practices. These in-office seminars give them a chance to meet you in a less intimidating fashion. Putting them more at ease today means they are more likely to return to see you again tomorrow.

Your marketing and promotional strategies to fill this event are similar to what I discussed in the patient appreciation party section. Internally you want to hand out flyers to your existing patients starting around three months before your event. You want to send emails about your upcoming event to all patients who've expressed interest in this procedure in the past or who have a treatment planned for this service but who haven't scheduled. Emails to them and the rest of your patient base should go out once a month. RSVPs should be requested to get an idea of how many will attend.

Externally you should target your efforts toward your target demographic, sending them a direct mail postcard promoting your event, displaying info about it in their neighborhood magazine or newsletter, and doing some online Google AdWords, Facebook posts, and lead generation funnels to spread the word about this event.

2. Off-Site Patient Education Seminars

Off-site patient education seminars are typically held outside of your dental practice and at a neutral location to you and your potential new patients. Most often these are held in conference or meeting rooms of popular Italian or Steakhouse restaurants. While this medium is fairly new to dentistry, those in the financial planning industry have successfully used this type of seminar to attract new clients for over 20 years. Your goal is to create a demographic of your target market and send out invitations inviting them to your educational seminar. The incentive you'll use to attract them and a guest will be an offer to educate them on some dental topic and buy them a nice meal in return.

Disadvantages

- **Reliance on a third party**: Because of the complexity of organizing these events, working with restaurants who'll host them, targeting a marketing list to promote your events to, you'll typically need to work with a third-party company to help you put on and fill these events. The company I use and who has the most experience in this type of seminar format is called Leading Response.
- **Cost**: Of the three seminar formats, this one is by far the most expensive in upfront costs. There are costs to create an invitation and send to your target market, costs to cover the call center that will be needed to handle and screen calls from potential new patients who respond with interest in attending, and cost of the dinner and tip after your event as you're paying for each person who attends as well as for any of your team members who participate.

Advantages

- **Time**: By working with a third party such as Leading Response, the time needed to organize and fill these events by you or your team is nonexistent. They take care of it for you by creating a qualified marketing list, so you know the people invited can afford your services, creating and mailing invitations, screening incoming calls, getting real commitments out of the most serious who'd attend, helping you decide which restaurant works best in your area to host this event at, and working with them on logistics for your event. Your team just needs to make confirmation calls to those who plan to attend. You just need to show up and give your presentation and then meet and eat dinner with your team after to debrief the night's challenges and successes.
- **Audiovisual and comfort needs met**: While your office may not be set up to comfortably seat people or to give a proper presentation, the conference rooms at these restaurants are built just for this purpose. Usually they have varying size rooms available, so if the number of people who want to attend surpasses your expectation and the room you had planned, they can usually move you to a larger room to accommodate more.
- **Quantity and quality of potential new patients**: For any given campaign, Leading Response was able to attract around 80–90 potential new patients. Many of them were targeted and needed high-end dental implant procedures, and most of them did not have dental insurance and were very receptive to our dental membership plan solution. I would typically give two or three presentations depending on the size of the room the restaurants had available, seeing those 80–90 people over two nights on a Tuesday or Thursday or adding in a third night on a Wednesday. On average I'd hold these events once per quarter as it took some time to fully accommodate all of these patients we converted into the practice, both on the doctor side and the hygiene side.
- **ROI**: Total expenses per campaign ran about $12,000. That covered everything from the marketing campaign to attract patients, all of their meals plus waiter tip at the restaurants, gift bags, and compensation for any of my team members for attending. On average, these events gave me a minimum 4:1 ROI, many times collecting that in the first month following an event and usually surpassing that number by the time we held the next event.

3. On-Site Patient Education Seminars: Go to Your Target Market Events

This type of educational seminar is held at locations where your target market lives, works, or socializes. Most commonly, I'd give these seminars where my target market lived, in active, independent living retirement communities. In my book *Grow Your Dental Membership Plan*, I go into a lot of detail on how to make these events successful. Of the three grassroots patient educational seminar formats I've mentioned, this one is by far my favorite. Using this medium I was able to successfully launch a dental membership plan for my practices and grow their combined revenue from $1.6 million to just over $6 million within a three-year period of time.

Disadvantages

- **Solicitation mindset**: In its most basic definition, the word "solicit" means to ask for. As such, the term "no soliciting" is the request and demand that no person comes to you, your business, or your home, or contacts you by other means, in order to ask for anything. Getting over the stigma that the purpose of your event is to solicit new business for your practice is one of the main hurdles you'll have to overcome to be able to host these seminars at senior centers or in retirement communities.

  That's why we are approaching this from an educational standpoint. It's also the reason why we're not asking anyone who attends our event to do anything. We're not directly asking them to purchase your dental membership plan. We're not asking them to make an appointment that night. Our purpose is to educate. One of the main areas I focused on was a presentation I called the "Top 5 Dental Issues Affecting the Aging Population," a presentation that tried to educate them on the dangers of sugar and acids present in the food and drink they enjoy and how to offset that risk and protect their teeth from gum disease or resulting decay that can occur. Approaching these communities from an educational standpoint should get you around the solicitation mindset, will present you as an authority to the crowd you're speaking to, and will, by its very nature, influence more new patients to your practice.
- **Availability of communities: Are they present? Which to choose?** Two of the challenges I see dentists face when attempting to give these seminars is understanding what type of community to choose and then finding those communities. When searching for these communities, remember they have to meet certain criteria. I want the majority of people who live or socialize here to be active and independent. That means they live by their own means. They come and go as they please, and they don't have anyone coming into their home to consistently help or assist them in any capacity.

  This is very different than what's called assisted living, nursing home, or long-term care facilities. Assisted living facilities have a professional nurse or attendant who aids the resident a minimum of four hours per week in some activity. Nursing home and long-term care facilities provide that care for their residents 24 hours a day. Not to say there isn't a need for dental care in these communities, but these are not the places that fit my target market or that fit with the strategies I'm discussing in this book.

  Instead, we're searching for active, independent retirement communities or graduated care facilities where the number of independent residents outnumbers the assisted and long-term care residents by at least 10:1. These are places similar to Del Webb Active

Adult Communities (www.delwebb.com). To find these in your area, you can use a simple Google search using the phrase "active, Independent living retirement community." While these communities are plentiful in and around my area of Charlotte, North Carolina, one disadvantage you may run into is that these places are not readily found or available where you live. If this is the case, then you might want to consider in-office seminars or hosting these events off-site at popular restaurants.

Advantages

- **Becoming the social event of the community**: I held my events at the nearest Del Webb retirement community near my offices, one that had over 3500 homes in the neighborhood, its own dedicated golf course, and one focused on creating activities for their residents to participate with. Using my educational seminar format, I was allowed to give a talk once a month, typically, on a Thursday evening at 6 p.m. On top of the gifts I'd raffle off, my hook to attract potential new patients was to provide high-end wines from the famous Napa Valley, California region. I'd promote my events in the community's neighborhood magazine and post flyers on a community board I learned residents looked at to see what events were being held on-site around that time. The more I did these events, the better the attendance became and the more repeat customers I noticed attending. Many of those who returned for multiple seminars had already become patients at our practice and had heard the seminar talk two or three times in a row. When I asked one of those patients why she had returned to hear the same presentation again and again, she knocked back the glass of wine in hand and told me that she loved these events because she got to see her friends in the community and meet new people as well. Without realizing it, my events had become one of the big social events that community held each month. With that reputation and influence came a whole host of new patients to our practice.
- **Attendance**: My events were consistently able to attract 40–60 potential new patients to each event, significantly more than any in-office seminar could accommodate and fairly close to the numbers I was drawing for the steakhouse seminars.
- **Costs**: Total costs numbered around \$300–\$400 per event, covering the wine, fruit, and cheese plate we provided and any gift cards, membership plans, or Sonicares I gave away. Because this had less upfront costs than the steakhouse seminar, it was easier to coordinate and do these events more frequently. Plus, I was able to attract more patients who needed basic preventative and restorative care to support my associate dentists, whereas the steakhouse seminars brought in patients who needed more expensive dental services.
- **ROI**: Within a six-month time frame, half of those who attended our monthly events purchased our dental membership plan that night while the other half made appointments to come and use their insurance or buy our plan, practically a 100 percent conversion rate at each event and without us ever asking anyone to make an appointment or purchase. If 30 people attended and each of them purchased our dental membership plan for \$299, then these events generated \$8970 in revenue for the \$400 and one hour of my time I invested in them, a 22:1 ROI that doesn't even factor in the dental work performed on these patients.

Grassroots marketing is one of the best media I've discovered to attract enough quantity and quality of new patients to grow my practice. Whether you do these events in your office, off-site at a restaurant, or on-site where your target market lives, it's hard to be successful and see an amazing return for your investment.

2. SYMBIOTIC MARKETING

Defined by the *Harvard Business Review* in 1966, symbiotic marketing is an alliance of resources or programs between two or more independent organizations that is designed to increase the market potential of each, the efforts of which translate into a win-win situation for both parties involved. In our focus, that means an increase in our brand awareness and ultimately new patient numbers. Let's review a couple of ways that you can tap into this medium in dentistry.

A. Chamber of Commerce

A chamber of commerce is commonly defined as a voluntary partnership of businesses and professionals working together to build a healthy economy and improve the quality of life in a community. Its goal is simple: to support local businesses and further their interests. There is a typically a nominal annual fee to be a member of the chamber, which gives you certain benefits:

- **Discounts**: Being a chamber member entitles you to certain discounts off services provided by other businesses who are members.
- **Credibility**: Consumers trust the chamber name, and membership implies that your business is more established and credible.
- **Professional development**: There are monthly luncheons that feature a prominent speaker discussing topics relevant to your business needs.
- **Networking**: Gives you access to other business owners, which might allow you to create a referral network, influencing these business owners to become patients at your practice while also referring others as well.

While the expense to join isn't usually that large, these groups have large membership numbers, which gives you the largest quantity of potential referral sources to attract new patients. The downside here is this is an investment of your time more than anything else, so there are some things you can do to help maximize your ROI.

Be the first to like them

These meetings are all about networking, and everyone present would love the opportunity to talk about themselves. Give them that chance. Cialdini's principle of reciprocity states that people tend to give back in kind what's been given to them. The principle of liking states that we tend to like others who like us or show us interest first. The monthly chamber luncheons give you a great opportunity to combine both. Work the crowd and meet as many people as you can. Be the first to show interest in their business. Find connections and point out commonalities that arise. Once you've done this, your business colleagues will reciprocate and ask about your business. Highlight any dental stories they have or any dental needs they or their clients may have.

Join a committee

Joining a chamber committee or running for a chamber position can be a great way to present you as an authority other members may look to for advice or counsel. It helps differentiate you from the other business members and keep you and your business brand top of mind at every chamber meeting.

Attend all new member events

New member reception events are a great opportunity to meet and connect with potential referral sources. New member meetings can be stressful for new attendees because there is so much unknown. They don't know anyone yet and have no real expectation if people will like them or their business offerings. Being the first ones to engage them, reassure them, guide them in this process of being a chamber member, you're giving them a great gift they will reciprocate on.

Be the first to support and refer to their business

One of the ways I had success influencing other businesses to refer patients to my practice was by leveraging the reciprocity principle and being the first to refer potential new clients to them. We are in the people business and talk to a lot of people each day who come from all walks of life. In your conversations with patients you may discover a need present for which a colleague in the chamber could be the solution for. Chiropractors are one example since we share some synergy between our target markets. I've taken the time to get to know several chiropractors from our chamber, each who practices some distance apart or in different areas of town who I could refer patients that needed additional TMJ/TMD therapies I couldn't provide. In return, I found these chiropractors to be some of my best referral sources for new patients.

Create a solution to their problem

The majority of chamber members are small business owners. A small business is defined as having 50 or less employees. One constant struggle every small business owner faces is how to retain good employees while keeping costs at a minimum. Out of all of the expenses a business must deal with, employee benefits probably account for one of their largest expenses. While offering medical insurance and some retirement benefits are an absolute necessity, many have chosen to offset these costs by not providing dental insurance in their benefits package. In fact, I've often found the majority of the small business owners themselves don't carry any type of dental insurance plan. This is a great opportunity for practices who offer a dental membership plan.

In my book *Grow Your Dental Membership Plan*, I discuss how this absence of having dental insurance is a mounting problem that is keeping many new patients from coming to the dental office. By offering a dental membership plan and tracking it with a service such as Dental Membership Direct, offices can help these patients get over this mindset barrier and come in for the preventative and restorative care that they need. While my main target market for these plans are active, independent living retirees, small business owners and their employees make up the second largest group that are receptive to the membership plan message.

Find out what your small business colleagues in the chamber are providing for their employees. If the answer is minimal to no benefits, show them how your dental membership plan can be an affordable option they can provide as part of their overall employee health benefit plan. Look for marketing or promotional activities that can help you spread this message to other chamber members. Many times those monthly luncheons have sponsorship opportunities that allow you to speak and address the crowd for 5 or 10 minutes. These are the best times to highlight the problem most of these business face and how many are choosing your membership plan as their solution.

B. Network marketing groups

Another cost-effective medium to promote and advertise your practice is through network marketing groups such as Business Network International (BNI). BNI is the world's largest business referral organization with over 270,000 members, spread out over 9,500 chapters worldwide. In 2019, members generated over $16.7 billion in revenue through referrals they received from fellow members.

Annual membership fees will be higher than you'll pay with your local chamber of commerce, but there are some unique benefits that can help provide you with a high ROI. The largest benefit I saw as being a member of this organization was that you were placed into smaller groups. With chamber meetings, I might be in a room with 100 other business owners, which can make it difficult to meet and interact with everyone or find the businesses that have the most potential to be a referral source to your practice. At a BNI breakfast or lunch, I would be placed with a group of maybe 10–12 people in total. This allowed ample time to get to know those in your group and form some strong connections.

Another advantage of BNI groups is the lack of competition present. Chamber of commerce meetings were open to any and all business owners. So in every category of business you would find several different companies present. For example, there were at least 15–20 other dentists who were members of my local chamber. Given the large overall number of members this didn't deter my efforts to meet with, connect with, and find success with all who were present, but it can potentially lessen your odds. With my BNI group, they limit the number of those who can be apart in each industry, so I was the only dentist member.

By limiting the total number in each group and limiting the number of those in each category, I found this medium as a higher-quality way to attract new patients over the quantity approach the chamber of commerce provided. It was much easier to connect and interact with those on a smaller scale, and it also aided in everyone's referral efforts. Instead of having 5 chiropractors to refer patients to, I now had one place to send my patients, allowing more referrals to come their way and in return seeing more referrals my way. The biggest thing I would caution you on here is that because you're limited to those in your group, you need to vet your fellow members and their business before you send referrals their way. Check out their Google reviews, send out an email to your patient base, and ask if any of them have used their business or service and ask for their feedback, and if possible, use their service yourself. The worst thing you can do is refer someone to a bad experience. That's a loss for you and your patient. Do a little homework and make sure this business or service is something you can put your name behind.

I was an active member in BNI for my first four years of clinical practice. I loved the people I connected with in my group and almost every one of them became my patient. I can't count the number of referrals they sent my way over the years, but I can tell you that it provided an extremely high ROI for the time and money I invested. As time went on, my schedule got too busy to step out and participate in the meetings, and I had found other pathways to attract new patients that didn't require my time. Ten-plus years later, I am pleased to say that many of those business owners who were members of my group are still patients at my practice.

C. Business-to-business (B2B) gift card program

One day I was with my wife and kids eating some frozen yogurt at a local establishment. While I was enjoying the time with my family, an interesting thought struck me. That was the first time our family had ever shared frozen yogurt together. You see, for the most part, we usually go to ice cream places, not yogurt shops, yet here we all were. When I asked my wife why she had decided for us all to come here, she reminded me that we had a $5 gift card, a card my oldest son had received for recently attending one of his friend's birthday parties. The principle of reciprocity was at play again. My son had brought the birthday boy a present, and in return he reciprocated by giving him a $5 gift card that thanked him for coming to the party. Because of that gesture, the gift card had brought us to a business we had never visited before, a place we actually all enjoyed and would now frequent again in the future.

Back in the general practice referral section, I discussed how a $5 gift card to places where people enjoy spending their money could set the stage for more patients to refer to your practice. The longer you give those $5 gift cards, an interesting thing occurs. Either through an accountant's influence or your own, eventually, you start looking at the money you're spending on those gift cards as an expense, something that needs to be reduced or eliminated. When that feeling occurs, I encourage you to remember that when using the principle of reciprocity, if your intent is genuine, you can always count it as in investment. More should come back to you than what you give. That one small gift card to the yogurt shop has now influenced my family to return as happy and frequent customers to that business. This got me thinking: Is there a way to leverage the influence power of the gift card but without having to actually pay for it?

The short answer is yes, there is. It's what is now known as my business-to-business (B2B) gift card program. The benefits to this program are simple:

- Promote local businesses to your patients by getting them to donate gift cards for you to give out;
- In return for you promoting their business, they allow you to have some exposure to their customers;
- By donating the gift cards instead of you paying for them, it removes the expense of paying for gift cards;
- Even though you didn't pay for the gift cards, you can still leverage the power of reciprocity with your patients to ask for Google reviews, referrals, or to schedule their next treatment.

No one likes to be the first

I've mentioned before that the principle of social proof states that many times we look to the evidence of what others are doing or have done to show us it's safe to do the same. The more businesses you have on this gift card program, the easier it will be to attract even more businesses to join. Having said that, the opposite is true in that no one likes to be the first.

If businesses don't see others as members of your gift card program, it will be a barrier for you to get this going because of the uncertainty being the first can create. To counter this, you have to approach those you have the best relationships with. They are the ones to start with because if it's a friend, someone they know or like asking, then it will be harder for them to say no to your request.

The first business I approached was an Italian restaurant called Arooji's Wine Room & Ristorante. On most Friday or Saturday nights you can find my wife and I here, enjoying some amazing food, wine, and the live music they offer. We come here so frequently that I've come to know the manager and the owner pretty well. After visiting several weeks in a row, I noticed a disturbing pattern where it seemed like the restaurant wasn't doing very well. Each week the number of patrons seemed to be less and less. I knew that Arooji's had recently closed their sister location due to a bad economic downturn, and I was afraid the same was happening here. After talking with the manager, it seemed that all of their marketing efforts were coming up short, and they weren't sure what to do. In my mind I knew I had a solution for them, but I also knew I had to ask some key commitment questions first, before I could make my request. These are the same questions I ask every business manager or owner before I discuss the B2B gift card program:

- Do you need more clients? If they said no, then the conversation would end there.
- Are you already spending money marketing your business? If they are already committed to this, then it would be a simple step to commit to the type of marketing venture that you'll offer them.
- How much is a new client worth to you? Here, we need them to commit to how much money a new client is worth to them: $100 a year or $500+ per year? Anchoring them to this value is key, and we'll discuss why in more detail later on in the "Acceptance" section of this book.
- How much would you pay to get one: $5, $10, more? In this case the manager said he'd pay $10 all day long to attract a new customer. Someone who might bring someone with them and who might become a frequent customer from there. See Figure 38.

Once they've acknowledged that they need more new customers and determined how much a new client is worth and how much they are already spending to attract them, our next request will seem nominal in contrast. Next, I'm going to be the first to give and offer to promote them to my patient base. "I'd like to help. Would it be okay if I promote you to my 3000+ active patients?" The manager of course gave me an emphatic yes. Once I had him committed, it was now time for me to ask for what I wanted to make this all happen. I advised him about my B2B gift card program, the rules of which were simple. I'd agree to use their logo and at my expense print up $10 gift cards to their business. I used an online printing company that creates custom gift cards for businesses. I also agreed to give this gift card to everyone one of the patients who came into my practice for the next three months to satisfy my offer to promote them to my patients. In return I asked that they do two things for me.

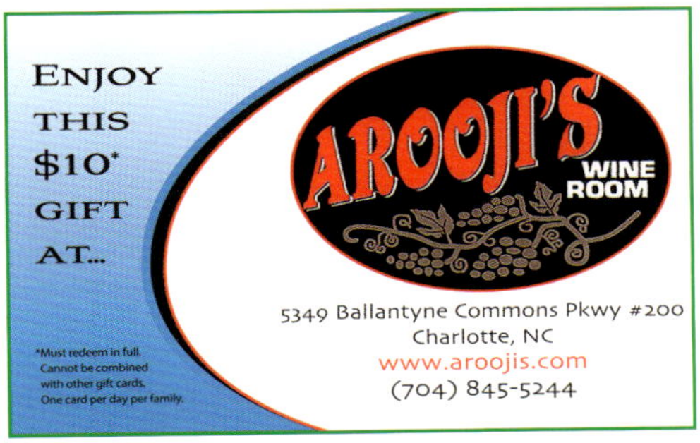

Figure 38. Example of business gift card.

First, I asked that if one of my patients brought in this gift card, then all they had to do was honor it and give them $10 off their meal. People had to spend more than $10 to use the gift card, so there wouldn't be any change to give back. There is no magnetic strip on these cards, so they have no real value except what is perceived and honored by all parties. The second request I made was that the restaurant hold all of the gift cards brought in for me to collect once a month.

Commonly Asked Questions about the B2B Gift Card Program

1. Why a gift card?

Why not a gift certificate? Why not do something simpler like a coupon? I chose a gift card because of how each of these are perceived. Coupons are viewed by many as cheap, and oftentimes people who use them feel entitled to the discount they are being given. Gift cards on the hand are perceived in an opposite way. People feel grateful for receiving them and reciprocate by spending more money on average than they do when using coupons. I like to use an online or local print shop to create these cards for me because their product looks and feels like a real gift card you'd get from any major retail store.

2. Why collect the gift cards from the businesses each month?

I do this for two reasons. First, I want to make sure that people value and are using the gift cards. If I give out 100 cards to patients and 0 use them, that tells me that they are not valuing the gift I'm giving them. Thus there is no influence power. That means this business is not going to be a good fit for our program, and I need to seek out another instead. The second reason I do this is because I want to recycle the gift cards. Eventually you'll get enough quantity of these in circulation that you will have to purchase very few moving forward, in essence making these gift cards a one-time purchase expense for the practice.

3. How much do these cards cost the practice?

Prices range based on the volume you purchase. I was able to purchase 1000 customized gift cards for around $240, or around 24 cents each.

4. What resistances do business owners have to this program?

Once they see that you have several businesses on the program, there usually isn't any resistance to joining if they've agreed that they need new clients and have paid a lot of money to attract them. If you do get a resistance, then it will most likely be like one the owner of Arooji's presented to me. His fear was that my patients would abuse the $10 gift card by only spending $11–$12 just to get $10 off. Since he was donating the $10 gift card that means he'd only profit $1–$2 on that dinner. Knowing the restaurant industry has tight margins, he reported that he couldn't afford to stay in business if this occurred in volume.

On the surface, this objection makes complete sense. If that occurred 100 percent of the time, then the math doesn't look good. The reality is that they are already spending that $10 and probably more with those other marketing efforts. So by replacing those efforts with this program, they are not really losing more money. They are just redistributing it to a new medium that should be more effective for them. The other thing I shared with him is that most people don't eat at this restaurant alone. They bring one or more people with them. So while he may be giving $10 off for one person, he'd make his full amount on the other 2–3 people in the group. The last thing I shared is the psychology of gift card users, which was that people who have a gift card typically spend more money per trip than those who didn't have a gift card. Think about your own experiences here. Maybe you don't normally get an appetizer, but because you have a gift card, now you do. Maybe you don't usually get dessert, but tonight we're all getting dessert. Add all of these items together, and it's rare that the business will actually lose money for participating in your gift card program.

In this owner's case, that logic still wasn't enough to get him over his objections. Given that this was my best chance to get this B2B gift card program off the ground and tested, I decided to remove his objection. I told him that if anyone of my patients came in and attempted to use the gift card off a total check purchase that was less than $20, then I would happily pay him $10 to help offset his perceived loss. I'm happy to report in the 8+ years they have been a member of our program, I've never had to reimburse him for a $10 loss.

On the flip side, he was pleased to welcome a ton of new customers from our promotional efforts. For every 100 gift cards we gave out to patients, around 34–38 were being used. This is well in line with what behavioral science studies showed in similar tests. Arooji's was ecstatic as that usually meant they served 68 or more new customers per month from the promotion, many of which returned as repeat customers. To help with promotion of our practice, I had given Arooji's some of the gift cards I had printed up that were good for visits at my own office. Gift cards that would equate to a free exam and x-ray. Perhaps the wait staff or the cooking team or someone in their families were looking for a dentist and wanted to use the gift card for themselves? If any of their customers reported that they were in need of a dentist, maybe because they couldn't fully enjoy their meal, then the waiters would give them one of our gift cards with their check, a great win-win for us both.

With the data I collected from Arooji's success, I was then able to approach other businesses about joining our program. Once you have one, you can leverage that to get another one on board. Once you have two, you can influence two more to join. Then the conversation becomes easier the more you have on your plan.

5. What businesses do I start with?

Start with the businesses that you potentially have the best relationship with. Like I did with Arooji's. These would be places you frequent on a regular basis. Places you may have a friendly relationship with a waiter or manager. If you don't have a place like this in mind, the next best place to look for opportunities is right in your own dental chair. Right now I bet you have several patients that are local small business owners. Because you are their dentist, you already have a relationship established, which should make the conversation go a lot easier. Plus, what better business to support with this program than one whose owner or manager is already supporting you by being your patient? Lastly, I'd approach businesses that you have connected with through the local chamber of commerce or BNI-style groups.

6. How do I know this business will be a good fit to be in our program?

First and foremost, this has to be a good thing for your patients. Like in the case for Arooji's, I really loved that restaurant and felt strongly that others would too if they knew about it and tried it. Remember, the worst thing you can give someone is a bad experience. So before you approach a business to be in your program, you have to vet them. You and/or your team need to try them out, use their service, and confirm that all feel comfortable referring and supporting this business. In thinking about this rule, one business comes to mind. I knew I

Business To Business Referral Plan

Would You Pay $5 or $10 To Get A New Client?
One that probably would become a repeat customer?

Would you like to put your Business in front of 2000 people this year?

Would You Like To Market & Promote Your Business To Potential New Clients BUT Only Have To Pay For Them If They Show Up To Your Business?

If you answered YES to any or all of these, you'll love our Business - Business Gift Card Promotion

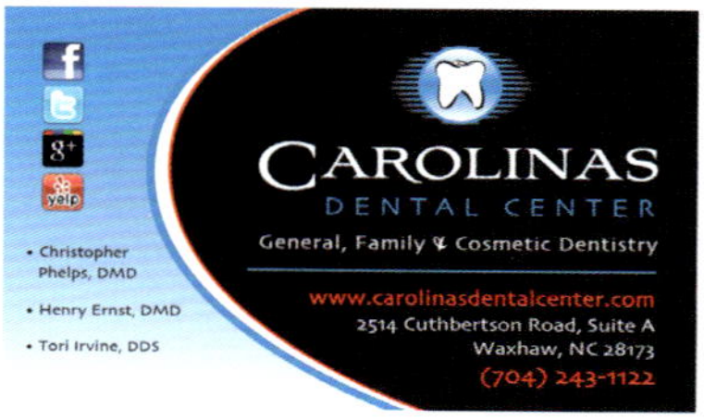

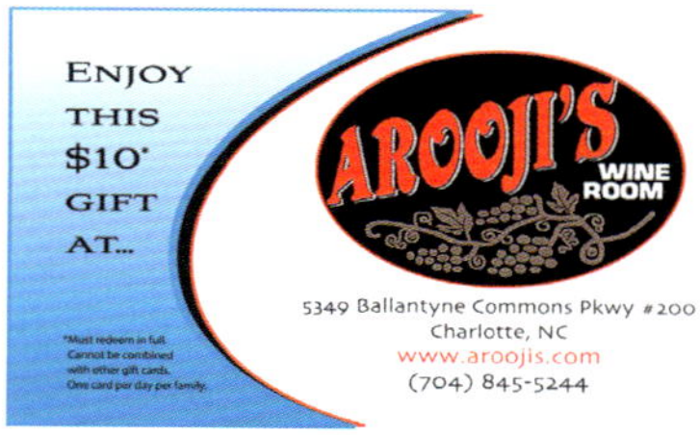

Business #1 Responsibliities

- Designs a Gift Card using your Businesses logo that includes an offer of $ 5 or $ 10 amounts
- Prints All Gift Cards
- Agrees to present Gift Card to every potential customer in the business & encourages them to try your business
- Touch base with Business monthly to collect used Gift Cards & track Success of the Program
- Includes an offer of $5, $10 or other custom amount.

Remember, it ONLY costs you $5 or $ 10 and only if the new client shows up to your business.

There is no contract, you can decide to stop the gift card at any time. The Business just requires a 30 day notice to alert their customers accordingly.

Business #2 Responsiblities

- Honor Gift Card if Presented for client $5 or $ 10 amounts, depending on your Business product or service. Potential New Client must overpay at your Business to receive the $ 5 or $ 10 off. Ex. must spend $ 6 to get $ 5 off.
- Decide what works best for your business $5 or $ 10
- Save Used Gift Cards and report back to Agent of Business #1 who will come by monthly to collect used cards
- Honor gift card in presented amount ($5, $10, or other) depending on your business product or service client must overpay at your business to receive the discount. Ex. must pay $6 to receive $5 off
- Decide what amount works best for you: $5, $10 or a custom amount.

I would like to offer gift cards in the amount of:
$5________
$10________
Other: $________

Figure 39. Example of business-to-business gift card contract.

wanted to have a nail salon as part of our gift card options as this is a gift some of our female patients might value. The problem was that I knew nothing about nail salons. Which are good, which are not good, and why? Luckily, I knew that my team would.

I told my team to take some time on a Saturday and try the nail salon across the street from our practice, thinking if it's convenient for our female patients to come here, then it might be equally convenient to get their nails done as close to us as possible. As a reciprocity gift to them, I paid for all of them to get their nails done. All I asked in return was feedback. Did you like them? Did they do a good job with their work? Was it clean? Did you approve of their sterilization techniques? Would you recommend this place to other women?

Based on their feedback, the consensus was that this place was not going to be a good fit for our program. Two months later I found a different nail salon just up the street from our practice. I sent my team in to get their nails done and covered their costs. Same outcome as the first business. Not a place they'd feel comfortable referring to. After a few more months I found Bubbly Nails. I sent my team with the same mission as before. This time all were in agreement that they'd found the place they all felt comfortable referring to. My team let me know this as soon as their visit had concluded. I immediately headed over to the nail salon to pay their combined bill and talk to the manager about the gift card program. Having just given them a gift of paying for 14 staff members to get their nails done, the manager was more than happy to reciprocate and listen as I described our gift card program. With similar results that Arooji's saw, the manager told me it was one of the most successful marketing things they'd ever done.

7. What kind of businesses should we approach?

I looked for a mix of businesses and services. Restaurants, local coffee and bakery shops, and services such as in-home maid and dry-cleaning services were my main targets. I then supplemented those with businesses like Bubbly Nails or local golf stores. Places that might cater to men vs women specifically.

8. What about approaching corporate or franchise businesses?

I think this would be a great idea. I'd love to get a company like Starbucks involved, which would benefit them and dentists all over the world. The problem I found with businesses that are not really owned or operated locally is that it is very hard to reach the real decision maker in the organization and describe this program to them. After six months and lots of time invested in climbing the corporate/franchise chain of command, I was able to accomplish this, but I don't recommend you spend too much of your time investing in this.

Let other people's giveaways be your gift card

Whether you realize it or not, the majority of businesses out there are providing some type of coupon or discounted offer to try to attract potential new customers. This is good news for us and gives us another avenue of business to approach for our gift card program. Going back to Cialdini's consistency principle, if these places are already committed to giving away an amount of money in a coupon or discount format, then why wouldn't they let you give it away to your patients on their behalf? If they are smart, then they should.

Look to industries that are desperate to attract new clients but who have competed so much on price that they are practically giving away their service as a "foot in the door" strategy, hoping that if people appreciated the deeply discounted service, they will return as a paying customer in the future. One that I researched was the maid or in-home cleaning services. In our area I repeatedly saw advertisements for a free one- to two-hour cleaning of your home. Having numerous businesses in our gift card program, I felt comfortable confronting one of these groups who I'd researched as having the best online reviews. I hired them to clean my house and a few of my team members' and once we agreed, I approached the owner about our B2B gift card program. We calculated how much a one- to two-hour home cleaning would normally cost a consumer and created our gift card to match that value. With similar results as our other businesses were receiving, it proved to be one of the most successful drivers of their business growth.

How is this a win-win-win for all involved?

When I was developing this B2B gift card program, I wanted to make this a win-win-win for all who was involved. First, it had to be a win for my patients. I mentioned earlier that I did not want to gift them a bad experience. Second, I wanted it to be a win for the businesses involved. I can safely say we achieved that goal as many told me it was the best advertising they had ever invested in. Yes, because it helped attract a lot of new clients to their business but most importantly for them because it didn't really cost them anything unless someone show up to use the gift card. There are not many things in marketing you can do where this occurs. You always pay up front and hope that it works. Now we've flipped the paradigm on that. Lastly, it was a win for my practice. Yes, it was a win in that each of these businesses became advocates of my businesses. Whenever any of their customers relayed a need for a dentist, there was no hesitation on their part to recommend us and pass on our gift card to them. A bigger win for me was that I was eventually able to stop paying for $5 gift cards and now had more than enough options to give my patients as gifts. Then leverage the reciprocity felt to ask for things like reviews, referrals, and to schedule their treatment.

How do I get these businesses committed to the program?

The best way to do this is by having some type of informal contract (see Figure 39) in place for them to sign. Something that outlines what your responsibilities are and what their responsibilities are, something that gives them a choice on what amount they want to give away in the gift card and gives you both a place to sign off your respective duties. Once signed, a copy is given to each party for reference. Below is an example of a B2B gift card program agreement I've used.

3. PARASITE MARKETING

A parasite is an organism that lives on or in a host organism and gets its food from or at the expense of its host. It implies a one-way benefit. Good for one party and not necessarily good for the other. A tapeworm may come to mind, which on the surface, doesn't paint a pretty picture. While they may not be a good thing in the biological world, from an advertising standpoint, parasitic marketing has proven to be a successful medium for many businesses. Picture a shopping mall. Most malls are anchored by large retail stores such as JC Penny, Macy's, and Neiman Marcus. These stores spend a good bit of marketing money to promote their name and attract customers to their store. This of course helps the smaller retail stores who don't have those kind of marketing budgets but can instead focus their efforts by feeding off the customers who were drawn in by the big retail stores.

In the dental world, dental specialists have historically tapped into this medium to fuel their practice growth, relying on the referrals of general dentists as their main new patient source. Using this model as a guide, I decided to use this medium to promote a unique service my practices offered: sedation dentistry.

At that time the number of general dentists in my state who were permitted to provide oral sedation dentistry was less than 200 dentists. Of those who provided IV and general sedation services in a general dentistry office setting, the numbers dropped to less than 3. At my offices, our dentists provided oral sedation while we had a dental anesthesiologist who came in and provided IV and general sedation. Given that sedation dentistry for general dentistry services were scarce and that specialist offices did not provide general dental services under sedation, I saw this as a great parasitic marketing opportunity. My hunch was that at some point, general dentists in my area had come across patients who needed extensive restorative work but would not move forward unless they could be sedated in some capacity. Since these patients had no options really available for them, maybe these dentists would refer them our way if they knew their patients had another option.

The first step I did was to have my team do a Google search for all of the dental offices who sat within a 5–7-mile proximity to my practice locations. Once that list populated, I had my team go to each of those office's websites to research if they provided sedation dentistry services of any kind. Of those, we finalized our list to 25 possible general dentistry sedation

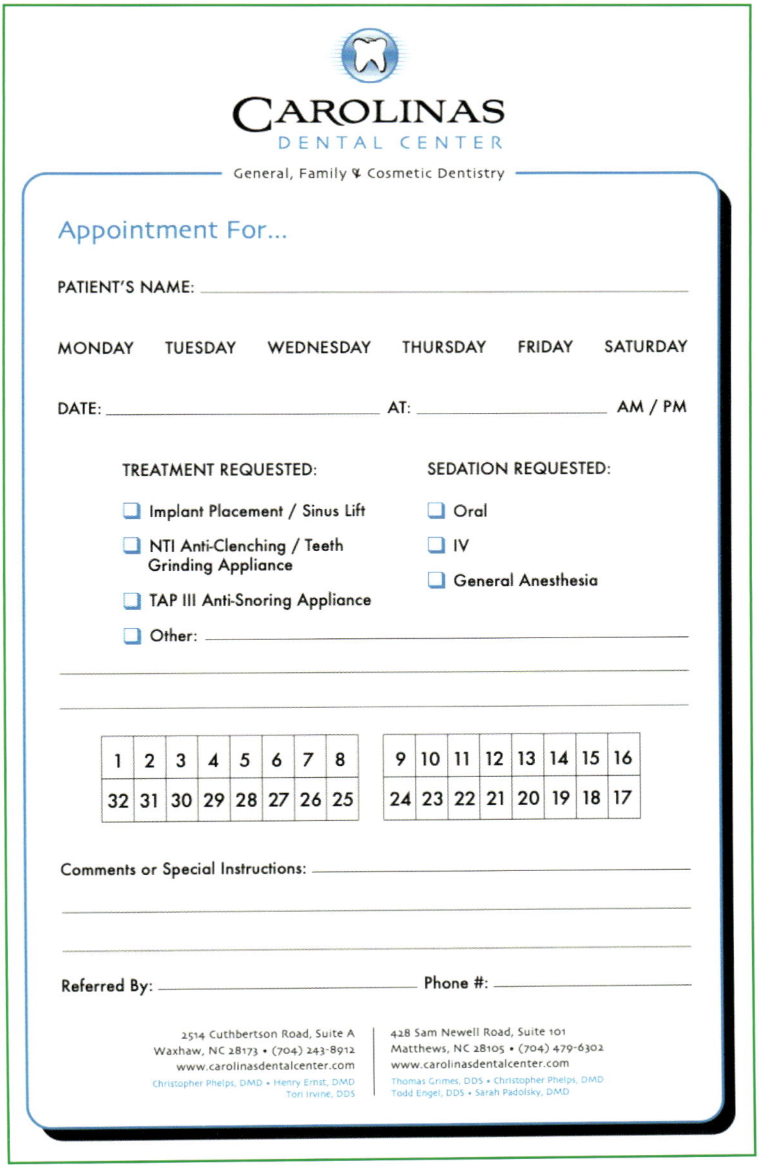

CAROLINAS
DENTAL CENTER
General, Family & Cosmetic Dentistry

Appointment For...

PATIENT'S NAME: ______

MONDAY TUESDAY WEDNESDAY THURSDAY FRIDAY SATURDAY

DATE: ______ AT: ______ AM / PM

TREATMENT REQUESTED:

- ☐ Implant Placement / Sinus Lift
- ☐ NTI Anti-Clenching / Teeth Grinding Appliance
- ☐ TAP III Anti-Snoring Appliance
- ☐ Other: ______

SEDATION REQUESTED:

- ☐ Oral
- ☐ IV
- ☐ General Anesthesia

1	2	3	4	5	6	7	8
32	31	30	29	28	27	26	25

9	10	11	12	13	14	15	16
24	23	22	21	20	19	18	17

Comments or Special Instructions: ______

Referred By: ______ Phone #: ______

2514 Cuthbertson Road, Suite A
Waxhaw, NC 28173 • (704) 243-8912
www.carolinasdentalcenter.com
Christopher Phelps, DMD • Henry Ernst, DMD
Tori Irvine, DDS

428 Sam Newell Road, Suite 101
Matthews, NC 28105 • (704) 479-6302
www.carolinasdentalcenter.com
Thomas Grimes, DDS • Christopher Phelps, DMD
Todd Engel, DDS • Sarah Padolsky, DMD

Figure 40. Referral pad example.

referral offices. With our list in hand, we created our own referral pad that these offices could use to refer patients who needed general dentistry services under sedation. Over time, we expanded our list of services to other procedures these offices didn't offer but may want to send our way.

With our referral pads (Fig. 40) and list of potential referring offices in hand, it was now time to create our marketing plan. For this, I wanted to use the principle of reciprocity, giving these dentists and their teams a gift they might value and then educating them on the sedation benefits mostly to one party. The gift I chose was to send a mobile car wash company to these offices that would wash and detail the dentist's and team's cars. My office manager would arrange this for their team, letting them know it was our gift to them and educating them about our sedation options for patients who needed general dentistry, encouraging them to send them our way if they came upon a patient who might need our services.

To offset my costs, I negotiated with a mobile car wash company and arranged a bulk pricing deal. In total, I spent just over $2400 on the car washes and $200 on printing of the referral pads and other miscellaneous items. A $2600 total investment. In the first month, we received two referrals. Each case committed and performed over $17,000 in treatment while under sedation. A 14:1 ROI in the first month alone. Each month we consistently treated 1–2 cases a month from our referral sources. While not a large quantity of new patients, these bigger cases definitely provided the quality and ROI I like to see from our marketing efforts.

4. PUBLIC RELATIONS

Public relations (PR) is the process of maintaining a favorable image and building beneficial relationships between an organization and the public communities, groups, and people it serves. Unlike advertising, which tries to create favorable impressions through paid messages, engaging in PR efforts does not typically require you to directly pay for this attention and publicity. Instead, PR strives to earn a favorable image by drawing attention to newsworthy and attention-worthy activities of the organization and its customers. For this reason, PR is often referred to as "free advertising" although it's not costless. It can require salaries to be paid to people who oversee and execute PR strategy. It also involves expenses associated with events, sponsorships, and other PR-related activities.

Public relations efforts should strive to do the following:

- Build and maintain a positive image;
- Inform target audiences about positive associations with a product, service, brand, or organization;
- Generate goodwill among consumers, the media, and other target audiences by raising the organization's profile; and
- Maintain good relationships with *influencers* – the people who strongly influence the opinions of target audiences.

In dentistry, one of the best ways I've found to help satisfy those first three points is by providing an annual day of free dental care for our community. This is a day where we offer free exams, cleanings, x-rays, and extractions to those in our community who can't afford this care. It's offered on a first-come, first-served basis and is limited to the first 100 patients who attend. Typically by 6 a.m. the morning of the event, the line for those interested would be wrapped around our building. Between my two office locations, we were able to provide over $750,000 in free dental care for our community, creating a lot of goodwill among our existing patients as well as others in our community.

To start this process, I knew we needed help. That's why I reached out to a PR firm called Dentistry from the Heart (DFTH), www.dentistryfromtheheart.org. Started by a dentist in New Port Richey, Florida, this nonprofit organization helps dentists and their teams organize and promote the free dental day events. To date, the dentists involved have donated over $25 million in care back to their communities.

One of the biggest advantages of using DFTH was the PR aid they gave us, which included promotional tools like branded t-shirts for the team to wear the day of the event, creation of banners to help us in promotion, and help reaching out to local newspaper, radio, and TV media outlets. Thanks to those efforts, we were able to get the word out over a large radius that we were offering a day of free care to those in need. In fact, on multiple occasions, I had patients tell me they drove over 100 miles to sit for our event. Routinely our office was featured on several local news stations for 3–4 days before the event, throughout the news cycles on the day of the event and then for the next week to follow. If there was a slow news cycle, then our office would be featured on the front page of our city's newspaper. On a busy news cycle, we'd at least be featured on the front page of the "Life" section of the newspaper.

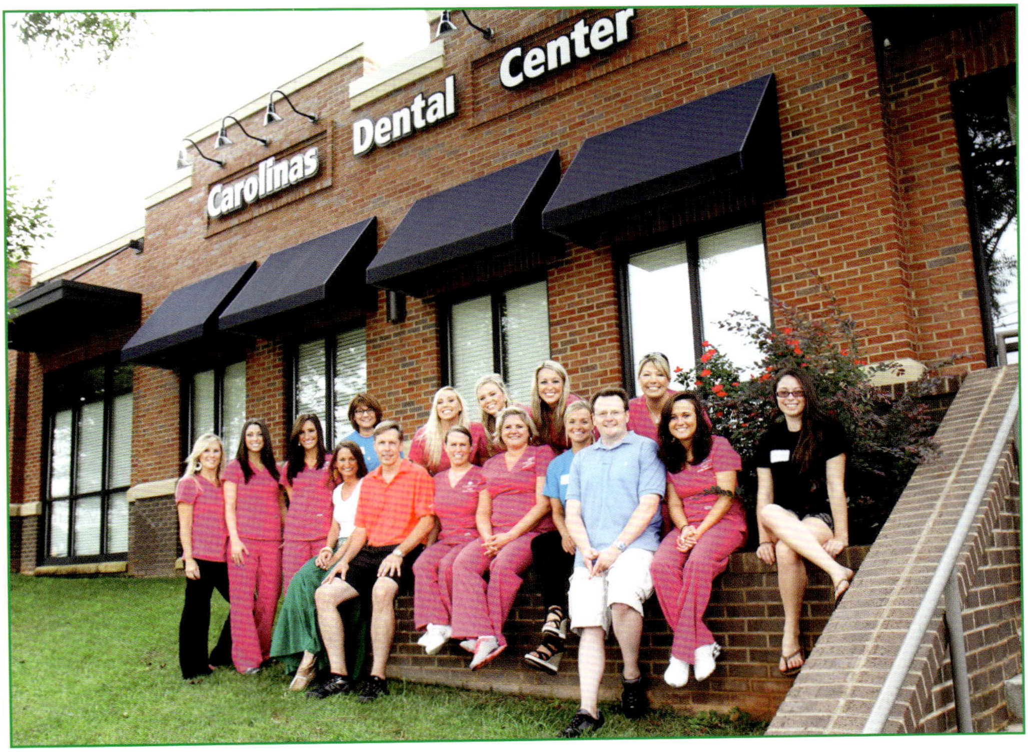

Figure 41. My team gearing up for a "Dentistry from the Heart" event.

There are so many great reasons to host your own day of free dental care. You can do it because it serves a great need for your area. You can do it because it creates a lot of good will with your existing patient base. Months after the event it was still a popular conversation with our patients in their hygiene chairs, praising us for our efforts and stating how much they appreciated being our patient. We made sure to let them know how supporting us as a patient allowed us to support others in our community. You can do it for the publicity and brand recognition. To this day I have people that recognize me from the newspaper and TV interviews I did around our events. You can also do it to attract new patients. We had several new patients report this activity as being one of the main reasons they chose our office over others in the area. In true reciprocity fashion, several patients who participated in these events returned to our office in later years as full-paying patients because of the kindness we showed them when they couldn't afford dental care.

PR activities also play an important role in identifying and building relationships with influential individuals and groups responsible for shaping market perceptions in the industry or product category where an organization operates. This has led to a burgeoning new area called "influencer marketing."

5. LEAD GENERATION

A "lead" is a traditional marketing term used to describe the consumer, prospect, or for dentists, a future patient. These titles of consumer, prospect, or future patient can be used interchangeably when talking about a lead. Lead generation is the marketing process used to *identify* and call these potential patients out, *qualify* them as truly interested and capable of paying for your services, and then *convince* them to become new patients. Lead generation is not just about reaching an established audience but creating a new or bigger audience. The wider the audience, the better the percentages are for growth.

One of the hurdles many dentists must overcome is the myth of the perfect patient. Every good marketer will help you create an *avatar* (or ideal patient) profile, but don't let the dream of a perfect patient keep you from nurturing leads/prospects who may not initially appear perfect or *ideal*. Make your sales process so good that you and your team can take a weak lead and turn it into a strong patient of record. A lot of times giving up on people too soon in the process is what kills marketing campaigns and results.

Marketing will take work on the team's side, whether they do the follow-up or it is outsourced. Cultivating a positive attitude towards potential new patients and guiding them through the process to accepting treatment is good work. Sometimes it is not about getting a prequalified lead as much as qualifying that lead once they are in your pipeline. It doesn't mean you lose time or money, but you build a marketing system that has the power to nurture people along the way!

Whether the lead has been prequalified before you speak to them or qualified after you speak with them, eventually you can quantify them as "good" leads, meaning they are interested in and can afford the goods and services you offer, or else they can be considered "bad" leads, those who are not interested in or do not qualify for your offer for a particular reason. Before you can conclude whether they are good or bad, we have to categorize them into three main opportunities and work to establish their true motivation or intent.

Three Lead Categories

- **Cold**: A cold lead is a consumer who has zero working knowledge of you, your brand, or your services. They may or may not be interested in what you are offering, but your lead generation marketing is designed to cold-call them out of the shadows by introducing yourself and your offer to see whether they may be interested since they would fit into your target market demographically.
- **Warm**: A warm lead is a consumer who is 40–70 percent closer to a buying decision because of some level of preexisting exposure or knowledge. A warm lead is someone who falls into your target market and has been exposed to previous or similar type of marketing efforts and/or has a working knowledge of the industry, service, brand, or product. Warm leads are more likely to respond to your lead generation efforts because of that personal interest or previous exposure.
- **Hot**: A hot lead is a buyer. They are 95 percent ready to buy on the spot and will respond immediately to your lead generation opportunity. They have previously been exposed to the brand, service, or product, most likely have done their research, been exposed to your industry/competition in some way, or are simply an opportunist with a decisive, quick-start personality who knows and feels ready to say yes when an opportunity presents itself.

As stated earlier, the goal of lead generation marketing for dentists is to convert interested and even uninterested or prospective consumers into new patients. When you break it down from a dentistry and business perspective, lead generation is designed to move the prospective patient into a dentistry buying position. To do this, a sales process/pipeline is required for an effective lead generation marketing process, a process that starts by attracting their attention.

Dental marketers understand you have less than eight seconds for someone to forget about you. This limited amount of time is because of the Internet and the advent of smartphones. Consumers are smarter, more connected, more influenced socially, and more informed than ever before. Everything they need is at the touch of a button. It is also important to understand that every buying decision, including dentistry, can have some emotional component to it. Regardless of the patient's intellect, logical approach, or endless research on comparison shopping, the decision usually comes down to what a patient wants.

The challenge, as it relates to dentistry, is that you – by no fault of your own – start out in a negative position in the mind of the potential new patient. People are afraid of you. They do not want to go to the dentist. In their mind, you're the person with "mouth weapons." They want a nice smile, they want to be out of pain, they want to pay less for obligatory dental care, they want their kids' teeth not to decay, but they don't want to come see you.

To counter this, we can leverage one of Dr. Robert Cialdini's principles of persuasion by putting yourself in the "liking" position through your lead generation campaigns. From a scientific standpoint, that means you don't just sell dental services, you sell you. When patients *like* you, it significantly increases the likelihood they will become a loyal, committed patient who is willing to pursue higher levels of treatment over a long period of time.

To relay this liking message, social media marketing has made this possible in ways never before seen in history. Digital social platforms provide the greatest opportunities for higher-performing call-to-action marketing. The demographic targeting and data tracking features of social media platforms allow for accuracy and precision of messaging to elicit a response and provide the opportunity to use digital tools to immediately move an interested lead into a curated sales funnel and elicits instantaneous action! Traditional lead generation has been around forever; however, the Internet and social media have brought about a fundamental shift in how lead generation campaigns are executed. Now you can directly and personally call someone to action and get an immediate response.

The key to successful lead generation is understanding you need both a comprehensive marketing strategy and delivery system. Choosing marketing solutions because "everyone else is doing it" is not the proper foundation for effective lead generation. Your practice is as unique as you, and your marketing should reveal that in every way. Inconsistency and discontinuity leads to disconnection with your desired audience. Choosing random marketing opportunities because it is a known or common practice or has a low price-point just so you can say you are doing marketing but has no connectivity to who you are, what you do, and what you're trying to accomplish will ultimately fail. Instead, focus on the following 5 unique areas to build successful lead generation campaigns.

5 Elements of Lead Generation

1. Make-up questions | (Storyboard): Lead generation requires you to know what makes you you.

- The lead generation strategy starts at the identity level.
- First, answer:
  - Who are we?
  - What makes us unique?
- Next, answer:
  - What do we do?
  - What do we do best?
  - List your top 3–5 *best services*. This will be part of the story you begin to tell over and over.
- Lastly, answer:
  - How do I want to present myself / my practice to others?
  - What do I want them to really know about me/us?
- Bonus question:
  - What will I say yes and no to? Know your level of resistance and openness to investing in lead generation marketing on the front end. There are many options and opportunities for lead generation – you have to decide how much or how little you are willing to try, experiment with, and pay in order to grow the practice. What is an acceptable ROI? What is an acceptable loss for trying something new? How much of my overall budget am I willing to commit to marketing?

2. Mindset | (Avatar): Understand the mindsets of your target audience.

- Start at the identity level again but this time with your target audience.
- Research the demographics of your target audience
- Answer the following questions:
  - Who are they? (buyers' persona)
  - What motivates them to buy?
  - What way do they typically buy (local, commercial, or online)?

- Understand the people in your community
  - Answer: What is *unique* about my community's buying habits?
  - Talk to local friends and neighbors
  - Constantly ask questions of people in the community to get insights and clues into what they want, like, dislike, etc.

3. Message | (Copy): Craft a main message. Craft marketing messages.

- First, craft your story (based on the make-up questions above)
  - Your marketing messages should never contradict your main message/story.
- Second, connect your story to your audience's story
  - *Use empathy.* Put yourself in the place of your audience, and then write from that perspective or point of view.
  - Ask: How do our stories connect or overlap? What do we have in common?
  - Ask: How are they disconnected from us? Do they understand us, dentistry, dental services? Why or why not?
  - Ask: What do they need to know about us in order for them to be motivated to engage with us?
- Third, time to do some copywriting – write a central message with an appealing offer
  - Use the consumer-first approach, meaning start with *them*, not *you*, and build a simple marketing message, better known as "copy" in the marketing world. Tap into their pain points or wants and how your offer or practice can meet their need/want or solve their problem.
  - Copywriting will be required for ADS and landing pages
- Write two types of copy for the same message:
  - "**Short form copy**" is delivering your message in as few words as possible to inspire and make the offer with a call to action. Clarity matters.
  - "**Long form copy**" is delivering your message with a long story that touches on a deeper level of behavioral science and psychology to educate and move the consumer through to action.
  - **Simple starter copy guide**:
    - → Set the problem
    - → Talk about the solution
    - → Say what's in it for the consumer
    - → Add a simple call to action
  - There are plenty of copywriting resources available to help you build effective copy
- **Warning**: Copywriting is *not* as *easy* as it appears on the surface. Don't be fooled – even with great coaching or tools, it will take a lot of time to become a proficient copywriter.

4. Medium | (Media buy): Choose the right social platform, channel, or marketing placement.

- There are **two types of lead generation**:
  - Traditional: *print media*
    - → Billboards
    - → Magazines
    - → Journals

        - Postcard mailers
        - Newspaper
        - Events
        - Community events: banners, practice merch/collateral, etc.
    - Modern: *digital media*
        - Facebook
        - Instagram
        - LinkedIn
        - Google Ads
        - Tik Tok
        - Twitter
        - YouTube
        - Blogs, email, etc.
- Traditional or modern media are *marketing delivery systems* that either help *create* or *reach* a specific audience.
- As a general rule of thumb, we recommend using modern marketing as the main driver and traditional as a supplemental tool in your overall marketing strategy.
- Each medium is unique in purpose, function, and audience. Choosing the right medium and crafting the right message (offer) to reach that platform's particular audience is critical in finding success in a lead generation campaign.
- **Some modern media examples:**
    - **Facebook**: Social media platform designed for personal social connection. Most engaged audience is age 30 and above.
        - **Organic**: Post daily to reveal the happenings of daily life in your practice. It is all about personality and content people want to see that helps them get to know you before they show up.
        - **Sponsored/paid**: Consideration or conversion ads can be customized to directly reach your specific targeted audience in their personal feeds with call-to-action offers.
    - **Instagram**: Digital window shopping. It is a photo/video-based platform designed for engagement. Built around followers, likes, and comments. Most engaged audience is age 30 and under.
        - **Organic**: Informal pictures of office life. Patient testimonial videos. Dental tip videos mixed with quality graphics are all positive ways to use Instagram for lead gen.
        - **Sponsored/paid**: Instagram is owned by Facebook, so paid ads can run simultaneously to Instagram to reach a younger audience with a unique message/ad carrying the same offer.
    - **LinkedIn**: A business-oriented social platform designed to reach professionals. Paid ads can be used to reach businesses or a professionals-centric audience. Both organic and paid/sponsored content is often centered around business, work life, and leadership content.
- Each of these platforms have back-end marketing and business managers where paid marketing can be managed. They also have digital training manuals and courses if you want to learn to run marketing campaigns on demand.

- **Traditional media examples:**
  - Mailers: Mailers are a traditional marketing solution. Call-to-action options for mailers are "visit the website," "call the number to schedule an appointment," or "bring the mailer with you to the visit."
  - Printed lead gen marketing materials are a challenge to track unless there is a secondary tracking system for calls and/or converted patients from the mailer.
  - Mailers are typically most effective for lead gen when there is a grand opening for a new practice or there is some big event / promo that is atypical.

5. Metrics | (Data analysis): Track audience behavior and response to your marketing.

- Modern marketing and social media platforms are uniquely designed for lead generation marketing.
- The biggest benefit of social media: ability to create and/or expand a **trackable audience**.
  - Social media allows you to build a database inside their platforms.
  - Retarget your custom audience based on positive or negative responses with new lead gen campaigns.
- Social media allows you to track behavior patterns.
- A/B split testing allows you to see what images, video, or copy your target audience prefers and responds to most.
- Social media allows you to track the decision points of the consumer through the entire marketing and sales process from AD to website.
- Social media allows you to set specific campaign goals and budgets to help you reach your new patient goals and measure your ROI in real time.

With the introduction of modern media, there has never been more lead generation marketing opportunities to drive new patients and new business to your dental practice. Those options can become a pro or a con, depending on your response. It is a pro when you maximize the opportunity to create, build, and grow a trackable audience that wants to hear from you consistently, an audience that you can build social equity with and sell your dentistry services. It is a con when all the options cause paralysis by analysis and you never jump into the marketing game, submit to the disillusioned learning that does sometimes happen, surrender to the fear of trying to learn marketing principles, platforms, or tools, or you capitulate to a negative view of marketing or marketers because of a previous bad experience or others' bad experiences or negative comments.

No lead generation marketing solution is perfect. There is no magic marketing platform. Every marketing campaign or system will require the practice's participation at some level and will need to be worked. Each lead generation platform serves a particular purpose, and when leveraged properly and put together strategically into a full marketing system, you can create a lead generation process that is capable of bringing abnormal levels of growth to your practice in a very short period of time.

Lead Generation Marketing Sequence:

Capture attention + nurture attention + qualify = buy

Social Media Lead Generation Marketing Sequence:
Ad (attention grab) + landing page (nurture/educate) + follow-up call / digital form (qualify) = new patient appointment

Tips to Ace Lead Generation

- **Agree**: You must start with total clarity and agreement on what constitutes a qualified lead before launching into a lead generation marketing effort. You must agree on what the handoff is from the marketer/front desk to the dentist/specialist. You must also agree on the process of qualifying a potential lead. Remember, more than 90 percent of consumers are not ready to buy instantly – they need to be nurtured and conditioned. This is the advantage of using a marketing company. Professional marketers understand the lead generation nurture process. Companies I've worked with such as tinyRHINO (www.tinyrhinomarketing.com) provide everything in their marketing system including a behavioral science methodology, social media campaign builds, custom in-office workflows, comprehensive team training, sophisticated sales scripts, and a custom digital dashboard for follow-up and tracking all to move the uninterested consumer from couch-to-treatmentTM.
- **Create**: Lead generation is about creating and driving content – relevant content. Think of content as the fuel for your lead generation marketing (traditional or modern) – event, email, and social media platforms. Building content should be part of your daily work life routine for you and your team. This is true whether you outsource to a marketing company or do marketing in-house. The more and better content you produce, the more effective your lead generation will be. Always remember: "content is king." If a dental practice is to remain relevant and seen in today's modern digital culture and e-commerce world, content building has to be on the forefront of a practice owner's mind, part of the actual business plan, and scheduled into your day-to-day operations.
- **Evaluate**: Lead generation is not a one-and-done effort. You must constantly evaluate your audience profiles, buyer journey, platform metrics, and copy/messages. Keep your lead generation goals and your customer concerns and challenges in front of you as much as possible. If you use a marketing company, don't go dark on them once you sign up for a marketing package. Stay in constant contact with them about your lead generation strategy, tactics, and performance. Keep sending them good content. Your practice's growth is your responsibility – not the marketing company's. Marketing companies provide you the road map and a delivery system for conversion, but in dentistry, you must become the expert at treatment presentation and convert these consumers into patients once they are in the chair!

6. PRACTICE ACQUISITION

A unique marketing medium that has gained traction in recent years is this idea of making someone else's existing patient become your new patient through practice acquisition. Historically when dentists were ready to retire or sell their practice, it was a packaged deal. It included the active and inactive patient base, commonly called the goodwill of the practice, along with any hard assets such as real estate, equipment, furniture and fixtures the practice had acquired. If you weren't interested in taking over both the goodwill and hard assets, most dentists weren't interested in talking with you.

As times have changed, so has the practice sale model. More dentists are employed in different dental service organizations (DSOs) throughout the country, leaving fewer to be interested in full practice purchase. Financial institutions have raised the requirements to loan the money needed to purchase a practice, oftentimes adding some type of down payment toward the purchase price. Couple this with rising costs of dental school education that has been financed, and again you have fewer dentists looking or able to make a full practice purchase. To adapt, some dentists have set their sights on selling just the goodwill portion of their practice, focused on some return for their practice investment over the risk of not being able to sell any portion.

These acquisitions make sense as most of the time you are acquiring a patient base with 1000–1200 patients, all of which are new to you. Many have outstanding treatment that needs to be completed and even more have treatment needed that hasn't been planned yet. If your goal is to attract 80 new patients a month, you could take the money you would have spent on marketing to attract those patients over a 15-month period and instead, invest it in purchasing a practice that has 1200 active patients. Same net number of new patients, but you're buying guaranteed revenue with patients who are committed to routinely coming in for preventative care as well as preplanned restorative work you could use immediately to start repaying your investment.

CASE STUDY

Dr. Richard Wyne, a practicing general dentist in Rockville, Maryland, received a call from a desperate dentist he had recently met a few months earlier at a local study club meeting. This long-practicing dentist had set up his practice in the basement of his home but due to a recent stroke, found himself in need of selling his practice and retiring. In the previous year, he had collected $180,000 in gross revenues. Because his practice was one with his home, a traditional approach to selling the entire practice as one asset was out of the question.

Dr. Wyne realized that the only viable option to help this dentist out would be to arrange some type of chart merger, or practice acquisition, as it's called. He offered the retiring doc $90,000 to take ownership of approximately 3000 patient charts, which accounted to 50 percent of his previous year's revenue or $30 per chart. In exchange, this doc would forward his main phone line to Dr. Wyne's office and would send out a letter introducing him to his patients and recommending that they continue their care in his office, located approximately 2–3 miles away.

In the first three months after this practice acquisition was completed, Dr. Wyne had collected over $90,000 in treatment generated specifically from the patients who came over in this acquisition, paying himself back for his initial investment. From this investment, he was able to double the revenue of his practice but without having to spend any other funds in marketing to do so. To this day, some 8 years later, Dr. Wyne is still working his way through all of the patients who came over during this acquisition, and his ROI is estimated to be greater than 16:1.

Seeing the power of this type of marketing investment, Dr. Wyne began to look for other opportunities and to date has completed 5 additional practice acquisitions, paying anywhere from 35 to 70 percent of that practice's previous year's collections, based on factors such as the distance away from his current practice, the active patient count, and number of periodic exams performed in the previous year. A major factor he uses to determine the sale price is whether the selling dentist will be staying on for some period of time. If they are willing to continue on as his associate for 1–3 years, then he's willing to offer them a higher percentage of their previous year's collections as the payout for the patient charts in question. Here are some of Dr. Wyne's recommendations about practice acquisitions that's allowed him to grow from $450,000 to over $3 million in practice revenue:

- Look for practices where the doc wants to stay on and continue practicing for some time, ideally for a 2–3-year window. In these circumstances, you can offer them a choice. Take a lower percentage to be done with the practice and the patients now or a higher percentage if they are willing to stay on 1–3 years.
- When evaluating these practices, be on the lookout for outliers in the data. Pull a "procedures by provider" report and look for anything that stands out to you as odd or perhaps filled with procedures you might not be able to continue with moving forward. For instance, one practice Dr. Wyne looked at, the office charged patient an "OSHA/HIPAA" fee for each visit. While this added to the overall revenue count, it would not be a fee Dr. Wyne would be able to continue as his status as an in-network provider for multiple insurance plans would prohibit.

Another practice he looked at charged out over a third of the total revenue for holistic or biologic dental procedures such as ozone therapy. Not being trained in these procedures, this loss in revenue would have to be factored into the purchase price for the patients' charts.

- Limit the area you'll consider acquiring practices from 3 to 5 miles away at the most. Once you go above 5 miles, the number of inconvenience factors and potential barriers for people to travel increase significantly, reducing the number of patients you'll actually get to see at these offices and thus limiting your ROI.
- Invest your time into this medium. With each practice acquisition, Dr. Wyne has been able to significantly increase the annual revenue of his practice, using that additional income to expand his facility from 4 chairs to now having over 12 chairs, creating new patient opportunities for his hygienists and associate doctors. Dr. Wyne actively searches for these opportunities by going to local study club meetings and seeking out those who've been in practice over 30 years. He sends letters out to all licensed dentists in that 5-mile radius, asking whether they are tired of running their practice and invites them to dinner to discuss a new opportunity.
- Consider investing some money into this medium by creating an incentive program that lets others become your advocates: those who already have a presence in different practices in the area but who could now actively seek out and find you opportunities. These could be people like your local dental supply reps, who still tend to have some presence in the majority of the dental offices in your area. This could also be dental hygienists or assistants who work as temporary hires around your area. Dr. Wyne's preferred incentive is to offer these people $50 for a name of a potential dentist who may be looking for a change or to retire in the near future. If that name and introduction leads to a dinner or meeting to discuss the practice acquisition opportunity, then he offers that $50 turns into $500. If the relationship leads to him purchasing that practice, that $500 becomes $5000, ultimately making this a win-win for all involved: A win for the doc who was looking for a way out or

new opportunity, a win for the person who found the lead and made the introduction, and lastly a win for Dr. Wyne as he knows how to turn these acquisitions into investments that will continue to fuel the growth and prosperity of his practice.

You can use the following market worksheet to strategically pick some media you would like to test.

Map Your Medium

Instructions: Now it's time to strategically pick the media in which you will place your message to attract your target market.

Check possible media to promote your message, content, and offer to your target market. Think of the survey you gave your top patients and referrals. What are they reading, listening to, and looking at? Where do they live or get together regularly where you could easily put your message in front of them. Check all that apply:

External Marketing Media

- [ ] Direct mail (postcards)
- [ ] Direct mail (3/4 panel brochure)
- [ ] Direct mail (newsletter)
- [ ] Direct mail (self-published magazine)
- [ ] EDDM
- [ ] Newspaper
- [ ] AM radio
- [ ] FM radio
- [ ] Radio: self-recorded
- [ ] Radio: announcer recorded
- [ ] Radio: celebrity recorded
- [ ] TV
- [ ] Satellite
- [ ] Streaming service
- [ ] Dentomercial
- [ ] Billboard with direct mail campaign
- [ ] Billboard without direct mail campaign
- [ ] Magazine (local or nationwide)
- [ ] Internet: SEO
- [ ] Internet: local search
- [ ] Internet: PPC
- [ ] Internet: Google Ads
- [ ] LinkedIn
- [ ] YouTube
- [ ] Facebook
- [ ] Instagram
- [ ] Nextdoor paid ads
- [ ] Other:____________

Internal Marketing Media

- [ ] General dentistry referral system
- [ ] Patient appreciation party
- [ ] Acquire Google business reviews
- [ ] Other: ____________

Symbiotic Marketing Media

- [ ] Chamber of Commerce
- [ ] Network marketing groups
- [ ] Other: ____________

Parasite Marketing Media

- [ ] Office referral pad, e.g., sedation dentistry
- [ ] Other: ____________

Lead Generation Media

- [ ] General dentistry services
- [ ] Niche services, e.g., dental implants
- [ ] Other: ____________

Grassroots Marketing Media

- [ ] Community forums. e.g. Nextdoor
- [ ] In-office patient education seminars
- [ ] Off-site patient education seminars, e.g., steakhouse seminar
- [ ] On-site patient education seminars, e.g., at retirement communities
- [ ] Other: ____________

List the top 5 media you want to try. Rank in order of your priority.

1. ____________
2. ____________
3. ____________
4. ____________
5. ____________

THE PHELPS INSTITUTE

8

Figure 42. "Map your medium" worksheet.

Chapter 8
Tracking Your Success

Earlier in the book I talked about the quote from the famous retail marketer John Wannamaker, who said, "Half of my advertising spend is wasted; the trouble is, I don't know which half." If only Mr. Wannamaker had spent more effort to measure the true effectiveness of his campaigns, then he might not have found advertising so frustrating. Proper tracking is key to understanding what's working in your marketing efforts, what's not working, and most importantly, understanding why. If we don't have the right data, then we can't make smarter marketing decisions. No one stated the benefits of proper tracking better than the famous British statistician Karl Pearson. Pearson's law states: "When performance is measured, performance improves. When performance is measured and reported back, the rate of improvement accelerates."

Despite the importance of collecting analytics and data on your marketing effectiveness, there seems to be a big discrepancy in the industry on those who use it. A 2015 study by *Forbes* magazine reported that only 22 percent of marketers use data-driven initiatives to achieve significant results. What's worse is they found that 74 percent of marketers can't measure or report on how their efforts affect their client's businesses. With so few who understand the importance of this, that puts the responsibility back on you to search out and work with companies who do follow data-driven initiatives to achieve their results. It also means having some systems in place to track these companies' results so you can have unbiased evidence of your return on investment.

AREAS TO TRACK

When it comes to tracking dental marketing, I focus my metrics and analytics in two key areas. Each relates to the two sides of the marketing coin this book centers on. On one side we need to track data concerning the leads generated by our marketing efforts. What quantity of potential new patients did we receive? What quality of new patients did our marketing attract? Quality we've defined before as those who pay our full fee and return for future treatment. Putting these together, did we have an ROI to justify what we invested over a defined period of time?

On this side of the coin, I use an ROI of at least 3:1 within in the first six months as the main measure of my marketing's success. In the dental world, it's been reported that a 3:1 return within the first year should translate to 20:1 return within five years. This increase is due to the additional treatment these patients will receive, family and friends they will most likely refer, and the additional revenue you'd collect as a result.

The other side of the marketing coin we need to have data from concerns what I call the lost opportunity side. We'll dive into this area in more detail in later chapters, but for our discussion on tracking, it warrants a mention here. For now, we'll define lost opportunity as any new patient opportunity that does not actualize. For example, maybe your advertisements generated a significant response leading to numerous new patient opportunities calling your practice to make an appointment, but what happened to those opportunities? Was the office able to answer each of those new patient calls? If answered, were you able to make them appointment? If we made them an appointment, did they show up? By not capitalizing on these new patient opportunity calls we can expect our marketing expenditures to skyrocket, our new patient goals to fall short, and a poor ROI.

This was the situation I found myself in when I had sold my two best, most profitable offices and took over my two struggling ones. During that time, I was spending $37,000 per month on dental marketing, all to get 60 new patients for those efforts, 30 new patients at each of my two offices. My ROI for that money spent was nowhere near a positive number. When I started tracking the results myself and stopped listening to the marketing companies who were not effectively tracking this for me, the reasons became readily apparent. My team was unable to answer 224 new patient calls per month, calls that came in specifically from external marketing sources. When my team did answer the telephone, we only made an appointment for that person around 24 percent of the time. In the coming chapters we'll discuss the strategies I used to correct this issue and how I made my marketing start to become an investment instead of a large expense for my practice.

SYSTEMS TO TRACK DENTAL MARKETING

Now that you understand the overall areas you need to track, let's discuss some systems you can use to acquire these key analytics. For websites, you can use a service such as Google Analytics, which tracks your website activity. Using it you can acquire information such as how many people visited your website, what pages did they navigate to while present, or your current bounce rate. Bounce rate is defined as the number of people who click to go to your website but then immediately leave without really navigating it.

When working with digital marketing media such as pay-per-click, the bounce rate metric is important to know since you're paying for each click and thus person who gets transferred to your website. Unfortunately, there are programs and people who click on these ads without any real intent to become a potential new patient at that practice, ultimately leading to more fees you pay to run your pay-per-click campaign yet getting few actual results.

Social media websites such as Facebook and Twitter have their own analytic capabilities built into their advertising services. If you goal is to use these platforms as well as others, you can look to services such as Buffer or Hootsuite, which offer a myriad of metrics you can track including likes, shares, and views of your social media posts or marketing pieces across all of the major social media platforms.

For off-line media such as direct mail, TV, or radio, the most widely system to track results comes from using unique call tracking numbers on your advertising campaigns. In the US, Canada, Australia, and the UK, call tracking numbers can be acquired from a service such as Twilio. It can have a local area code assigned to it to look more familiar to potential new patients in your area or it can have a more universal area code like a 1-800 prefix.

Once acquired, you'd use a single, unique number and assign it to each of your different marketing campaigns. Each number can be set up so that when dialed, it automatically forwards to your main office telephone number. For example, if you wanted to track your results from a direct mail campaign and radio advertisement, you'd want to have three distinct tracking numbers: one for the direct mail piece, a different number for the radio ad, and a third number to host on your website. Any calls that come in from these unique numbers are logged, so you have an idea of how many people responded from each of these media, giving you info on the quantity of calls received from each source.

Having a unique number on your website is also important to help you capture information about the people who viewed your site and called. Many times those who see your direct mail piece may choose to go to your website to look up more information before they feel comfortable to call. Those who heard you on the radio may not have been able to write down your phone number as they were most likely driving but may remember your website and find your phone number through that route. Ultimately you'll want to capture as much data as you can as to what are the ad sources through which your new patients are learning about you and responding.

Another benefit of using call tracking numbers is that each phone call is recorded and available for you to listen from a dashboard the call tracking company will set up for you. This is key when it comes to evaluating how effective your team is with making appointments, helping you identify any barriers the patient is putting up when it comes to scheduling these appointments but also identifying any roadblocks your team may be putting up that are preventing more patients from scheduling.

For digital marketing channels such as pay-per-click, Facebook, or Google Ads, call tracking numbers can also be deployed with great success. While discovering how many people click on an ad or like your post is important, when it comes to ROI, the only thing that really matters is how many of them actually picked up the phone and made an appointment in our office. For those who did over some period of time, how much did they spend with us versus how much did we have to spend on that marketing medium to acquire them? To help us with tracking online marketing media, your call tracking number should have "dynamic number insertion" capabilities.

If a potential new patient is looking at a pay-per-click ad and calls directly from the number they see, then you'd have an accurate log that the new patient call came in from this marketing source. If they don't call from that number but instead click to go to your website, then they may end up calling your office from your website tracking number. So the call would be logged through the website and not the pay-per-click ad that was the real reason why this call was generated. Without knowing the true ad source, you can't properly calculate the ROI for your pay-per-click ad.

With dynamic number insertion, you can change this. The company who provided you with the call tracking number can provide you with a special code that you would have embedded onto every page of your website. This code is specifically tied to that telephone number and how that number is shown in the digital advertisement. Normally numbers are displayed in a static fashion. So there is no link embedded into the number that a mouse could click on and that might take you to another site. When the number is dynamic, it shows up as blue in color and underlined, meaning someone could click on it and travel to your website to learn more. With the special code embedded into your website, if someone clicks on your dynamic number, by the time they reach your website, the telephone number displayed here has completely changed. It's no longer your original website tracking number but now the number shown is the same as the one they saw looking at your pay-per-click ad. So if they decide to call your office at this point, even though they got the number from your website, the call will be logged as coming in from your pay-per-click ad.

With these calls being recorded, you can follow the sequence to learn how many scheduled, what were their names, and ultimately track how much they spend in your office. Before dynamic number insertion, digital marketing was tracked by the number of likes, clicks, and other metrics that showed people were interested but not necessarily committed to making an appointment. Now, we can use this technology to accurately calculate your ROI from how many people scheduled appointments and how much money they spent in your practice.

POTENTIAL METRICS AND OTHER KEY POINT INDICATORS TO TRACK

With an understanding of the importance of why you need to track your marketing efforts, let's now look at some potential metrics and other key point indicators you can choose to focus on.

General Marketing Metrics

- **Brand awareness**: Measures the level of familiarity your target audience has around your brand or product.
- **Customer lifetime value**: How much revenue a business will generate per customer over that customer's lifetime.
- **Customer acquisition cost**: The expense of activities required to earn one customer.
- **Return on investment**: How much revenue is generated per dollar spent on marketing.
- **Conversion rate**: The percentage of calls compared to appointments made or visits that result in a desired action (like completing a form or making a purchase).
- **Leads generated**: The raw number of sales leads brought in by marketing.

Website and Blogging Metrics

- **Referral traffic**: Traffic referred to your site through another source (search engine, email, social media, etc.).
- **Organic traffic**: Unpaid traffic driven through search engines.
- **Total visits**: The aggregate number of hits over a given time period.
- **Customer attrition/churn**: The rate of customer loss over time.
- **First visit**: The number of new potential customers who land on your website for the first time.
- **Returning visits**: The number of hits from visitors who have been to your site before.
- **Traffic sources**: Places that refer traffic to your website or blog.

- **Click-through rate**: The percent of search engine queries that result in a click to your site.
- **Time on page**: The average amount of time visitors spend on a web page before leaving.
- **Bounce rate**: Tracks visitors who only view one page on your site before exiting.
- **Downloads**: The number of times downloadable assets and freebies are downloaded (like e-books, templates, and other gated content).
- **Page views per session**: The number of pages an average visitor views on your site before leaving.
- **Unique visitors**: The number of individual users that arrive on your site.
- **Sessions by device type**: How many visits a site receives, broken down by the type of device people used to access it (e.g., Mac, Windows PC, iPhone).
- **Page views**: The total number of pages that have been viewed on a site.
- **Top pages**: The pages that are driving the best performance, either by traffic or conversion rate.

SEO Metrics

- **Keyword rankings**: How high a page ranks in search engines for a given keyword.
- **Search traffic**: The amount of referral traffic sent to a site through a search engine.
- **SERP (search engine result page) visibility**: The share of traffic that a website receives from its rankings in the organic search results.
- **Total back links**: The number of links pointing at a web page from other sites.
- **Domain authority**: Measures how authoritative search engines view an entire website.
- **Page authority**: Measures how authoritative search engines view a single web page.
- **Page load speed**: How fast a website loads (which may affect search engine rankings).
- **Organic click-through rate**: How often searchers click a given page when it appears in search engine results.

Social Media Marketing Metrics

- **Likes**: The number of clicks on post's "like" buttons.
- **Comments**: The number of comments on your posts.
- **Shares**: The number of times a post has been shared, also called retweets on Twitter or "repins" on Pinterest.
- **Engagement rate**: Measures the level of interaction happening between a social media profile and its audience.
- **Follower growth rate**: How quickly a profile is gaining new followers.
- **New followers**: The number of new fans or followers earned over a given period of time.
- **Social media traffic**: Website or blog traffic driven by social media platforms.
- **Social media conversions**: Website or blog conversions from social media referral traffic.
- **Page demographics**: A breakdown of demographic data based on a profile's followers, according to age, sex, location, occupation, etc.
- **Sentiment**: Measures how social media audiences feel about your brand.

PPC Metrics

- **Cost-per-click (CPC)**: The cost of getting one click on an ad.
- **Click-through rate (CTR)**: Measures how many people click an ad, based on how many times it appears.

- **Quality score**: Used to determine an ad's relevancy based on keywords, search intent, and the quality of the destination page.
- **Impression share**: The number of impressions ads receive, measured against the total number of impressions they were eligible to receive.
- **Total conversion value**: The total monetary value of all conversions over a period of time.
- **Return on ad spend (ROAS)**: The amount of revenue generated measured against the amount spent.
- **Call tracking**: The number of calls placed after clicking an ad. Tracked using dynamic number insertion technology.

Paradox of Choice

With an abundance of tracking metrics, analytics, and data points we could focus on, where should we turn our focus? Do we need to look at them all to be effective with our dental marketing efforts? The good news is that the answer is no. We don't have to focus our attention on all of the metrics available to us. We just need to narrow our focus to the most important ones.

In his book *The Paradox of Choice: Why Less Is More*, Barry Schwartz outlines the psychology behind choice and the paradox it creates. On the one hand, people do prefer to have a choice, to have at least two options in front of them when making a decision. Without a choice, they tend to feel more coerced, intimidated, or forced into a buying decision, setting the stage for many to say no as a result. When at least two options are presented, that person feels more in control of their situation and is now more likely to say yes to one of the choices in front of them.

The problem comes when there are too many choices. The more choices we have in front of us, the more options to play, the more metrics or key point indicators we turn our attention to, it seems the less likely we are to focus or decide on any of them. You see, our brains lose the ability to differentiate between all of the different things in front of us. If our brain can't tell the difference or discern the real importance of the options at hand, then it chooses to ignore them all, resulting in inaction or a rejection to our request. Studies show this tends to be the case when we have more than 5 items to choose from.

This paradox of choice plagues us in the dental marketing arena as well. I know of several inexpensive call-tracking companies that give you some basic metrics but force you to listen and evaluate all of the marketing-based phone calls. This could mean hundreds of phone calls you have to go through and evaluate to get the whole truth on what happened with those new patient opportunities and calculate your true ROI.

With dentists spending the majority of time on patient care, that makes it a next to impossible task, forcing dentists to take shortcuts, relying solely on basic data such as the total number of calls that come in from each tracking number and ignoring the fact that not every one of these calls could be new patient calls. From our data at Call Tracker ROI, some are usually existing patient calls. They saw your advertisement, remembered they had a dental issue, and then just called from the number on the ad. Sometimes these calls come from solicitors who saw your ad and felt like you might be willing to buy something they had to sell.

From the total number of calls that came in, did they actually make an appointment or spend anything at your office? If we just rely on this basic data point, we'll never really know what our ROI was.

Many dental call tracking companies have tried to alleviate this problem by having software programs that listen to and analyze your telephone calls. In doing so, their programs provide you with a dashboard of 100+ call tracking metrics in an attempt to provide value for the service you pay them for. With this robust dashboard with all of these metrics, we as practitioners are stuck in that paradox of choice. Too many metrics to focus on, so we tend to ignore them all because we can't tell which ones really are the most important that warrant our attention.

Another aspect many docs don't understand is that there are no true artificial intelligence–based software programs listening and analyzing our marketing calls, despite many of the claims otherwise out there today. Instead they are still just static programs, which struggle with issues such as the use of slang, translating foreign languages, distractions from loud background noises that occur in busy dental offices, and other issues that prevent these programs from accurately telling you what happened in your telephone calls. Instead of alerting you to this fact, these programs altogether ignore the data from these calls, so they are absent from their reporting feature. Thus, you're missing out on getting the whole truth of what happened with your new patient opportunities and won't get a true measure of your ROI.

Top 5 Most Important Metrics to Track ROI

When I discovered I was spending $37,000 per month in marketing but was not getting a return for that investment, I tried every call-tracking program available on the market at that time, finding many of the frustrations I outlined above. Too many calls to analyze myself. Those programs that did analyze calls only gave me the half-truth but not the whole truth of what happened with those opportunities. I realized technology was important, but it wasn't enough. It still had to be supplemented with live people. I didn't have time to listen to and evaluate all of those calls, but the data from them was too important not to have someone do it on my behalf. That's when I created my Call Tracker ROI platform, a company dedicated to providing dentists with an unbiased assessment of what's working with their current marketing efforts, what's not working, and why.

With the service, we would assign our clients with call tracking numbers to use on their various marketing campaigns. If they were for digital advertising media, then we'd turn on the dynamic number insertion feature and walk the website team on how to embed the code required for their proper function. I'd have a dedicated listener assigned to their account to listen to every call that came in and document what transpired in that call. Reports were then generated on any time frame the dentist chose to review the data collected from both sides of the marketing coin, what I defined as the top 5 most important metrics to track ROI:

1. Missed New Patient Calls

If you can't answer a significant number of new patient calls, then your ROI will suffer as a result. For missed new patient calls, I define this as any potential new patient call that goes unanswered, meaning it went to voicemail, the caller just got a busy signal, or the call just rang and rang and the caller hung up before anyone could answer. From the data we've collected from our Call Tracker ROI clients across the US, Canada, Australia, and the UK, those spending anywhere from $0 to $2000 per month in dental marketing are missing one third of their new patient calls. When an office spends over $2000 per month, the rate of missed new patient calls rises to almost 55 percent. In the case of my own practice, I mentioned how we didn't answer over 224 marketing-based new patient calls per month.

For tracking purposes, I want to collect enough data at critical times to identify any patterns or trends. To capture these patterns properly, I recommend you have these calls tracked by hour of the day, day of the week, week of the month, and month of the year. Since every office can have a busy day, I prefer to look for these patterns over a longer period of time such as monthly or quarterly. Across the board, our client's data shows us an important trend where 99 percent of missed new patient calls happen during normal business hours, not after hours or on weekends when you are closed.

There is a popular misconception among dentists and the feedback they are receiving from their teams that the majority of their missed new patient calls are occurring after the office is closed. While that may be many people's opinion, the facts and data just don't reflect that. Instead, it shows an interesting pattern where many of our new patient calls go unanswered 30 minutes after you open your office, the hour during your lunch break, and 30 minutes before you close for the day.

2. New Patient Appointment Conversion Percentages

In addition to answering the new patient phone call, we need to place some emphasis on tracking what happened to that new patient opportunity. Did it end with an appointment? For this, I recommend you track this at two levels: total new patient appointment conversions across the whole office and then broken down by individual team member. While learning that my total office phone conversion rate was 24 percent was troubling, it didn't tell me if the problem was coming from one team member who happened to handle the majority of our calls or if it was systemic to all of the team members answering the phone. By tracking this percentage at both levels, you'll get the whole truth on what's going on and where you should turn your attention to provide additional support and training.

From our Call Tracker ROI data, the average fee-for-service general dental and specialty office is only converting around 34 percent of the phone calls answered into appointments. The average in-network or PPO-based dental office converts around 47–49 percent of their new patient calls into appointments. This is an interesting trend since if the office is in network with that patient's insurance carrier, there should typically be less of a barrier present to get them to schedule.

Since we provide our clients with an unbiased assessment of what's happening with their dental marketing across all media, we've been able to acquire data on how successful or unsuccessful many of the major dental marketing companies have been in the results they've delivered. The same is true for many of the current dental call centers our clients have used to help answer and schedule more of their new patient calls. On average these dental call centers are only able to schedule an appointment 17–24 percent of the time for fee-for-service offices and have similar percentages as most dental teams when it comes to in-network-based calls.

3. Reasons New Patient Calls Went Unscheduled

While understanding the new patient conversion percentage for the office and each of our team members is important to identify areas of lost opportunity, it is equally important to understand why the team was unable to make that patient an appointment. Sometimes there are instances where the team had no chance to schedule an appointment, a situation where it really wasn't possible, and thus they shouldn't be responsible for. Other times maybe they could have scheduled the appointment, had a few things been said differently. Regardless, knowing why they didn't schedule the appointment is the #1 piece of data you need to train your team and improve their performance on the telephone.

Let's look at some examples of when it might be out of our team members' hands, and they have little to no chance of scheduling an appointment. Perhaps the patient is being referred by a friend, but they got confused and mistakenly called the wrong office. Sometimes patients call asking to schedule for specific procedures, but your office doesn't provide those procedures. We hear this often with people calling to schedule to get their wisdom teeth removed, but that office doesn't offer wisdom teeth extractions. What if the patient needs a Medicaid- or Nationwide- or state-supported dental insurance provider, but your office doesn't participate in these programs?

On the flip side there are definitely situations where had our team member handled the call differently, an appointment could have been made. Price shoppers, for instance. People who call you up and ask, "How much is your crown?" or "How much for a cleaning?" Most teams tend to have a poor conversion rate on these patients, scheduling less than 20 percent of them into appointments.

The single biggest reason why the team doesn't schedule more appointments is centered on the insurance question that inevitably comes up during their conversation. Most notably when you are an out-of-network provider and the patient asks, "Do you take/accept my insurance?" Most of our team members have not been trained to understand the mindset of who this person is and why they are completely different than the person who asks, "Do you participate with my insurance?" or "Are you in network with my insurance?" We'll discuss my strategies on increasing your team's conversions during these challenging calls in the attendance section to come.

4. The Half Truth vs. the Whole Truth

This is all about giving credit where credit is due, to the best of your ability, figuring out what advertising source was responsible for attracting your new patient. It's a critical metric to track because it's the only way you'll be able to calculate the actual return on your marketing investment. Let's go back to the example I used earlier. A patient hears your advertisement on the radio. They like what they hear, but they were unable to write your number down because they are in their car driving. Luckily they remember your website address and are able to pull up your phone number from that site. When the call comes in, it gets logged as originated from your website, not from the radio. Who should get credit for this?

Did they do an organic Google search and find your website through these means? Did they see a Facebook ad or post? Did they get referred by another patient and went to your website to get your office information? In this example, it was the radio that was the lead source, not the website, but when you pull up your call tracking analytics, that's not what you'll see. This is why I call this the half-truth. Just looking at the total calls that come in by each marketing source is telling, but it doesn't tell you everything. Instead we need the whole truth. To the best of our ability, let's give credit where credit is due and track these leads back to the original source responsible for generating them.

To get the whole truth, we need to rely on our team's help. It is critical that for every potential new patient call – that means the ones they make an appointment for and the ones they don't make an appointment for – our team needs to ask each of these people a simple question: "How did you hear about us?" Once asked, they need to document this answer. Now since it's not in the team's habit to ask this question, I recommend printing the question out and putting it right in front of the phone as a reminder that they need to ask the question. That's a small thing you can do to remind them of its importance and increase the chance the question gets asked.

At Call Tracker ROI, our team tracks how often the team asks this question, as it should be 100 percent, and we track it by team member as well. The answers are factored into our reporting. For website calls, for instance, when people answer the question with, "Oh, I heard you on the radio" or "Matt and Ramona recommended you on their show," then my team knows to take that credit away from the website and give it back to the radio ad.

Before I started factoring in the whole truth, I was disappointed at the results my radio ads were generating. By looking at the calls from the radio tracking number alone, it was only 4–5 calls per month. Given what I was paying for those ads, the ROI didn't make sense, and I was almost to the point where I thought it wasn't working and was going to stop doing them. After I realized we were missing out on the whole truth and we started asking that question, it turned out that we were getting 20+ new patient calls per month because of those advertisements. By tracking the names of those who scheduled and figuring out the actual ROI, it suddenly changed from something that wasn't working well to something that worked extremely well. With the half-truth I found a go-to marketing medium that consistently provided me with a high ROI for over 10 years.

5. The Actual ROI

When most marketers talk about ROI, they are referring to the estimated ROI or the anticipated ROI. Dentists are surveyed and asked how much a new patient is worth to them. This is calculated by taking the total production or collections generated by your new patients for some specified period of time such as the first year. That amount is then divided by the total number of new patients who generated that revenue. Currently in the United States, the average new patient spends around $500 in the first year with that practice, an average calculated across all government-supported programs, dental insurance, and out-of-network providers.

Using this average new patient value, they will take the total number of calls that were logged to the tracking number associated with that advertising campaign and then project out that annual new patient value compared to the amount of money invested in that marketing piece. Example: I once ran a direct mail campaign for three months and then sat down with the marketing team to review my ROI. They showed me that I had 60 total calls that came from that advertisement over the three-month period of time. In my practice our average new patient value was over $1000 in the first year, so 60 new patient calls, each worth $1000 in year one, meant I could expect around $60,000 in total production. Given the ad campaign cost me $15,000 in total, that would give me an ROI of 4:1 based on their estimation.

This is another example of the half-truth in dental marketing analytics. On the surface, this estimation seems good, especially considering my benchmark for success of having a 3:1 ROI within the first six months. The reality is just the opposite. When I dug into the data on those phone calls, the story changed dramatically. Of those 60 calls, my team didn't answer 18 of them, leaving only 42 potential new patient opportunities. Of the 42 calls we answered, 5 were existing patients, people who called the wrong number, or were solicitors trying to sell us something, leaving us 37 potential new patient opportunities. Of those, we only scheduled 22 percent of them into actual appointments, meaning eight made an appointment, six of which actually showed up for their appointments over that three-month period. All in all, we collected just over $5000 on those patients. So when considering the $15,000 I spend on that campaign, our actual ROI was 1:3. Not to say that all of the fault of this fell on the marketing company, but if I didn't recognize the reality, then my new patient goals would have continued to elude me, I would not reach the production goals established for the practice, and I would have continued to waste marketing dollars in my attempts.

To calculate the actual ROI you must get the whole truth and know how many new patient opportunities really did come in from each ad source. As I mentioned in that radio ad example, the story can change dramatically once we have more complete and accurate information. Once you know the number of patients who came in from these sources, you should also have their name listed out with each source. Your team can do this with a Google or Excel spreadsheet or you can use the one Call Tracker ROI provides you. With each person's name listed by the ad source that attracted them, you want to document what they spend in your practice over some period of time. Typically, I use six months. In addition, I want to monitor any referrals they are responsible for. If they refer their spouse or kids, then any revenue generated from that should also be factored in and credited under this person's name. Once you have an accurate list of those who came into the office and what they spent, then you can calculate your actual ROI.

CONCLUSION

To truly making marketing a science instead of a mystery, you have to focus on getting data in these 5 areas, getting to the truth of what your actual ROI is and understanding what is and isn't working in your marketing efforts and why. Once you have the data, you can start making smarter decisions.

Let's look at an example of this from my celebrity endorsement radio ads. With this medium, I worked with Matt and Ramona, who ran the popular drive home from work radio show on a local FM station. Their program ran Monday through Friday from 2 p.m. to 6 p.m. With my advertising package, Matt and Ramona had recorded 30-second commercials on our behalf that aired throughout the day, night, and on the weekends. Three times a week they would pause their normal program and do a live one-minute commercial endorsement of my practices. All in all, there were 18–20 commercials that ran per week with an investment of $14,000 per month.

From the Call Tracker ROI data collected from my ads, it was clear that the spots were bringing in opportunity, but my team wasn't able to capitalize on it due to the missed call and poor phone conversion issues. Once I made changes to correct this, we went from seeing a couple of new patients each month to seeing well over 20 new patients a month from this source. Using the data on what these patients spent in my office over the next few months I was able to see a change in my ROI from a ratio less than 1 to a very solid 3:1.

As the next few months passed, the 3:1 ROI continued. Now that I was able to consistently count on this source for a good ROI, it allowed me the opportunity to test this medium to see if any changes would positively or negatively affect it. When doing a test in marketing, the goal is to change one variable per test and then track the effects of that one change and measure if the effect stays consistent before making any other changes.

When thinking about the mindset of the patients who came in from the radio ads, I discerned that they were definitely impulse shoppers, people who heard our advertisement, got excited, and immediately picked up the phone and called to schedule their appointment. You could look at the data on when our call volume from the radio ads spiked and correlate that with when our radio ads aired. One pattern that stood out to me was that we seemed to be capitalizing on these calls during business hours of Monday–Friday but were not answering the calls coming in on Saturdays or Sundays since we were closed.

As my first experiment, I decided to cut out all radio ads on the weekends. Based on the pattern of the patients we'd seen during the week, most likely these people were looking for same-day appointments, which we would not have been able to accommodate. By eliminating those weekend spots, I was able to reduce my monthly cost down to $11,000. After two months of tracking, the total number of new patients stayed consistent at 20+ per month, but because I had spent less overall to attract them, my ROI increased to 5:1, a significant change and improvement.

Next I decided to drop all radio commercials that aired before our offices opened or after our offices closed, reducing my monthly investment down to $8500. Again, the total new patient count stayed above 20 new patients per month, and the ROI rose again to just over 6:1. Over the next couple of months I continued the test and settled on a light schedule. I ran Matt and Ramona's recorded commercials during the drive into work show from 6 a.m. to 10 a.m. on Mondays, Tuesdays, and Wednesdays, on average running 2–3 times on each day during that time window. On these days, Matt and Ramona would do a one-minute live commercial for us during their normally scheduled program. My monthly investment decreased to $6000 with my new patient number not decreasing and the ROI rising to 8:1.

While there are many factors that helped me take my overall marketing budget from $36,000 per month and reduce that cost by 74 percent, tracking the actual ROI of my results was critical. Not only did it allow me to identify areas of improvement, but it also allowed me opportunities to make strategic changes, changes that could be well tracked and ultimately help me to become more efficient with all of the marketing media I was investing in.

Creating a Return for Your Marketing Investment

Throughout this book, I have discussed a myriad of ways to create new patient leads and opportunities, both their quantity and quality. This started with understanding how you can attract the potential new patients' attention by truly defining your brand and identifying what target market you'd like to promote that brand to.

In addition, I talked about how to take that brand and pair it with unique and differentiating messages, messages that speak to patient problems and the solutions you have to those problems. I discussed why it's important to know what stage of the buying cycle your potential new patient is in and how to add visual, written, emotional, and color content to garner their attention to your marketing pieces. At multiple times I commented on how you can add the behavioral science research of Dr. Robert Cialdini to influence more potential new patients to respond and how to leverage different types of call-to-action offers to incentivize them as well.

Once all of these points have been addressed, I turned your attention and outlined the different types of marketing media you could use to attract your target market, ultimately tracking five main areas to know what's working, what's not working, and why. If you follow the steps I laid out like a road map, you should be able to generate as many new patient opportunity leads as you desire and give yourself the best chance to achieve a significant return on your investment (ROI).

But as I originally mentioned at the start of the book, marketing is not a one-side coin. There is another side we need to consider. To create an opportunity is one thing, but if we can't capitalize on that opportunity, then it's lost to us, becoming a wasted marketing expense. To be truly effective and maximize your ROI, you also need to understand and have a plan to minimize your lost opportunity.

Part 3

Turning a Prospect into a Patient

There are four main areas where a new patient opportunity can be lost: on the telephone, at the chair, when they don't return, and in times of uncertainty. In this section I'm going to cover these critical touch points as they are vital to helping you maximize your marketing ROI. Let's look at this first area, which comes on the telephone.

Chapter 9
Converting Them on the Telephone

While technology such as online scheduling has made it easier for patients to make appointments with us and bypass communicating with our team altogether, the vast majority of opportunities still take place on the telephone. This means that we must have a good understanding of what's happening on these telephone calls and a clear directive on how we can maximize these leads, for if we fail in our efforts here, then our ROI will suffer and our marketing dollars will be wasted. To counter this effect, let's look at the three main areas in which lost opportunity is created on the telephone:

1. **Unanswered new patient calls;**
2. **Poor appointment conversion ratios;**
3. **Patients who don't show up for their appointments.**

From the data collected by my call tracker ROI service, the average dental office is not answering 33 percent of their marketing-based new patient phone calls. When they do answer, the team is only able to make an appointment approximately 34 percent of the time. If an appointment is made, the average no-show rate in most dental offices in the United States ranges between 17 and 24 percent. If the advertisement came from an online marketing source, that no-show rate can be well above 24 percent. The higher these percentages with any or all of these three areas, the less return you'll see for your marketing investment and the more money you'll have to spend to hit your new patient goals. Let's get into each of these three areas to define the challenges seen in more detail and discuss solutions to maximize your marketing ROI.

1. UNANSWERED NEW PATIENT CALLS

As mentioned earlier, even though we're in the age of technology and there is a shift to communicating with one another via text, email, or webchat, the telephone is still the predominate form of communication patients choose when contacting a dental office. While many like the conveniences of these nonverbal communication platforms for simple matters such as making a cleaning appointment, studies show that over 61 percent of consumers still prefer the old-fashioned phone call when they see their issue as being more complex in nature, such as when they have a specific dental issue or need. Of these, 75 percent believe that calling your office will get them the fastest response to their immediate concern.

This makes answering every new patient phone call critical to the success of your practice and to maximize your marketing's ROI. For our purposes, I'll define these unanswered or missed new patient calls as opportunity calls, where a potential new patient called your office but was unable to talk with one of your team members. Perhaps they got a busy signal, maybe the phone just rang and rang until they hung up due to frustration, or worst case it went right to voicemail. Regardless of the reason, the end result is the same. When calls go unanswered, it's a lost opportunity that will stifle the growth of your practice.

Voicemail is a great option for our existing patients, the ones we've already established a relationship with, as it allows patients who'd missed out on talking to your team to leave a message, advise us to their issue, and request a call back. With new patients, we don't have that relationship in place yet. Couple this with their limited time to search for a solution, and you can see the problem from their point of view. They're at work, with their kids, they're in the car running errands, or they have a thousand other to-dos on their list to complete today. They have a limited window of time to solve the problem at hand; this is, to find a dental office and make their appointment, which is now their top-of-mind focus, only to discover that when they call, your team doesn't answer.

From our data at Call Tracker ROI, we've tracked that 78 percent of new patients that call your office will not leave a voice mail. Of the 22 percent that will, almost 100 percent of those were patients that were referred to your practice. Overwhelmingly, regardless of why you couldn't answer, the end result is the same and was echoed in a popular study conducted about a year before Apple launched the first iPhone. This study showed that when a potential new client called your business, you had around seven minutes to return that call before they had moved onto to calling your competitor. More than 10 years of smartphone development later and with so much information available to us in a blink of an eye, that time to return those phone calls has diminished even more. Our best defense? To answer that call when it first comes in.

A. Popular Misconceptions about This Missed Call Issue

1. **My team answers all of our new patient calls**: When speaking to dentists at different dental meetings and conferences this is probably the most common response I get when I try to educate them about this missed new patient call issue. This is a feeling dentists have because they've made a mandate that their team must answer all new patient calls, and so it must be occurring. Sometimes it's because their team has informed them that they are answering all of their new patient phone calls. When I follow up their response with asking how many of them have actual tracking data to support their feeling, it's rare that I find someone who does. If you're not tracking this to get to the actual fact, then "you don't know what you don't know."

   Our worldwide data from Call Tracker ROI shows this a problem that plagues the vast majority of dental offices we've tracked. The average office, spending $0 to $2000 in marketing per month doesn't answer around a third of their new patient phone calls (Fig. 43). Those that spend over $2000 per month in marketing miss out on over 55 percent of their new patient opportunities (Fig. 44). This was worse in my own offices when I first started tracking my marketing results and I discovered we didn't answer over 224 new patient phone calls each month.

Day of the Week	Missed Calls	Answered Calls
Monday	6	10
Tuesday	1	11
Wednesday	4	10
Thursday	2	7
Friday	4	4
Saturday	2	0
Total	**19**	**42**

32% Not Answered

Figure 43. Call tracker ROI missed call by day example from a real office.

Day of the Week	Missed Calls	Answered Calls
Monday	11	7
Tuesday	6	12
Wednesday	12	10
Thursday	8	7
Friday	15	4
Saturday	8	0
Total	**63**	**41**

61% Not Answered

Figure 44. Call tracker ROI missed call by day example from a real office.

2. **I have 100 VoIP phone lines, so we don't miss calls**: In contrast to the standard analog phone line associated with your office telephone number, VoIP, or voice over Internet protocol, is a technology that converts your voice into a digital signal, allowing you to make calls directly from your computer, a VoIP phone, or other data-driven device. It allows an office to have an unlimited number of phone lines that ring to their office for a low monthly rate. With these additional phone lines also comes a false sense of security. The reality is that it doesn't matter how many phone lines you have or how sophisticated your phone system is to handle those calls because if you only have one person to physically answer that phone, you really only have one functional phone line that can be handled at any given time. Of course you could put numerous callers on hold while you attempt to answer more incoming calls, but this diminishes the patient experience and more are likely to hang up and find another dental office who can talk to them now.
3. **All of our missed calls happen when we're closed**: When doctors believe that their team is handling all of the new patient calls during business hours, that must mean that any unanswered calls occur when they are closed, after normal business hours or on the weekend. This is a natural assumption to make, but the facts from the tracking data paint a different reality. For the majority of offices, over 98 percent of their missed new patient calls occur during their normal business hours (Figs. 45, 46, and 47).

Missed Calls	
6 a.m.–7 a.m.	5
7 a.m.–8 a.m.	6
8 a.m.–9 a.m.	14
9 a.m.–10 a.m.	4
10 a.m.–11 a.m.	7
11 a.m.–12 p.m.	6
12 p.m.–1 p.m.	9
1 p.m.–2 p.m.	10
2 p.m.–3 p.m.	3
3 p.m.–4 p.m.	5
4 p.m.–5 p.m.	7
5 p.m.–6 p.m.	3
Total	**79**

Figure 45. Call tracker ROI missed new patient calls by hour of the day. Real office example.

Day of the Week	Missed Calls	Answered Calls
Monday	6	10
Tuesday	1	11
Wednesday	4	10
Thursday	2	7
Friday	4	4
Saturday	2	0
Total	**19**	**42**

Figure 46. Call tracker ROI missed new patient calls by day. Real office example showing the majority of calls go unanswered during days the practice is normally open, not when they are closed.

Day of the Week	Missed Calls	Answered Calls
Monday	3	27
Tuesday	2	30
Wednesday	8	25
Thursday	3	22
Friday	6	41
Saturday	2	13
Total	**24**	**158**

Figure 47. Call tracker ROI missed new patient calls by day. Real office example showing the majority of calls go unanswered during days the practice is normally open, not when they are closed.

B. Why Is It Happening?

1. **You don't know what you don't know**: For most offices there is a lack of evidence-based tracking to identify if a problem exists. That means the responsibility falls onto the team to become aware of any issues.
2. **Human nature**: Truthfully our team members don't bring this up because they are not aware of it either. Even if they were aware, it's typically not in our nature to shoot ourselves in our own foot. It would be rare to find a team member who come forward to bring up a potential missed call issue for fear they might lose their job. How would you respond if your team member came up to you this month and said, "Doctor, last month I wasn't able to answer 40 new patient phone calls." That probably would not be a good conversation for you or the team member who brought it up.
3. **Understaffed**: Many offices are understaffed at their front desk position. Hiring for revenue-generating positions such as the dental assistant and dental hygienist tends to become a priority, but we understaff the front desk in an attempt to keep our overhead and staff payroll under control.
4. **Increased call volume during high-demand times**: Most will find a pattern of unanswered calls when they first open their office (Fig. 48), during their lunch break when everyone is out of the office, and just before they close down for the day. At each of these critical points in the day, the team at the front desk is busy taking care of a flurry of other activities, leaving those new patient calls to go unanswered.
5. **Existing patient calls**: I've stated earlier that if a new patient call goes unanswered, the vast majority will not call you back. They will move on in their search until they find an office to accommodate them. Existing patients, on the other hand, will do just the opposite. If they call your office and don't get someone, many will hang up and call you right

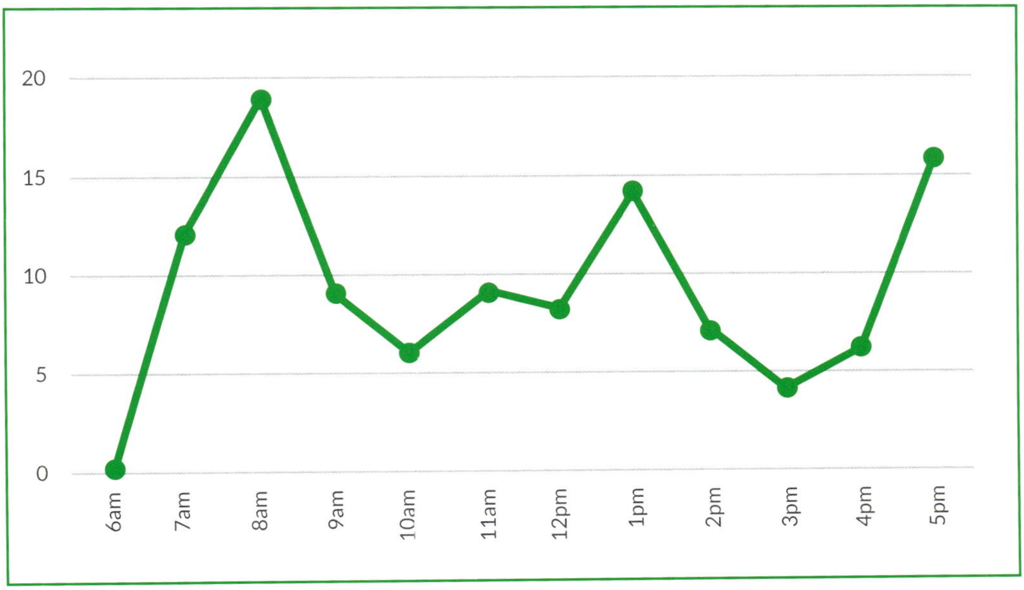

Figure 48. Call tracker ROI report graphic showing missed new patient calls by hour.

back, hoping they'll get through to you with a second call attempt. If not, maybe a third. In continually calling and trying to break through, they are actually making the problem worse for your team and for your chances of any potential new patient call getting through. From our studies at Call Tracker ROI, it seems that for every new patient call that comes in at any given moment there are three existing patients trying to call you at the same time. Remember, regardless of how many phone lines you have for them to call, there is still only one person directly working that phone, leaving your new patient with a 25 percent chance of reaching someone to discuss their dental need. With two team members up front, you've increased the odds so the new patient call has a 50 percent chance to be answered. I think most of us would prefer to increase these odds to much higher levels than that of a simple coin toss.

6. **Overworked**: Think of all of the duties the front desk team is responsible for at any given moment during the day. It takes this idea of multitasking to a whole new dimension. They are responsible for answering and scheduling new patient and existing patient phone calls, making confirmation calls for upcoming appointments, and calling insurance companies to verify dental benefits only to be left on hold for 20–30 minutes at a time trying to complete their task. Then there are the patients in the office to contend with: checking them into the office, possibly even presenting them with financial options concerning the treatment diagnosed and planned by the dentist. Then they must be checked out, taking their payment for today's visit and making sure they are scheduled for their next visit.

C. What Can Be Done to Correct This Issue?

1. **Get the data you need to make smarter decisions**: Either through your current phone system or using a call tracking service, track your incoming new patient calls and get the facts on what's happening with your new patient opportunities. Don't assume it's all good and being handled. Know it.
2. **Understand it's not your team's fault**: As the leader of the practice, it's ours for not recognizing this is a problem and giving our team the tools they need to correct it. When I realized my own team was struggling to answer our new patient calls, I discovered the root cause of the problem was out of their control entirely because of all of the activities they were forced to juggle throughout the day.
3. **Let the data justify your next expense**: When my data showed me that my offices couldn't answer 200+ new patient calls a month, the first thing I did was hire an additional team member at each office and dedicated them to answering those calls. With three people answering the phones, now we had a 75 percent chance of answering a new patient phone call when it came in. Yes, it increased payroll, but my profitability increased. Why? The ROI is simple. If each new patient is worth $1000 to your practice in the first year and a new team member can help you bring in 20 more of those a month, that additional revenue you'd generate will more than justify the increase in payroll that results. If you have one person at the front, maybe your data justifies hiring a second. If you have two team members at your front desk, like I did, maybe the data can give you confidence to hire a third. If it's an investment, you should see an increase in new patients, an increase in your marketing ROI, and an increase in your monthly revenue.

4. **Eliminate the check out**: If we decrease the volume of patients who need to check out at the front desk, we'll free up the team's time so they'll have more opportunity to answer any new patient calls that come in. We can eliminate this check out in two ways. First, we can make sure we schedule any future appointments for them at the chair. Second, consider having the patient prepay before you schedule their appointment, or perhaps you can collect their portion due for today's visit at the chair. Credit card processing services such as Square allow you to use a smart phone for patient purchases. The account can be set up with ease and purchases completed anywhere in your office. So why not do it at the chair? If their next appointment is scheduled at the chair and the financial responsibility for today has already been taken care of, either through prepayment or taking the patient's payment at the chair, then the patient can bypass the front desk altogether, improving their overall experience. At the same time, by eliminating the wait at the front desk to check out, you free up your team's time to be ready to handle those new patient phone calls.
5. **Leverage technology**: Let people communicate with you in the way they want to communicate with you, not the way we're currently forcing them to. By giving our patients other ways to schedule their appointment beside calling our office, we'll decrease the amount of phone volume traffic and further increase the chance a new patient call can be answered. Let's look at a couple of ways we can do this:

a. **Live chat**: Studies show that 78 percent of consumers below the age of 50 prefer to chat with someone to make an appointment versus having to call them. By offering a HIPAA-compliant live chat feature on our website, we're giving existing and potential new patients the opportunity to communicate with us in their preferred route, making them an appointment but without having to tie up the phone lines in the process. Offices that we've tracked are consistently scheduling 8–12 new patients a month through this chat feature. What I find most significant here is the number of existing patients scheduling via this route. That means less of them calling in and tying up your new patient phone lines and answering capability.

b. **Online scheduling**: There are numerous online scheduling platforms available that can directly communicate with your office's practice management scheduling system. These portals can be embedded into your website, just as a live chat module would. You can assign certain blocks of appointment times for the dentist's chair or hygiene and you can open these up to new and existing patients who prefer making their appointments through this medium. I highly recommend using one of these services and want you to encourage your existing patients to schedule their future appointments through this route. As I stressed above, if we can decrease the volume of existing patients trying to call in to us, we'll reduce the amount who hang up and continue to call back, further increasing the chance that any new patient calls that come through will be answered.

c. **Recapture missed calls**: Leverage technology to put yourself in a position to be able to recapture any opportunity call that was missed. Caller ID is a service most major phone carriers provide for your phone line. With it, you'll be alerted that a call was missed and what that telephone number was of the person who tried to call you. If your team gets tied up, say being on hold with a dental insurance company, once their call ends, they should immediately check to see if any calls went unanswered. There are also some dental technology companies that can be tied into your phone system and will tell you if the call that came in was from one of your existing patients or a potential new patient.

At Call Tracker ROI, we patented a unique missed call text alert feature (Fig. 49) to help teams recapture these missed new patient call opportunities. If a call that comes in from one of our tracking numbers is unanswered for any reason, a text alert goes out to the dentist and any of their team members at the front desk within seven seconds of that occurring. Included in this text alert is the caller ID data, so you'll know the name of the potential new patient who called, their telephone number, and what advertising source they called from.

If the potential new patient called you from a cell phone, as most people do nowadays, then they would receive a customized text alert on behalf of your office within seven seconds as well. Remember the study I cited earlier that told us if you miss a new client call that you only had about seven minutes to reach out to recapture them before they'd moved onto looking for another office. With the data we've collected from those using our missed call text alert feature, we've found that potential new patients will wait 20 minutes and up to an hour for you to call them back.

Why? Because you satisfied their search. That's what was top of their mind and important in that moment. They needed to find a dentist and make an appointment. When they received your text alert that told them you were sorry you missed their call but would call them back shortly, that communication stopped their search and allowed them to move their focus to other items on their current to-do list. It's unrealistic to think that your team will be able to answer 100 percent of your new patient phone call opportunities. With this technology, regardless of what led to them being unable to answer the call when it first came in, it's 100 percent realistic that they can now attempt to recapture any lost opportunities.

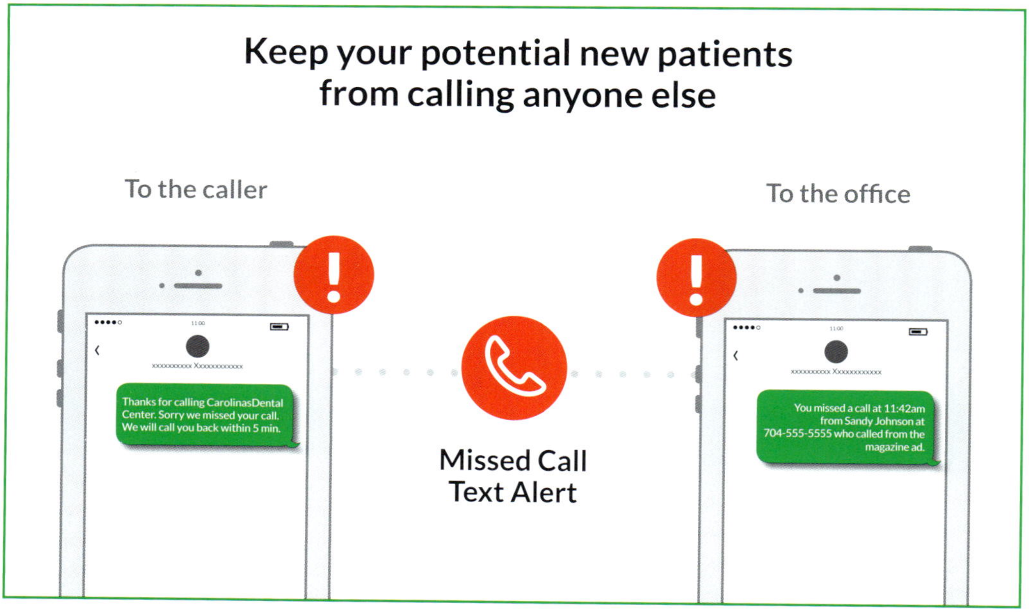

Figure 49. Graphic demonstrating Call Tracker ROI's dual missed call text alert feature. Within seven seconds, if a call goes unanswered for any reason, the team at the office and the potential new patient all receive a text alert.

d. **Outsource responsibilities**: There are few people who have a real talent for multi-tasking. The act itself is impossible as there is no way to actually do two things at once. Behavioral science studies tell us what actually is happening during multitasking events is that people are constantly shifting their focus and attention between the items they're working on. Even those who are instinctively built to have more energy to shift their focus between their tasks eventually will fall short, compromising their productivity in the process. Instead of putting our team members in a position to constantly fail, consider outsourcing or automating some of their duties. By taking certain items off their plate, you're freeing up their time, mental energy, and capacity to be more productive at the remaining items they have to focus on.

In my office, I automated all of the upcoming patient confirmation calls. We had a software program that would review our schedule and then send out text and email confirmations to those who had upcoming appointments. When a patient texted or emailed a confirmation, the software updated our practice management system so we could see that confirmation reflected in our schedule. In addition to the texts and emails, this software program recorded the voice of one of our team members and then used that recorded voice to make phone calls to our patients, asking them to punch in the #1 if they would be able to make their appointment or the #2 if they could not make it, again updating their status in our system once complete. Using this automated platform, our team went from spending 60–90 minutes performing these tasks themselves, to now less than 5–10 minutes to make phone calls to the few who didn't confirm their appointment through one of these three automated means, freeing up more of their time to answer new patient phone calls.

I mentioned earlier about the significant amount of time that was needed for my team to verify dental insurance benefits for patients, many times being left on hold for 10–20 minutes until they could talk to a live person and get an answer. If you're only getting five new patients a month, this may not seem overwhelming, but when your new patient numbers rose to over 150 per month, suddenly it was no small task to be completed. Fortunately, I found a company that could take all of the insurance tasks off my team's plate, from the verification of benefits to filing of the claims as well as follow-up if any claims went unpaid by the insurance carrier. Before using this group, I had a dedicated insurance coordinator who handled these tasks. When she decided to leave her position, many of the responsibilities fell to my other team members. After outsourcing all of these tasks, I freed up over 30 hours per week for my team, avoided having to hire someone to replace the team member who moved on, and ended up spending less per month than what I was paying out in salary for that position. A win-win by all accounts.

Whether you automate or outsource, taking away time-consuming tasks will improve your team's morale and will increase their happiness and productivity levels. You'll also give them back more time to answer and schedule any new patient phone calls that come in while simultaneously freeing up more of their time to focus on what I consider to be one of the most important aspects of their job: making sure the existing patients in the practice are taken care of, that they are communicated with and leave with their next appointment scheduled.

6. **Utilize a patient-scheduling service**: Generically, these services are referred to as dental call centers, but I break them down to differentiate them as call centers (CC) and scheduling services (SS). Call centers are services that take your calls. They'll answer calls for you when your office is closed, and they handle overflow calls that ring to them only after two or three ring attempts at your office. Most of the time they are not directly tied into your practice management software, so if it's after hours, they'll take messages and relay them to the dentist on call or leave messages for the team to return in the morning. If during business hours, they'll talk to the patient while they attempt to connect that person to one of your team members in the office. While these centers can provide a valuable service to dental offices, without an ability to schedule appointments, there are still numerous new patient opportunities that are lost.

   Scheduling services, in contrast, not only answer your new patient phone calls, they are tied into your practice management software and can physically make an appointment on your behalf. These services can schedule new or existing patients. They can be second in line to your team, which is a backup position. If a call rings two or three times at your office and goes unanswered, the call automatically forwards to a dedicated line at the SS for them to answer. You could also choose to have the SS be first in line to your team. In this capacity, when a call comes into the office, it forwards directly to the SS first and only rings at your office if the SS is unable to answer it.

   With any SS you use, you still have to be aware of the results they are providing for you. If they do their jobs well, utilizing these services should be investments that provide a great ROI on top of their cost. If they are able to help you answer and schedule more new patient phone calls than your team could have done on their own, the revenue generated by the practice should automatically rise. If they are able to schedule more new patients from your advertising sources, then your marketing ROI will only improve. In short, SS should make all of your marketing efforts more productive, but just as we discussed in the attraction stage, you must track and have data on the results they are providing you.

   About five years ago, I turned my attention to studying the results of all the major dental call centers and scheduling services operating at that time. Fortunately, I was able to get an inside look at these companies' real results by using my Call Tracker ROI (CTROI) service. My clients were dentists who were using CTROI to track the effectiveness of their marketing campaigns as well as track how well their team answered and scheduled new patient phone calls. A large percentage of them were also outsourcing their new patient

Week of the Month	Missed Calls	Answered Calls
March 1, 2016 – March 5, 2016	9	4
March 6, 2016 – March 12, 2016	9	8
March 13, 2016 – March 19, 2016	12	9
March 20, 2016 – March 26, 2016	2	11
March 27, 2016 – March 31, 2016	12	3
Total	**44**	**35**

Figure 50. **Call tracker ROI report showing missed calls by weeks of the month.**

calls to the various CC and SS. With the CTROI data, I was able to study how effective these companies were handling new patient phone calls, to discover their missed new patient call rate and identify how effective they were at making patient appointments from these calls they answered. Across the board, the data was disappointing at best.

Figure 50 is an example of new patient data from one of the popular dental scheduling services we tracked. This SS was second in line. If a new patient call went unanswered after ringing three times at the dentist's office, the call was forwarded to the SS to be answered and an attempt was made to make an appointment. Out of the 79 total new patient opportunity calls that came in during the month of March, the SS was unable to answer 55.7 percent of the calls. Being second in line should have meant less call volume the SS would have to attend to compared to being first in line and handling all of the incoming calls. Less call volume should have meant that they should have been able to handle most of these incoming calls. The reality, time and time again from our analysis showed that these services were unable to do this consistently for their clients.

3/23/16	Wed,	23 Mar	2016	14:00	0	1 8772528569	0:00:00	0:00:28
3/23/16	Wed,	23 Mar	2016	17:00	0	1 8772528569	0:00:00	0:01:10
3/24/16	Thu.	24 Mar	2016	07:00	0	1 8772528569	0:00:00	0:01:02
3/24/16	Thu.	24 Mar	2016	10:00	0	1 8772528569	0:00:00	0:00:15
3/24/16	Thu.	24 Mar	2016	10:00	0	1 8772528569	0:00:00	0:00:29
3/24/16	Thu.	24 Mar	2016	10:00	0	1 8772528569	0:00:00	0:00:27
3/24/16	Thu.	24 Mar	2016	10:00	0	1 8772528569	0:00:00	0:00:33
3/24/16	Thu.	24 Mar	2016	11:00	0	1 8772528569	0:00:00	0:00:24
3/24/16	Thu.	24 Mar	2016	12:00	0	1 8772528569	0:00:00	0:01:13
3/24/16	Thu.	24 Mar	2016	14:00	0	1 8772528569	0:00:00	0:00:05
						261		
3/19/16	Sat,	19 Mar	2016	09:00	0	1 8772528569	0:00:19	0:00:36
3/2/16	Wed,	2 Mar	2016	18:00	0	1 8772528569	0:00:24	0:00:39
3/2/16	Wed,	2 Mar	2016	13:00	0	1 8772528569	0:00:31	0:00:52
3/14/16	Mon.	14 Mar	2016	15:00	0	1 8772528569	0:00:33	0:01:04
3/21/16	Mon.	21 Mar	2016	14:00	0	1 8772528569	0:00:39	0:01:02
3/2/16	Wed.	2 Mar	2016	15:00	0	1 8772528569	0:00:53	0:01:02
3/9/16	Wed.	9 Mar	2016	11:00	0	1 8772528569	0:00:54	0:01:16

Figure 51. Report from a dental call center showing they were unable to answer 261 total calls for their client dental office.

In a different office around the same time period, one of our CTROI clients was using a popular SS to answer existing and new patient phone calls on their behalf (Fig. 51). The SS was second in line again and should have provided backup to the dental team if they were unable to answer the call. Again they were unable to do so. In this case the SS was unable to answer 261 out of a total of 305 new and existing patient calls that month, an 86.2 percent missed patient call rate. Adding existing patient calls in addition to answering new patient calls only compounded the fundamental problem these SS have and led to a massive lost opportunity for this practice.

Staff Efficiency Analytics				
Staff Name	**Total**	**Booked**	**Not Booked**	**Closing%**
Abraham	1	1	0	100.000%
Jennette	1	1	0	100.000%
Nicole	1	0	1	0.000%
Shey	2	0	2	0.000%
Usenia	1	0	1	0.000%
Yaseni	1	0	1	0.000%
Total	**35**	**17**	**18**	**48.571%**

Figure 52. Call tracker ROI report showing the appointment scheduling rate of a popular call center's scheduling agents. The office's team members are blocked out in the green area.

In this office example (Fig. 52), I looked at the appointment conversion ratios of the SS agents assigned to my CTROI client's account. The SS was assigned to the second in line or backup position to the dental team. The green bolded boxes were data on the team member's appointment conversion percentages. Those remaining were agents of the SS. Some showed great results while others struggled. Overall, the dentist's team was able to make an appointment for 53.7 percent of these new patient opportunities. The SS agents only made an appointment 28.6 percent of the time, producing the overall average of 48.57 percent conversion rate shown above.

After reviewing hundreds of examples like these above, it was clear that the dental call centers had some major flaws. Yes, it was probably still better to use them over no one attempting to answer the phone call, but with these results I don't believe it was much better. That's why I decided to create Golden Goose Scheduling, a scheduling service dedicated to quality, built to actually solve this new patient phone call lost opportunity issue that's plaguing our industry. Regardless of what CC or SS you use, here are my tips on what criteria is needed to make these services a productive investment for your practice.

a. **Focus solely on new patient calls**: As we saw in the example above, every time the dentist used a service that attempted to handle their new and existing patients, the number of missed calls for both skyrocketed and the conversion rates for making appointments plummeted. Existing patients will continue to call you back to try to schedule their appointment. They'll leave you a voicemail asking you to call them back. There is no real need to outsource these calls, unless you physically don't have enough team members working for you at your front desk. If you have enough team members and have freed up their time by automating and outsourcing other tasks, they should have more than enough time to address your existing patient call volume. With existing patients handled, you can now turn your attention to look for a scheduling service that has a team who only focus on answering and scheduling your new patient calls, whether first in line or as backup to your team.

b. **Focus on quality control and training**: The average dental SS reviews less than 10 percent of the calls their agents handle. One of the largest SSs I talked to informed me that they only review 2 out of 200 calls each agent receives per day. That's only 1 percent of their total calls, many of which were picked at random and were used to determine that agent's pay via a bonus system that is based on their performance on those calls. After listening to 1000s of recorded phone calls from all types of dental offices, it's abundantly clear to me that there are different challenges to scheduling. Those challenges are directly related to that practice's business model and the type of patients they serve. A practice that is a provider for state-supported insurance plans such as Medicaid, for instance, will have a fairly low barrier to scheduling these patients because everything is paid for by the government.

On the other end of the spectrum, an office that is fee-for-service or out-of-network with all insurance providers may have a larger barrier to scheduling patients who have dental insurance of some kind to use. Unfortunately for these scheduling agents, it's the luck of the draw on how their performance is measured. With only 1 percent of the data being considered, it's the half-truth, telling part but not all of the story. Some agents may have had calls evaluated from Medicaid-based practices they answered while others may have been evaluated on insurance-based or out-of-network offices. Ultimately, you're not getting a true sense of what that scheduling agent is telling their dentist client's potential new patients or how successful they are or what challenges to scheduling they are facing.

Instead, look for an SS whose focus is on quality control and training from the whole truth. At Golden Goose Scheduling, we have quality control managers who listen to and review every call where our agent does not make an appointment for our dental client. These are the most critical calls that need to be analyzed and then reviewed with the agents, ones that have the biggest opportunity for training and growth and can help our agents schedule more new patients for the dental offices we work with.

c. **Don't throw bodies at the problem**: In general, the more agents you have trying to make appointments for an office, the worst the results for the whole group tend to be. We saw an example of that above. Some of the SSs I interviewed told me that they could have 15–20 different agents answering the telephone on behalf of a dental office. If the focus is on existing patient calls, then this makes sense. If the focus is on new patient calls, there is no way all of these agents have a good understanding about the office they are scheduling for. If they don't really know anything about the dentist or the team, how can they connect with the new patient calling and help guide them to an appointment? Instead, look for an SS that will limit the number of agents responsible for your office. Four agents should be more than enough to handle the capacity of your practice. Especially if it's a second in line or backup position to your team. Each of these agents can be well versed and understand exactly who they are scheduling for.

d. **Select an SS that understands the science of scheduling appointments**: Scheduling a new patient appointment is not necessarily an easy thing. I assumed it was until I discovered my own team members were only scheduling 24 percent of our new patient opportunities. The more I researched why this was, the more I realized that just because they called interested in getting a new patient appointment doesn't necessarily mean they're committed to making one. Instead, we need team members trained in the barriers patients put up to scheduling and how they can help them get around them. They need to learn how to connect with the caller to invoke the liking principle and promote and endorse the dentist's authority as a dental expert in their community. They need to understand how to leverage social proof while drawing attention to the scarcity of appointment times available, all while asking strategic commitment questions, which set the stage for the person who schedules to show for their appointment. We'll cover this topic in more detail in the coming sections.

When you find a scheduling service that excels at those points, the results for your practice can be game changing. Let's look at a couple of examples from some Golden Goose Scheduling (GGS) clients. At an office outside of Tampa, Florida, a dentist was investing $5000/month into a three-panel brochure-style direct mail campaign. Through those efforts, the practice was seeing about nine new patients per month, giving that office just over a 1:1 ROI. When the CTROI data was analyzed, it became clear that there were opportunities being lost from answering and scheduling the new patient calls. Knowing that our team have the highest appointment conversion rates of any SS currently in the industry, the office hired Golden Goose Scheduling and routed us all of the new patient calls from this marketing source tracking number. In the first month, with no additional advertising dollars spent, GGS scheduled 32 new patients from that same direct mail piece. By the third month, we scheduled over 61 new patients per month from that same marketing medium, taking their ROI from 1:1 to over 7:1. With the average office only scheduling 34 percent of their new patient opportunities into appointments, having an SS that is well trained can have a huge impact on your marketing ROI.

In this example (Fig. 53) we have a different practice that was spending a similar amount but spread out between two marketing media: $5000 a month divided between direct mail

Tracking Ad Source	Opportunities
Website - Direct Landing	2
Yelp	9
Website - Organic Search	5
New Patient Flyers Mailer	1
Total	**17**

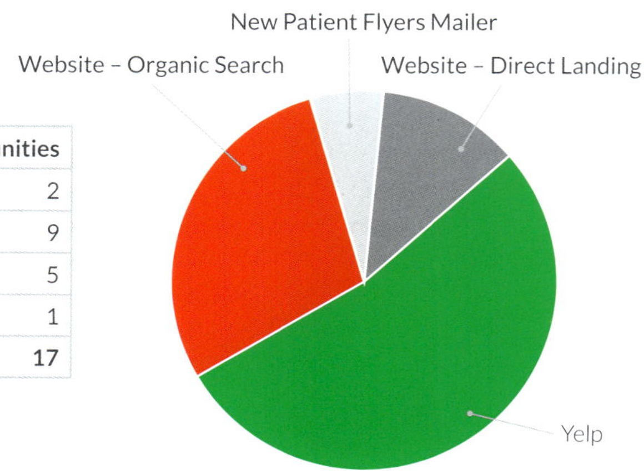

Figure 53. Call tracker ROI report showing only 17 of the 59 new patient opportunities made an appointment.

flyers and digital SEO efforts. This office had hired another popular SS to help them capitalize on the new patient opportunities created. From these efforts, approximately 59 new patient opportunities were generated. Of those the SS was able to schedule 17, or 28.6 percent, into appointments. After using CTROI to track the results of this SS, the dentist decided to try Golden Goose Scheduling. Using our dedicated new patient scheduling service, GGS scheduled 78.3 percent of the new patient opportunities that came from these ad sources the following month, scheduling 47 new patient appointments as a result. This was a 280 percent increase in new patients, which amplified this dentist's marketing ROI from the same amount of marketing dollars invested.

Dentists everywhere are looking for ways to attract more new patients. While spending more money and investing in additional marketing media is one option, the smart dental marketer looks for other areas of opportunity. Using the strategies outlined above, you can take steps to recapture some of this lost opportunity by answering more new patient phone calls. Doing so will automatically help you get more new patients and prevent you from wasting your marketing dollars

2. POOR PATIENT CONVERSION RATIOS

By implementing the above measures, your team is sure to be in a position to answer more new patient calls. Now comes the real challenge, one that the majority of dental offices across the world seem to be facing: that daunting task of making a new patient appointment.

On the surface, it seems as if it should be pretty straightforward. You've taken the time to create quality content in your advertisements to generate their interest. They've most likely

New Patient Opportunities	135	Ratios
Appointments Booked	48	35.56%
Appointments Not Booked	87	64.44%

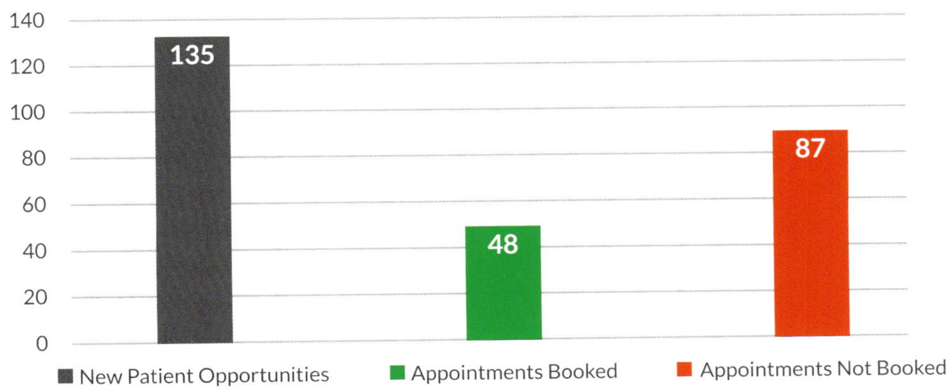

Figure 54. **Call tracker ROI report showing total office new patient appointment conversion percentages.**

taken the time to research your practice, looking at your website, checking for testimonials, and searching for other patient reviews on Google, Yelp, and other similar platforms. By picking up the phone to call you, they have made a commitment to getting their dental needs addressed somewhere. Right now you're the likely candidate. They've taken the time to find your phone number and are calling you because they want to schedule. Making the appointment at this point should be a given.

At least that's what I thought about new patient call conversions for my team. The reality was quite the opposite. As I've mentioned, when my team was able to answer these calls, they were only able to make an appointment around 24 percent of the time, meaning over 7 out of 10 patients who called and were interested left the call without scheduling an appointment. Across the United States, the average new patient phone conversion rates still hover between 34 and 36 percent (Fig. 54). This is for the hardest category to schedule, the patient who has dental insurance but the office is not a provider or in their dental network.

For offices that are in-network providers with a patient's insurance plan, there is one less barrier to overcome, so you'd expect the averages to be significantly higher. On average, these offices make an appointment between 47 and 49 percent of the time, still not a majority. In offices that are in network with state-supported insurance plans such as Medicaid, the lowest barrier to scheduling, they are booking at a rate above 97 percent.

A. Why Offices Struggle

1. **Lack of training**: In a popular dental survey taken in late 2010, less than 5 percent of all dental offices across the United States had some kind of formal telephone training given to their teams. For most, it was on-the-job training, meaning we hired them, put them up at the front desk, and instructed them to "schedule the patients" when they called, assuming it was an easier task than it actually is.

2. **Patient objections**: Because of this lack of training, our teams don't have a good understanding about the patient's mindset who is calling to make an appointment. Many times that patient may be afraid due to past anxieties, they may be concerned about getting the work done for the cheapest price, they may be wondering if they've selected the right office for their care, or they might be focused on getting in as soon as possible. Regardless of the reason, when they are calling they have a mindset pre-established. That mindset might create barriers to scheduling if the team isn't prepared to handle them.

3. **Team bias**: With enough time working in a dental office, there is a trend to start to classify people in certain categories. Good patient vs bad patient. Shows up on time vs always late. Accepting of treatment vs resistant to treatment. A person who is concerned about their dental insurance vs a person who isn't concerned about dental insurance reimbursements. Someone who knows what's wrong with their teeth, who understands their current tooth situation vs someone who is clueless about their current dental state. The more experience team members have interacting with patients, the more natural it becomes to start to classify who you're speaking with into one of these categories. The problem with these assumptions is that often they can be wrong, and it's our team that is responsible for putting up the barriers to scheduling these appointments.

4. **Distractions**: At any given time the front desk team member could be splitting their focus between multiple tasks at the same time. Perhaps they are checking a patient into the office or trying to check someone out of the practice, and the phone rings. Maybe they are on the phone talking to an existing patient trying to schedule their next treatment appointment, and a new patient call comes in. What are they to do? Put the existing patient on hold, as they may be more understanding of this? If so, the longer they put that person on hold, the more upset they may become, ultimately leading them to rush through the new patient phone call.

   They might not really be in the right mindset or have the time in their mind to handle potential questions this new caller may have. Regardless of the reason, the team up front is constantly having their focus pulled in multiple directions. When distractions are present, the likelihood of the appointment going unscheduled is high. The good news is this can be remedied hiring more team members and having them focus on a small number of responsibilities vs having them be responsible for everything, all at once. You could consider outsourcing certain tasks altogether and get more off their plate, limiting the distractions and freeing up their time to be ready to properly handle these new patient phone calls as they come in.

5. **No accountability**: "Out of sight, out of mind" is a popular phrase that comes to mind in this circumstance. Just like with the missed call issue, if you're not tracking your new patient phone calls, then you will be completely unaware of any conversion issues present. Plus, without tracking, you're not fully aware if your conversion problem is with all of your team members answering the phone or is it just one of them who struggles, the one who happens to answer most of your new patient phone calls.

Staff Name	Total	Booked	Not Booked	Ratio
Rachel	13	11	3	84.62%
Janis	23	3	20	13.04%
Paula	7	2	5	28.57%
Krista	30	13	17	43.33%

Figure 55. Call tracker ROI report showing average scheduling success by team member.

In the example of Figure 55, one team member is having great success while the other team members are struggling to some extent. The good news is that tracking systems can get you all of this data so you know with certainty how your new patient phone calls are handled and help identify any bottlenecks that need to be addressed.

B. Becoming a Telephone Maestro

A maestro is an artistic master: someone who is skilled enough to be considered an artistic genius. In music, we think of them as being distinguished musicians, usually the conductor of large symphony orchestras. Taking one music class or art class can teach you a lot, but it won't make you a maestro. "Maestro" (which comes from Italian) is reserved for people with an enormous amount of skill and talent. It's not achieved overnight but through time, experience, and having a fundamental knowledge of the ins and outs from the different elements that make up their craft.

In dentistry, it should be our goal to have anyone handling our new patient calls become maestros at scheduling. New patients are the catalyst for growth in your business, they can make or break your marketing ROI, and they are too important to not put your greatest effort into capturing. Let's look at the six elements your team needs to master to get the new patient phone call scheduled, the key factors my scheduling agents at Golden Goose Scheduling use to maintain the highest conversion rates in the dental call center industry—the training I gave my own team back in the day to satisfy objections and overcome any personal bias they had toward who they were speaking to, the principles that helped them raise their conversions from 24 percent to consistently being above 80 percent, helping me increase my new patient count from 60/month to averaging over 300 fee-for-service patients per month. To get the phone call scheduled, your team will need to become a maestro in these areas:

- **Get the basics;**
- **Get control of the phone call;**
- **Get their concerns answered;**
- **Get them from interested into committed;**
- **Get any additional info needed;**
- **Get it all together.**

1. Get the Basics

Be in a state of readiness

If you don't know when your available appointment times are, how can you effectively guide your patient to them? With readiness, I want my team to have a written out list of the next available appointment times for both the doctors and hygiene schedules for the next two weeks. Before the start of each day, the list is updated and a new two-week period selected. I have my team write this out and have it in front of them so they are ready when new patients call. Once an appointment is taken, it's scratched off their list and updated with any other team member's list who may be scheduling that day.

I also informed my team to let me know when they are unable to offer any appointment times during a two-week period. If we start booking patients out further than two weeks, then the practice is most likely suffering from a capacity issue, which may need to be addressed first before new growth can be seen. By keeping their focus on this important metric, they will help alert me if we begin to have a consistent problem that needs to be addressed.

Since distraction is a major causative factor that decreases your chances of scheduling, it should be the team's goal to limit these as much as possible. Avoid multitasking, especially during the high call volume times when the office first opens, during lunch, and just before closing. By eliminating distractions during these times, you'll be ready to focus all of your attention on the new patients calling in.

Another way the team can be ready to handle the new patient call is to know when it's actually a new patient calling. When the phone rings, you really don't know until you answer it. It could be an existing patient calling, it could be a vendor, or someone making a sales call to your office.

Of these, there is no greater priority than the new patient call. Today's VoIP technology and new phone systems allow you to segment out your new patient calls from all others in two ways.

First, you can turn your main phone line into an IVR tree: An interactive voice response (IVR), also known as phone tree, allows customers calling your telephone system to interact with voice menus using their phone's keypad. You can have your team members record the messages heard by patients who call in: "Thank you for calling Carolinas Dental Center. Press 1 if you are an existing patient. Press 2 if you are a new patient. Press 3 for all other calls." Each of these options can forward to your main office line or a dedicated scheduling service.

Once you have the new patient callers separated out, you can have a unique ring set up, one for the existing patients and other calls that come in and another one for the new patients. Now the team can be more aware when a new patient call rings through. For example, if they are on hold with an insurance company and the new patient ring is heard, they'll know to put that call on hold or hang up so they can move over to answer the priority call coming in. When your team is in a proper state of readiness, more new patient calls will get scheduled.

Identify the call type

If your office is not set up or capable of having a unique ring for new patients, the team's first priority when answering an incoming call should be to identify why they are calling. Is it a sales call that needs to end as soon as possible or is it an existing patient or potential new patient? Let's say the phone call goes something like this:

***Team*: Thank you for calling Carolinas Dental Center. This is Amber; how can I help you?**

Patient: Hello, this is Sally Jones, and I'd like to make an appointment to get my teeth cleaned.

Is this an existing patient calling or is it a new patient? If it's an existing patient, we'd like them to feel recognized and acknowledged as such and not made feel like a stranger at the practice. If you're not sure if they are new or existing, you can ask this question to quickly decipher their status:

***Team*: Great, I can help you with making that appointment, Sally. When was the last time you visited us?**

From here, the patient will alert you of their last appointment time, clueing you in that they are an existing patient or they'll let you know that this will be their first visit:

Patient: Oh, I've never been to your practice before. This will be my first time.

Now you can be better prepared to continue this call to completion.

Avoid providing poor customer service

First impressions are critical on these new patient calls. Established early on in the conversation, they can make or break your chance of successfully scheduling the appointment. To increase your chances of scheduling, you want to avoid providing a poor patient experience. One mistake offices make that will ruin that experience is putting the new patient on hold.

According to research from Velaro, all it takes is waiting on hold for one minute, and almost 60 percent of customers will hang up. In a different survey of more than 2500 consumers, nearly 60 percent of respondents believe that one minute is too long to be on hold, PRWeb reports. In addition, 32.3 percent of consumers reported that they believe that customer service departments should be answering immediately—with no hold time. When asked how long they were willing to be put on hold, about a third of respondents said they're not willing to wait at all, 27.6 percent said one minute, and only 4.1 percent said they'd wait as long as it took.

If you find yourself in a situation where you have no choice but to put the caller on hold, you should instead end the call and offer to call that patient back. A marketing survey that polled over 1100 consumers found that the majority, 63 percent, preferred a callback over being put on hold. I discussed another example of this in the previous section with Call Tracker ROI's dual missed call text alert feature. When a call goes unanswered by the office and the patient receives a text alert message from your team, that communication satisfied their search, and they were happy to wait for you to call them back.

Attempt to provide good customer service

Providing a great customer experience helps ensure a great first impression and sets the stage for more appointments to be scheduled. If possible, avoid using negatives such as "I don't know" or "that's not my department." Instead, put a positive connotation on it. Instead of "I don't know," try saying, "I will find that answer for you or find someone who can answer it for you." Instead of "that's not my department", try saying, "I'd be happy to transfer you to the person you need to speak with."

People can hear and sense harmony and chaos. When you answer the phone, what are your potential patients hearing? Someone who sounds unhappy or annoyed? One who feels bothered that you're taking them away from other things they are working on? If so, this will not be a great patient experience. Instead, we want to put our best foot forward. Patients should be able to hear our smile, meaning we should be positive and sound upbeat and excited to be talking to them. One way we can do this is by welcoming them to your office: "Let me be the first to welcome you to our practice." A little kindness and positivity goes a long way. Remember Cialdini's principle of reciprocity. You get back more of what you put out there. If you're the first to be welcoming, to show an interest in that potential new patient, then they are more likely to return the favor and schedule that appointment with you.

Always give the patient your name

It seems too simple to even mention, but in tracking offices around the world, I am often surprised at the large number of them whose team members do not share their name with potential new patients who call the office. Which of these sound better? "Thank you for calling Carolinas Dental Center. How can I help you?" or "Thank you for calling Carolinas Dental Center. My name is Amber; how can I help you today?" To me, the choice is simple.

Feeling that one way is better than the other may seem like a personal preference on the surface, but from our tracking data at Call Tracker ROI (Figs. 56 and 57), we've seen a definitive pattern emerge. When team members share their name with potential new patients, statistically they are more likely to schedule that person into a new patient. This makes sense when you think of it in terms of building relationships. Of course we'd share our name with a friend, someone we want to see and talk to again.

New Patient Booked Calls	Number Times Staff Gave Their Name	%
37	37	100

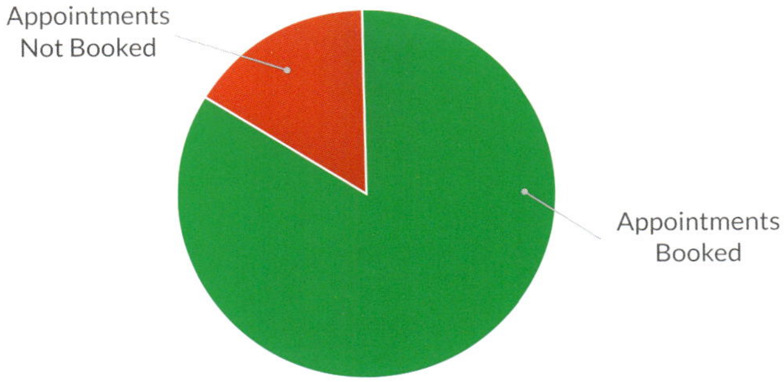

Figure 56. Call tracker ROI report showing an office a correlation of when the team member gives their name, 100 percent in this example, then the majority of time they schedule an appointment. Green shows the percentage scheduled.

When the team does not give their name to the potential new patient calling, our data shows that around 60 percent of the time the caller does not schedule an appointment. Why give your name to someone who you don't plan on seeing or talking to again? You wouldn't, right? That's not the mindset or perception we want our potential new patients to be in when considering choosing our office for their dental care.

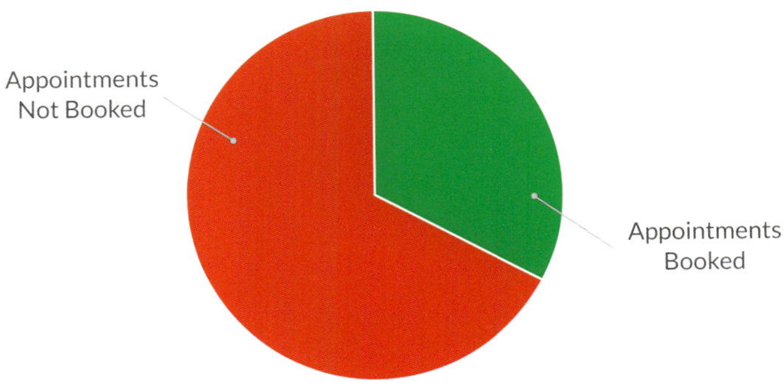

Figure 57. Call tracker ROI report showing when the team doesn't give the potential new patient their name, the majority of time they don't schedule an appointment. Red shows the percentage that went unscheduled.

2. Get Control of the Phone Call

After you've established that you are speaking to a new patient, it's now time to turn our attention to taking control of the conversation. If we let the patients control the calls, there are an endless number of paths they could take us down, getting bogged down with dental insurance questions, asking clinical-related questions, and attempting to get a diagnosis over the phone. Ultimately if we let them control the conversation, more often than not the call ends without scheduling an appointment. To counter this tendency, we can take control by asking questions that lead the conversation. One I recommend asking is: "How did you hear about us?"

Staff Name	New Patients – Apt. Booked	Asked "How did you hear about us?"
Alina	18	18
Megan	8	5
Mila	19	17
Ashley	3	3
Total	**48**	**43**

Figure 58. Call tracker ROI report tracking the percentage of times each team member asks: "How did you hear about us?" This is an important question needed to track the whole truth.

***Team*: Thank you for calling Carolinas Dental Center. This is Amber; how can I help you?**

Patient: Hello, this is Sally Jones, and I'd like to make an appointment to get my teeth cleaned.

***Team*: Great, I can help you with making that appointment, Sally. When was the last time you visited us?**

Patient: Oh, I've never been to your practice before. This will be my first time.

***Team*: Fantastic; let me be the first to welcome you to our dental family. How did you hear about us?**

Not only does asking a question like this help you control the direction of the conversation, it can also provide the practice with valuable data to help us calculate your marketing ROI (Fig. 58). With traditional call tracking phone numbers, you'll get a register of how many people called from that specific marketing source.

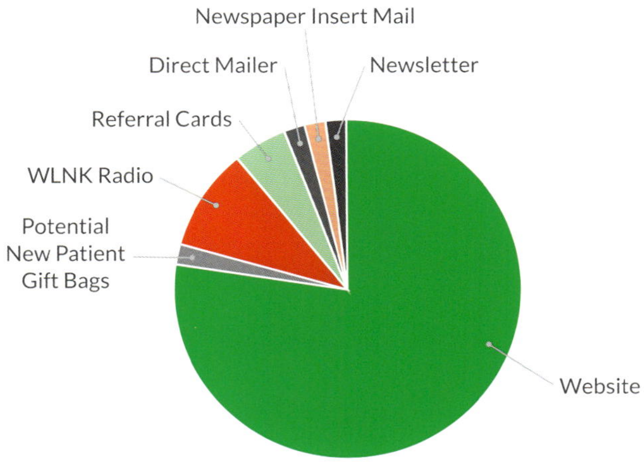

Figure 59. **The half-truth graphic showing the total number of calls, by percentage, that came in and which tracking number and ad source was responsible.**

REPORTED AD SOURCE: HALF-TRUTH	
Tracking Ad Source	**Opportunities**
Website	61
Potential new patient gift bags	1
WLNK radio	5
Referral cards	3
Direct mailer	1
Newspaper insert	1
Newsletter	1
Total	**73**

Figure 60. **Data table showing the total number of calls that came in per tracking source.**

While this is great info, say, if they are calling from the origin source directly, our radio ad for instance, the bad news is that this doesn't give us any insights about more generic areas such as those who come from the website. That's why I call this information the half-truth (Figs. 59 and 60). If we can ask potential new patients how they heard about us, it can help us track down the original marketing source that led them our way. I call this the whole truth and define it as the total number of new patients who came in from a specific ad source.

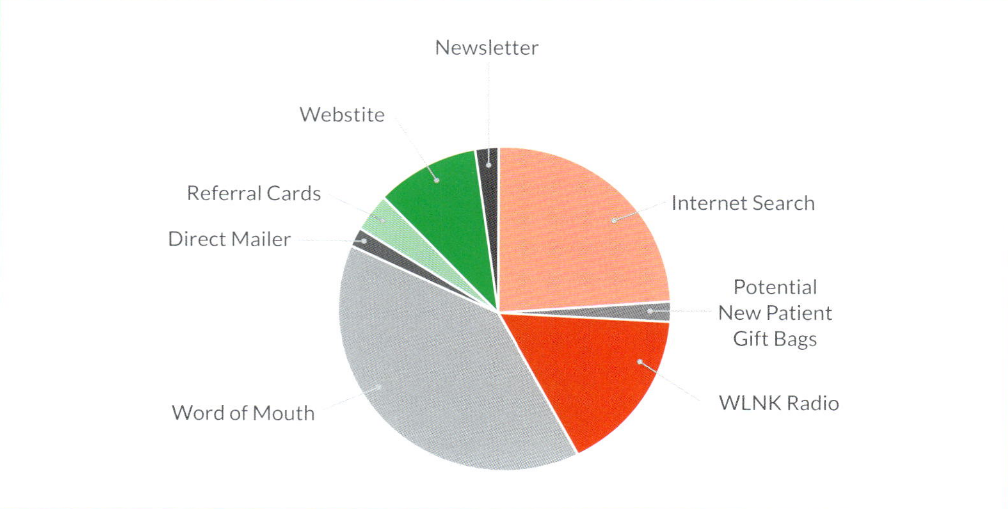

Figure 61. **Graphic representation, factoring in the "How did you hear about us?" question, to give us the whole truth: the total number of new patients scheduled from the true ad source responsible for them calling.**

REPORTED AD SOURCE: WHOLE TRUTH	
Tracking Ad Source	**Opportunities**
Internet search	12
Potential new patient gift bags	1
WLNK radio	6
Word of mouth	21
Direct mailer	1
Referral cards	2
Website	4
Newsletter	1
Total	**48**

Figure 62. **Data table representation, factoring in the "How did you hear about us?" question, to give us the whole truth: the total number of new patients scheduled from the true ad source responsible for them calling.**

Notice how in this example (Figs. 61 and 62) the story changes when you factor in the whole truth. Originally it looked as if the majority of the new patient opportunities were coming in from the website, something that might make our web designer or those doing SEO for us very happy if doing a generic search for office is what led them to us. When we ask, "How did you hear about us?" we can trace these website calls back one step further to get a better idea of the true ad source responsible. Once we know where they really came from, our ROI calculation becomes a lot more accurate. In this case, we see that more new patients are being scheduled due to our internal marketing efforts: encouraging those patients to pass on those new patient gift bags, intriguing them enough to look at our website to research us more, and once satisfied, calling us from the website number that was in front of them.

After we've asked this important ROI tracking question, we can continue controlling the flow of the call by invoking the liking principle and trying to find a connection and commonality with the caller. After the connection is made, the team should focus on endorsing the doctor and reinforcing that the patient made a great decision in calling to become a patient:

Patient: Oh, I've never been to your practice before. This will be my first time.

***Team*: Fantastic. Let me be the first to welcome you to our dental family. How did you hear about us?**

Patient: My sister gave me a gift bag from your office and said that I had to become one of your patients.

***Team*: Who is your sister?**

Patient: Tina Jones.

***Team*: Tina is your sister! We love Tina and always enjoy it when she's here. You know? I have a sister as well. She reminds me a lot of her. Well, you've made the right choice. Dr. Phelps has been practicing for over 17 years, and we offer the latest advancements that dentistry has to offer. I know you'll be in great hands with him. Let's get you scheduled and find a time that works for you.**

From here it's time to get to why they most likely called you in the first place: to schedule their appointment. We'll discuss this in more detail in the next section on how to present the patient with choices, but the goal is to get more commitments for them to make and show for their appointment. Here's an example:

***Team*: Let's get you scheduled and find a time that works for you. Would you prefer this week or next week? Morning or afternoon?**

Ultimately you continue presenting options in a "this or that" format until you funnel the patient down to one of your available appointment times. With each choice made comes a stronger commitment, and they are now more likely to schedule than our standard approach of just telling them our individual times we have open.

3. Get Their Concerns Answered

If you've successfully incorporated all of the aspects we've discussed thus far into your marketing media, most of those calling at this point will be willing to make an appointment. For some, there still may be some questions that need to be answered or objections that need to first be satisfied before they will move forward with making their appointment. There may also be some team bias about who they are talking to that may need to be overcome. Let's review the two main categories of potential patient questions or objections that are shown in the data from Call Tracker ROI, which is keeping many offices from scheduling more new patients: one that relates to price shoppers, those who ask about the cost of things, and one that relates to those asking questions about dental insurance.

- Price shoppers asking about non-hygiene-related services;
- Price shoppers asking about hygiene-related services;
- Patients who ask if you "are in network or participate with my insurance";
- Patients who ask if you "take or accept my insurance."

Each of these areas present with unique mindset challenges, which means our strategies to overcome them need to be different. Let's get into each one individually.

Price shoppers asking about non-hygiene-related services

Non-hygiene-related services are procedures done in the doctor's chair. In this circumstance the potential patient may call up your office and ask you, "How much is a crown at your office?" or "How much for an extraction?" The first thing to understand about this person is that their mindset in this moment is committed to an idea that it's all about the price, and this will be the sole factor they'll use to decide which dental office they need to schedule with.

Once they come into your office and go through your new patient experience, which we'll talk about more in the next cycle, you'll be able to change this mindset that's focused on the cost of your services. Given the limited amount of time you have available to speak with them on this call, it will be nearly impossible to change this mindset in this moment. So instead of fighting the mindset, we're going to work with it. The patient's focus is on the cost, so let's use two strategies to overcome this barrier.

Our first strategy is to offer this person a complimentary exam and x-ray. If they are worried about the cost, let's eliminate that altogether so it doesn't have to cost them anything to find out what their dental issue is and to get a plan to correct it.

Patient: How much is an extraction?

***Team*: Well, every tooth is different, and without seeing you, it's hard for us to know what you need. Let's get you in for a complimentary (free) consultation and x-ray. This way, it won't cost you anything to come in, talk with the doctor, and find out exactly what your tooth needs, and then we can go from there. Would you prefer today or tomorrow?**

Right off the bat we understand the patient's focus is on price, and we've satisfied this potential objection by offering them this initial visit at no cost. It's also important to point out that the price shopper is the only type of patient that I'll offer a free exam and x-ray to. All other type of patients will be charged for any exams and x-rays they receive because their focus isn't solely on the price as this one is. Secondly, note that after we offer them a complimentary exam and x-ray, you immediately go into presenting the "this or that" structure and attempt to schedule their appointment. From our Call Tracker ROI data on offices that have gone through my telephone training and use this approach for this type of caller, around 33 percent of the time they'll make them an appointment.

What do we do about the remaining 67 percent who are still hesitant to schedule? Let's go back to their mindset for a moment. For many of these patients, they are not only focused on finding the best possible price, but they are also focused on discovering what your actual price is. These patients won't schedule after you offer them the free exam and x-ray but instead will continue to push your team until they get them to tell them the price.

Team: Well, every tooth is different, and without seeing you, it's hard for us to know what you need. Let's get you in for a complimentary (free) consultation and x-ray. This way, it won't cost you anything to come in, talk with the doctor, and find out exactly what your tooth needs, and then we can go from there. Would you prefer today or tomorrow?

Patient: I appreciate the offer, but I really need to know how much you charge for an extraction. How much is it?

For those who continue to press to hear your actual cost, I want you to anchor them to your "starting at" price. We'll talk more about this anchoring principle in the case acceptance section to come. What I mean here is that I want you to give them the lowest possible priced item in that category of service they are interested in. In my practice, we have a range of extractions we can offer, each with a varying price. We have a price for bony impacted teeth that need to be removed, soft tissue impacted teeth, surgical extractions, and simple extractions. Our simple extraction costs around $175 per tooth while the other extractions range from $225 to $450. But the simple extraction fee on an adult tooth is not the lowest-priced extraction we offer in this category. We also offer extractions of pediatric teeth for around $75 per tooth. So at this point, we're going to anchor the caller to our "starting at" price, offer them the complimentary exam and x-ray, and then reattempt to schedule them.

Patient: I appreciate the offer, but I really need to know how much you charge for an extraction. How much is it?

***Team*: Well, they start at $75 and go up from there depending on the type of tooth you have and the level of difficulty and destruction present. Why don't you come in for the complimentary exam and x-ray? The doctor will sit down with you and come up with a customized plan, and you'll know exactly what will be needed from there. Would you like a morning or afternoon appointment? Today or tomorrow?"**

With the "starting at" strategy, you should schedule another third of price shoppers, increasing your overall performance on them to 67 percent. The one barrier that dentists and their teams have with this strategy comes from their own personal bias. They feel like they really understand what the caller is asking about or they believe the caller really understands what their dental condition is, so they want to give them the correct answer as a result.

The truth of the matter is, it's still just an assumption. An assumption based on past interactions and experiences with other patients who've shaped your expectations and perceptions, good or bad, which affect future patients as a result. The fact is that you really have no idea what that person on the other side of the phone line needs or what their condition really is. This is what I alluded to earlier when I said that sometimes it's our team who puts up the barrier to scheduling the appointment. How do you know that the person even needs a tooth to be extracted? Maybe it could be saved, but the patient doesn't know or understand that yet. How do you know they have an adult tooth that needs to be taken out and that it's not a pediatric tooth? I've taken out enough retained primary teeth on adults to know that you can't rule this out as a possibility. If they are asking about your price for a crown, how do you know if the tooth they have can even be restored with a new crown?

The purpose of the "starting at" strategy is to anchor them to the lowest possible thing it could be in that category. By limiting the cost and then reoffering the free exam and x-ray, we significantly increase our chances of overcoming this scheduling mindset barrier. Let's look at some other examples of this.

- **Crown**: I give them our onlay fee. "They start at $795 and go up from there."
- **Denture**: I give them our lab reline fee because maybe they have an existing denture, and that's all they need. "They start at $500 and go up from there."
- **Scaling and root planing**: I give them our gross debridement fee. "It starts at $105 and goes up from there."

Let's look at the remaining third of callers who will not schedule after offering the free exam and x-ray or after mentioning the "starting at" price. The mindset of those in this group were committed to not only finding out what your price is but also with discovering where they can find the best possible price. That means speaking to you alone isn't enough. Since they probably talked with you early on in the search, that means they must now call around and talk with three or four other offices, find out what their price is for the service in question, and then compare who has the best price for their immediate dental need.

What do you think they will hear when they call those other offices and ask, "How much is your extraction?" They'll hear something like: "Well, the limited exam is $75, the x-ray is $50, if you need an extraction, it's most likely surgical so that'll be $225." Other offices will probably continue to diagnose and treatment plan this patient over the telephone and add in things such as: "Oh and once the tooth is out, you'll need it back so that's a dental implant, which is $2000, a custom abutment for $700, and a crown for $1300." Remember this, every number you give to someone over the phone, because of the contrast effect, they are adding each and every one of them up, whether they are actually related or not. In doing so, here is what the caller is thinking after they've exhausted their search for the best price. "One of the offices was like $4500, two of the offices it sounds like it will cost me $500, but that one office seemed much less compared to these. I'm going to call them back. We'll discuss this contrast effect in more detail in the coming sections."

By anchoring them to your "starting at" price, you let the contrast effect work in your favor, making your office stand out among any others they may speak with. This is why a large percentage of that last group do end up calling our office back to make an appointment. Once they come in and go through our new patient experience, we change their mindset and focus away from the price. We show them what their true dental situation is and they are part of the process of creating the plan to fix it, influencing them to want the treatment they've chosen. That's why I've never heard a patient question the treatment plan or cost moving forward. I've never heard them say, "I thought it was $75?"

Instead, we've gotten over our personal bias of prejudging who we think we're talking to on the telephone and what their dental condition may be. We've identified their biggest objections to scheduling and worked with their mindset to overcome them. When applied successfully, your team should be able to achieve over 80 percent conversions of these callers into appointments scheduled, and if you learn to influence them properly, like we'll discuss in the coming sections, they can be some of the best, longest-lasting patients in your practice.

Price shoppers asking about hygiene-related services

Hygiene-related services are procedures done in the hygiene chair. This caller will identify themselves by asking questions such as "How much is a cleaning at your office?" Notice in the previous section that we did not bring up dental insurance before we attempted to schedule them an appointment. With this caller, it's going to be important that we do discuss dental insurance earlier on in the conversation as their insurance status will dictate the strategy and language we'll use. In the US, we have three main categories of practice providers. Practices can fall solely into one category or offer a mix of the three:

- **In-network (IN) providers**: These are dentists who have signed a contract with a specific dental insurance company. Under their agreement, there is a set fee schedule for all procedures and a reimbursement schedule established for those procedures. Preventative treatments such as prophylaxis cleanings are usually paid 100 percent by the insurance company. After the services are performed, the office would file an insurance claim and wait on the insurance company for payment. With these preventative treatments, there is little to no out-of-pocket expense to the patient.
- **Out-of-network (OON) providers**: Also called assignment of benefit providers, these are dentists who have not signed contract agreements with any specific dental insurance companies. They are free to charge whatever price they choose for dental services. Many times these offices will estimate what the insurance company will pay based on their OON status, they will file a claim on behalf of the patient, and wait on the payment to come in. The patient's only out-of-pocket expense is the balance due after the assignment of benefit payment has been applied.
- **Fee-for-service (FFS) providers**: These are technically OON providers as they are not contracted with any insurance companies. The difference here is that they do not accept the assignment of benefit payment from the insurance company. Instead, they ask the patient to pay their full fee for any service rendered, preventative or otherwise. While they may help the patient by filing the insurance claim to aid in their reimbursement, many times this act is left up to the patient to handle. Once a claim has been received, the insurance company will send whatever amount is covered back to the patient for reimbursement.

When it comes to price shoppers asking about your hygiene-related services, it's important to understand which of those three categories applies to the caller you're speaking to. Let's look at an example:

***Team*: Thank you for calling Carolinas Dental Center. This is Amber; how can I help you?**

Patient: Hello, this is Sally Jones. I've never been to your practice before but I wanted to make an appointment to get my teeth cleaned.

***Team*: Hello, Sally, let me be the first to welcome you to our dental family. How did you hear about us?**

Patient: I got this flyer in the mail that had information about your practice. I went to your website and read some reviews, and I think you're the office for me, but I wanted to know, how much is a cleaning?

***Team*: That's a great question. Before I answer, let me ask you a question. Do you have dental insurance?**

Responds yes to having dental insurance

- **In-network (IN) provider**: If they tell you that they have a dental insurance plan that you are an IN provider for, then there is no potential barrier to scheduling this patient. You can move right into offering your available appointment times in the "this or that" format.

***Team*: That's a great question. Before I answer, let me ask you a question. Do you have dental insurance?**

Patient: Yes, I have dental insurance with Metlife.

***Team*: Great. We have hundreds of patients that use that insurance here as well. What works best for you, this week or next week? Morning or afternoon?**

- **Fee-for-service (FFS) provider**: If you are out of network, won't accept the assignment of benefit, and require the patient to pay in full at the time of service, be prepared as this presents a big potential barrier and is one of the most challenging to schedule.

***Team*: That's a great question. Before I answer, let me ask you a question. Do you have dental insurance?**

Patient: Yes, I have dental insurance with Metlife.

***Team*: Okay, Dr. Phelps's goal is to maintain the highest quality of care for our patients. To do that, there is a cost, so the bad news is that we are not accepting any dental insurance plans at this time, but the good news is that we have hundreds of patients with that insurance plan that**

still choose us for their care. When you come in, the initial visit fee is $175. We'll file a claim to your insurance company on your behalf, and they will usually send you a check covering most if not all of your payment within a couple weeks. Does that work for you?

If they answer yes, then proceed to schedule them using the "this or that" framework until you find a time that works for them. If they say no, that's okay as well. Better to find out that they are not a good fit for your practice and philosophies now than when they are in your office. This avoids a potential confrontational situation in the office, protects them from having a bad experience, and most likely protects you from a negative online review. If they say it doesn't work for them, remember to thank them for calling and invite them back if their situation changes.

***Team*: Okay, Dr. Phelps's goal is to maintain the highest quality of care for our patients. To do that, there is a cost. The bad news is that we are not accepting any dental insurance plans at this time, but the good news is that we have hundreds of patients with that insurance plan that still choose us for their care. When you come in, the initial visit fee is $175. We'll file a claim to your insurance company on your behalf, and they will usually send you a check covering most if not all of your payment within a couple weeks. Does that work for you?**

Patient: No, I think right now for my situation, I need to find an office that works with my insurance company.

***Team*: I understand completely. Please remember that if you can find an office that works with your insurance plan but you're not happy with your experience there, just know that you are always welcome here. Thank you for thinking of us.**

Some patients do get stuck in a mindset that they must find an office that fully utilizes their dental insurance, meaning they pay as little as possible out of their own pocket. Your office policy just happens to be in complete opposition to their current focus. Many times we've seen that when patients don't have a great experience at the office that is in network with their insurance plan, their mindset and priorities on what's really important to them will change. When that happens, they will return to our office because we anchored them to a great customer service phone experience and welcomed them back. When they do come back, they are willing to wait on their dental insurance payment to come at a later date and pay in full for the service and experience you provide them today.

- **Out-of-network (OON), assignment-of-benefit provider**: To me, this is the best-case scenario to be in. You get to charge your full fee for both preventative and restorative treatment, yet you're still willing to work with the patient, estimating what the insurance company might pay, filing their claim, and then waiting on that assignment of benefit to come in, minimizing the patient's out-of-pocket amount due at today's visit. A win-win. This is how I operated my two dental practices.

In my experience, even though I was out of network, more often than not, the insurance company still paid us 100 percent of the fee we charged for the patient's exam, prophylaxis cleaning, and x-rays. At worst, the reimbursement amount was short $10–20 below our total fee. By not being under contract with these insurance companies, I had the freedom to collect that amount from the patients or I could choose not to collect it and write it off their balance. My strategy was to eliminate the out-of-pocket costs altogether for these patients toward these preventative treatment visits. Doing so gives your team the best chance to schedule this appointment but still allows you to collect most if not all of your preventative fee as well as give you the freedom to charge out and collect your full fees on the restorative side of things. These calls might progress something like this:

***Team*: That's a great question. Before I answer, let me ask you a question. Do you have dental insurance?**

Patient: Yes, I have dental insurance with Metlife.

***Team*: Well, if you have that insurance plan, then it should be $0 out-of-pocket expense for your initial visit with us. Does that work for you?**

Patient: It does.

***Team*: Great, then let's get you scheduled. What works best for you, this week or next week? Morning or afternoon?**

- **Exceptions to the OON strategy**: The out-of-network strategy I outlined is a highly effective way to increase your team's new patient scheduling percentages, especially when the dental insurance companies pay 90–100 percent of the fee we charge for these preventative treatment visits. But not all insurance companies are equal. Most have decent rates they'll pay for OON preventative services, but what happens in situations where the insurance company won't pay a lot toward the treatment? Let's say they only pay a total of 50 percent of total charged fee. How do we handle these situations?

First, before their treatment visit occurs, you have to identify the potential problem, not after they have come in and had the services. That means your team or a company you outsource to has to have verified their dental insurance benefits before the patient comes into the office. After the visit has occurred, your team will have a hard time collecting the large balance due from that patient. The patient won't understand why there is a balance to start with, and they won't feel responsible for paying it. The more you press the issue, the more likely you are to lose the patient over it and end up with a negative online review for your efforts.

Instead, get ahead of it before it's an actual problem. Let's look at two scenarios to help illustrate this point. One where you figured out the insurance problem before their visit and one where you discover it during their visit, assuming the insurance wasn't verified until that day they came into the office.

- **Problem identified before patient comes into the office**: Once you've discovered that the amount the insurance will pay you as an OON provider is too low for you to write off, you should immediately call the patient and let them know. The goal of this call is to put the onus of responsibility where it belongs: on the dental insurance company whose policies are vastly different than other similar companies and are thus causing this to be an issue. Once we've told the patient about the problem, we're going let them know they still have a choice in the matter of who their dentist is, and we're going to use social proof and let them know that others like them chose your office despite the lack of benefits their insurance plan offered.

> ***Team*: Sally, hello; this is Amber calling from Dr. Phelps's office. We're looking forward to seeing you at your visit this Thursday at 10 a.m., but I have some news. We just got done verifying how your dental insurance benefits will work at our office, and the bad news is that they just won't work. In fact, this is some of the lowest reimbursement rates I've seen from a dental insurance company in some time. What that means is that when you come in for your visit, your out-of-pocket expense that day will be $80 instead of the $0 we expected. Do you need to cancel your appointment and try to find an office that might work better with your insurance, or are you okay with keeping your appointment and covering the additional amount?**

Whatever path they choose is good. If that $80 amount is too much for them to pay, then better to find that out on the front end instead of trying to chase after them for it on the back end. If it's not an issue for them, then they know what to expect, and you can continue your relationship on from there. If they do decide to cancel their appointment, be understanding and remember that they are always welcome to return if they are not happy with their experience at the office that works well with their insurance company.

- **Problem identified once patient is in the office**: Let's now look at how to handle the situation if we are not aware of the insurance payment problem until the patient is physically at our office. Option one is to try to collect that shortage from the patient and explain the situation to them when they are checking out. Given their expectation was to pay $0 out-of-pocket costs today, it's usually not a pleasant conversation to have with someone and can totally ruin an otherwise positive experience they've had with you thus far. In these circumstances, I don't put the blame on the patient, I put it on myself and my team for not discovering the problem sooner. As such, I'm going to solve this problem for everyone involved, using the principle of reciprocity in the process. Once my team discovers that we'll get little to no OON payment benefit, I've given them permission to write off whatever balance is present, which should then be presented to the patient as my gift to them.

***Team*: Hello, Sally. Did you enjoy your visit with us today?**

Patient: Yes, I did. You guys are amazing.

***Team*: Thank you. We love hearing that. Sally, I have some bad news. We just got done verifying your dental insurance benefits, and unfortunately, the way your insurance works at our office is that it doesn't really work well at all. In fact, it's some of the lowest dental benefits I've seen an insurance company offer in some time. While we expected them to pay for the majority of your visit today, it looks like they will only pay half. That means your portion would be $80.**

Patient: Oh no, that's terrible, what are we going to do?

***Team*: I know. I've spoken to Dr. Phelps, and here is what he wants to do. He told me that he's going to forgo collecting that $80 from you. As a gift from him, we'll wipe the slate clean so you don't have an account balance with us.**

Patient: Wow, thank you so much, I was not prepared to pay anything today, and I really appreciate it.

***Team*: You're very welcome. You are part of our dental family now, and we take care of our own. The only problem is what to do about the next cleaning appointment you made in six months. Do you need to cancel that appointment and try to find a different office that might work better with your insurance company, or are you okay paying that $80 difference and keeping that appointment?**

Whatever path they choose is the right path for all involved. If you've done a good job building the relationship during their visit, then more often than not people will be glad to pay the difference and keep that appointment. They now see the value for what they'd be paying for because they've experienced it. If you offer a dental membership plan, this could be a good time to compare costs and coverage from your plan and their current dental insurance policy. If that money is going to be a problem for them, then better to resolve it now before it becomes a source of conflict down the road. Remember, if they do cancel their next appointment, thank them for being a part of your practice and let them know that if their situation changes or they are not happy with their experience at their next office, they are always welcome back with you.

Responds no to having dental insurance

Let's pause for a moment and look at what our language should be for those who ask about the price of hygiene-related services but do not have any dental insurance. Here there are two strategies you can employ, one to use if your office offers a dental membership plan (DMP) for patients who do not have dental insurance and one route to take if your office doesn't currently offer a dental membership plan.

If your office does not offer a DMP, then we want to use the same "starting at" strategy that we used for price shoppers asking about non-hygiene-related services and then attempt to make them an appointment.

***Team*: That's a great question. Before I answer, let me ask you a question. Do you have dental insurance?**

Patient: No, I don't have dental insurance at this time.

***Team*: Well, that's okay. We have hundreds of patients we serve who don't have it either. For them, our cleanings start at $79 and go up from there depending on the level of bone and gum destruction that has occurred. We'll go over your situation in detail with you when we see you in person. What works best for you, this week or next week? Morning or afternoon?**

If your office does offer a DMP, which I highly recommend you do, then we want to anchor the patient to the total cost of what's included in that plan and contrast that with the discounted price the plan offers.

***Team*: That's a great question. Before I answer, let me ask you a question. Do you have dental insurance?**

Patient: No, I don't have dental insurance at this time.

***Team*: Well, if you paid for all the cleanings you'd need this year, the x-rays we have to take, and your exams by the dentist, you'd be looking at $475. The good news is that if you have our dental membership plan, you get those two cleanings, two exams, and the x-rays you need for only $299. Plus you get a 10–15 percent discount off any dental work you may need. How does that sound?**

Patient: Wow, that sounds like a great deal.

***Team*: Agreed, that's why so many of our patients without insurance choose it. We can go over more of the benefits and get you signed up when you're here. What works best for you? Would you like this week or next week, morning or afternoon, etc.**

By using this approach, we are scheduling appointments for more than 80 percent of the patients in this situation.

Patients who ask if you "are in network or participate with my insurance"

Now that we've discussed how to handle those in the price shopper categories, let's turn our attention to those patients who place an emphasis or strong value on the insurance question.

These could be price shoppers or they could be patients who aren't concerned about any specific price per se, but they are more concerned with finding an office that works with their dental insurance company, people who want to minimize their out-of-pocket expense as much as possible. Usually, if dental insurance is a priority for them, then it will come up early on in the conversation, phrasing this concern in one or two ways by asking: "Are you in network with my insurance?" or "Do you participate with my insurance?"

Team: Thank you for calling Carolinas Dental Center. This is Amber; how can I help you?

Patient: Hello, this is Sally Jones. I've never been to your practice before, but I wanted to make an appointment to get my teeth cleaned.

Team: Hello Sally, let me be the first to welcome you to our dental family. How did you hear about us?

Patient: I got this flyer in the mail that had information about your practice. I went to your website and read some reviews, and I think you're the office for me, but I wanted to know, how much is a cleaning?

Team: That's a great question. Before I answer, let me ask you a question. Do you have dental insurance?

Patient: Yes, I have Metlife Insurance. Are you in network with them?

Someone who specifically asks whether you're in network or participate with their insurance plan is someone who may have had a bad experience related to their dental insurance at an out-of-network provider's office, an experience that has turned finding someone within their dental network into a top-of-mind priority. If you are a provider in that network, then there should be very little barriers to scheduling this patient. Use the "this or that" framework approach of offering them appointment times and schedule them.

If you're out of network, either as an assignment-of-benefit office or a fee-for-service office, then there is a large barrier to scheduling, one that typically gives you, at best, about a 20–30 percent chance of making this person an appointment. The language we use goes something like this:

Patient: Yes, I have Metlife Insurance. Are you in network with them?

Team: Unfortunately we're not in network with them, but we have hundreds of patients with that insurance who still choose us as their provider anyway. You do have a choice in the matter, just like they did, and I'm hoping you chose to make an appointment with us today. What works for best for you? Morning or afternoons? This week or next week?

Those truly committed to finding an in-network provider for their dental insurance plan will stop you right there and choose to end the relationship. There is little you could say or do to change this mindset. If they came into the office and really experienced what it was like to be a patient at your practice, then you have a real chance to change this mindset, but doing so on the telephone is very difficult. If they do decide not to schedule an appointment, I'd remind you to thank them for calling you and let them know that if their situation changes or they are not happy with their in-network office experience, they are always welcome to call you back.

Patients who ask, "Do you take or accept my insurance?"

At my call tracking company, not only do we track the office and individual team member's success rates or challenges on the telephone, we also track why they did not schedule the appointment. Was it because they bungled the price shopper call opportunity? Because the caller wanted a specific day and time that couldn't be accounted for? Maybe it was because the patient wanted a service that the office didn't offer?

By far, the #1 reason why offices fail to schedule a new patient call applies to out-of-network provider offices and early on in the conversation the potential new patient asks, "Do you take my dental insurance?" or "Do you accept my dental insurance?" After listening to thousands of recorded phone calls across the world that concern this question, it's clear to me that there is a disconnect from what the patient is really asking versus a bias as to what our team hears them asking. The patient asks, "Do you take/accept my insurance?" but the team only hears "Are you in network or participate with my insurance?" It's another great example of how sometimes our team can put up a barrier to scheduling the patient because of assumptions made from past, usually uncomfortable situations they've experienced.

From my experience and analysis of those recorded phone calls, it's fair to say that 80 percent of the patients who ask, "Do you take or accept my insurance?" actually have little to no idea what their insurance benefit is or what it means. They are not like the callers we previously talked about who ask if you are in network with their insurance. Instead, the focus and mindset of this caller is just that they want to know if you're going to file their insurance for them so they have little to no out-of-pocket expense for their cleaning. That's it, they just want to know if you'll work with them and try to maximize their insurance benefit as much as you can toward their dental treatment needs. That means this is a great opportunity for practices who are out of network but are still willing to accept the assignment-of-benefit payment from the insurance company for these preventative visits.

How do I know this to be true? How can I be so confident that this person asking whether you take or accept their insurance doesn't really care about your in-network or out-of-network status? I'm sure because of listening to thousands upon thousands of calls on how your team answers this question and how the patient responds in confusion, time and time again.

Team: Thank you for calling Carolinas Dental Center. This is Amber; how can I help you?

Patient: Hello, this is Sally Jones. I've never been to your practice before, but I wanted to make an appointment to get my teeth cleaned.

Team: Hello, Sally. Let me be the first to welcome you to our dental family. How did you hear about us?

Patient: I got this flyer in the mail that had information about your practice. I went to your website and read some reviews, and I think you're the office for me, but I wanted to know, how much is a cleaning?

Team: That's a great question. Before I answer, let me ask you a question. Do you have dental insurance?

Patient: Yes, do you take Metlife's Insurance?

Team: I'm sorry. We're not in network with them.

Patient sounds surprised and off-put: Oh, really? What does that mean? I can't be a patient there?"

Team: That's right, I'm sorry. You'll have to find a different office, someone who is in network with them. Goodbye!

Just like that, the call ends with the patient wondering what just happened, confused about why they can't come to see you because they chose to call you for a reason. Let's look at how we can change this outcome as many offices that have used my strategy have seen. These can be great patients in your OON practice and don't have to be turned away, costing you more in marketing expense to get a positive ROI and reach your new patient and practice growth goals as a consequence.

Team: Thank you for calling Carolinas Dental Center. This is Amber; how can I help you?

Patient: Hello, this is Sally Jones. I've never been to your practice before, but I wanted to make an appointment to get my teeth cleaned.

Team: Hello, Sally. Let me be the first to welcome you to our dental family. How did you hear about us?

Patient: I got this flyer in the mail that had information about your practice. I went to your website and read some reviews, and I think you're the office for me, but I have Metlife for dental insurance. Do you guys accept that?

Team: We do. We work with most major insurance carriers and will do everything we can to maximize your dental insurance benefits. For most of our patients that means little to no out-of-pocket costs for their

preventative visits such as their biannual cleanings, x-rays, and exams by the doctor. What works best for you, this week or next week? Morning or afternoon?

If you're an OON provider who accepts the assignment-of-benefit payment and you follow the strategies I laid out above, attempting to eliminate the patient's preventative out-of-pocket costs, you'll find that your team will be able to schedule 80 percent or more of these patients. In our next section on acceptance, we'll expand on this topic more and talk about how to ethically use the science of persuasion to eliminate dental insurance becoming a barrier to them saying yes to your treatment recommendations.

For now, the challenge will be to remove whatever feelings you have on this topic and look at the facts and understand that there is a big difference between the mindsets of someone asking, "Do you take or accept my insurance" versus the one asking, "Are you in network or participate with my insurance?" With understanding comes listening. Listen to what the patient is really asking you. Don't assume you know what they are asking you. Once you really hear what they are asking you, respond in kind.

One question I get asked often around this topic comes from why the team misinterprets who they are talking to. Why do they turn these patients away instead of embracing them as the opportunities that they are? Typically, the reason dates back to a bad past experience they had with a patient in the office or in a conversation they are having with a patient after their visit is complete, but there is a balance due on their account because the insurance company didn't cover the full amount of their preventative treatment. At some point, the team brings up the fact that the patient's insurance paid less than expected. When asked why, the team usually responds by telling the patient it's the difference between the out-of-network fee you charge compared to what fee the insurance company will pay as a result. Once the patient hears the reason is insurance related, it gives them a great excuse to get angry and yell at the team member they are speaking with. After that experience, most team members have told me that they made a vow to themselves to never be put in that situation again. So to protect themselves, anytime a patient mentions insurance, they treat them as if they have to have an in-network provider.

I can sympathize with team members who've gone through this experience and wouldn't wish that upon anyone. The real problem in this scenario is that the office didn't have a good system to address how to avoid conflicts such as these from occurring. One way to avoid this is by eliminating the words "in network" and "out of network" from your vocabulary altogether, which makes sense since dental insurance is confusing and most patients don't understand all of the details of it anyway. In my offices, we tried to simplify it to our patients in this manner: "After your insurance pays its part, your portion due is $X."

Another way you can avoid conflict is by making it little to no out-of-pocket expense when it comes to their preventative hygiene visits. Most people have been anchored by past experiences of not having to pay out of pocket for these visits, so it stands out to them when they do, especially if it's a large amount that is suddenly due. Next, you can make sure your team has a plan to handle these conflict situations. By verifying their dental insurance benefits and identifying those plans who really won't pay a significant amount toward their cleaning visit, you can avoid conflict by addressing this with the patient as we've previously discussed, before they arrive at the office. If by chance this happens to come up while they are in the office or if you're following up with them after their visit has occurred, consider leveraging the principle of reciprocity and eliminate that potential source of conflict altogether.

By training my team on the barriers patients put up to scheduling appointments, teaching them about the mindset of those calling, and how their own personal bias could be costing the office real opportunities, I was able to help them increase their new patient scheduling rate at our OON offices from 24 percent to consistently averaging 80 percent. This was a major factor behind why we were able to go from 60 new patients per month to then averaging over 300 per month, helping my ROI go from a very low to a large positive number instead.

4. Get Them from Interested to Committed

When patients call up your office, they are generally interested in making an appointment. The challenge is that being interested doesn't necessarily mean that they are committed to making or showing up for the appointment. When we've progressed in the conversation to the point where it's time to make them an appointment, we can turn their interest into something more substantial by getting more active, voluntary, and public commitments out of them. To do this, we can lean on Dr. Cialdini's consistency principle to aid us. We're going to cover this principle and these commitment scheduling strategies more in the next section as they are also critical factors that can help us ensure that these patients who scheduled these appointments actually show up for them. Here's a sneak peek at how we're going to get patients from being interested in making an appointment to being more committed to making and showing up for one.

Team: Great, let's make you an appointment. What works best for you? This week or next week? Wednesday or Thursday? Morning or afternoon? 2 p.m. or 4 p.m.?

Patient makes an appointment.

Team: Excellent, so I have you down for this Wednesday at 2 p.m. Do you have any dental insurance information we should know about?

Patient provides information.

Team: Thank you for providing me with that information. Looks like we have your appointment all set. Will you please call us if you need to cancel or reschedule your appointment?

Patient: Of course.

Team: Thanks! I'll let the doctor and other team members know you'll call us if you can't make it. Before you go, would you mind repeating back the day and time of your appointment just so I make sure I have it right in my system?

Patient reads back the information.

***Team*: Thank you. That's what I have as well. We all look forward to seeing you then.**

5. Get Any Additional Info Needed

At this point in the conversation, you've already made them an appointment. Now it's time to gather any additional information that you may need to complete this appointment. To minimize the amount of time this phone call should take, I recommend you limit your requests to getting the following:

- **Name**: If they haven't given you their full name at this point, now is the time to ask for it.
- **Telephone number**: Don't try to get too many phone numbers, just ask them for the best number to reach them and ask what type of number this is. Work, home, or cell phone number?
- **Email address**: You'll likely want to email them a welcome letter and/or new-patient paperwork and forms to fill out before their appointment.
- **Dental insurance**: If they have a dental insurance plan, now is the time to ask for the details of that plan. At least the details you'll need to verify they have coverage and what their benefits are as it relates to your practice's IN vs OON status with them. This could include their group number, subscriber number, and/or date of birth.
- **Answer any remaining questions**: Confirm that the patient doesn't have any other questions before ending the call. If there are unique instructions they need to know about when it comes to access your office, now is the time to relay that information to them. This could be special parking instructions and directions on finding your office if you're in a large office tower. It could be providing them with landmarks to look for if your office is tucked away and hard to see from the main roads.
- "**Is there anyone else we can make an appointment for?**": Before the call ends, ask this important question. Oftentimes, people get so focused on making their own appointment that they forget there are others they could make appointments for as well. One of my agents at Golden Goose Scheduling was able to schedule 10 new patient appointments for one of our client offices from one phone call. What if for every potential new patient that calls in, you could schedule two appointments per call instead of one? In essence it would double your marketing's effectiveness, significantly increase your ROI, but without costing you more money in the process.

6. Get It All Together

I want you to think of the things discussed here as guidelines and not necessarily scripts that must be followed word for word. There are multiple ways the conversation could go and multiple variations that can occur during them. For instance, you may have someone who starts out being concerned about the price of certain procedures but then shifts that focus to finding an office that works with their dental insurance. They key is not to be able to memorize scripts for these situations but to remember the core tenets and goals behind them. What mindset is this patient in at that moment? Listen to what are they really asking you. How can you simplify your answer and make them an appointment, to establish a connection with them and present the doctor as the authority that they are? How can you get them from interested to committed to making this appointment and gathering whatever info you need to make this appointment complete?

From here it all comes down to tracking your new patient phone calls and getting as much data out of all of those calls as you can. Listening to and evaluating some of the calls can be helpful, but the reality is it will do you no good when it comes to identifying the real issues plaguing your office or help you calculate your actual marketing ROI. So find a call tracking service to do this for you or make the commitment and budget the time for your office manager or yourself to do it. For me, it's one of the most important areas of practice growth and success that you must pay attention to.

Sit down with your team and let them know that you are going to be tracking their results, not to fire them or yell at them but to give them the tools they need to be more successful at their jobs, to provide better customer service for your potential new patients so that everyone wins. Set realistic goals for them and explain what your expectations are in this area. With my own team, when I met with them and shared that they were converting only 24 percent of our new patient opportunity calls into appointments, I let them know the blame fell solely on me, not them. I didn't understand the challenges they faced and the barriers both sides were putting up to scheduling, and by not training them properly, I had put them in a position to fail, not succeed. But moving forward, that was going to change.

As a team, I told them my long-term goal was for them to consistently schedule at least 70 percent of the new patient calls into appointments. Based on the worldwide tracking data I've seen, I think this is fair and definitely attainable by any team, regardless or whether you're an FFS, OON, or IN provider or some combo of the three. While the most successful teams out there took around four to five minutes to schedule their new patient calls, I wanted a short-term goal of seven to nine minutes. Our average at that time was 13 minutes. I gave them leeway by telling them it was okay to take as long as they needed to connect with that patient and schedule that appointment, if that's what it took, but our goal should be to use language that help us become more efficient with the time we had.

As a team we talked about certain factors that were out of their control but that led to an appointment not being scheduled, things such as patients asking for services that we didn't offer or asking for a specific day and time, maybe like a Saturday appointment, but we can't accommodate their request because we weren't open or available on that specific day or time. Our plan was to not count these appointments against the team as to me they weren't really viable opportunities the team had to scheduling the appointment. Not like the price shopper or insurance-focused patient. Instead, I wanted them to keep me apprised of whether these issues started coming up randomly or the majority of the time. Using their input and the data collected, it might help me justify my next move if there is an opportunity present. If my call tracking data consistently showed me that we're missing out on 20–25 new patients a month because we're not open on Saturdays, then maybe I would consider figuring out a way to be open that day. Since our new patient value was worth over $2000 that first year, that's a lot of opportunity we're missing out on.

I remember a time back when the television show *Extreme Makeover* was at its height of popularity. Because of the promotion on that show, the Zoom, 1 Hour Tooth Whitening system blew up in demand. I remember being at the front desk of my practice one day, and five straight phone calls came in from our radio ad, each one asking the same thing: "Do you guys offer Zoom whitening?" After the fifth time hearing my front desk person tell these people that we did not, I got online and ordered the Zoom Whitening system. Remember, when your target market speaks, this one interested in cosmetic dentistry, then maybe we should listen. We did over $100,000 in production that year by offering Zoom, all because the data showed me a demand for something we didn't currently offer but could.

What production opportunities are potential new patients asking you about that you are missing out on because you don't currently offer them? If the data shows they're calling to ask about whitening, dental implants, sedation dentistry, Invisalign clear aligner therapy, and so forth, then maybe that data would tell you where you needed to invest your continuing education dollars this year, to bring a service to your existing patients that they may find valuable but that also has shown some high potential new patient demand. If you don't want to offer these services yourself but don't want to continue to miss out on these opportunities, maybe that means you look to bring on another dentist or dental specialist to provide those procedures for you.

For those items that are within our team's ability to control and can help them schedule more new patient calls, such as how to handle the price shopper and what to do with patients who bring up the dental insurance question, I reminded my team about Pearson's law, which states: Whatever is measured increases, but whatever is measured and reported on, increases significantly.

To capitalize on this statistical law, I scheduled monthly accountability meetings with my office manager and anyone who handled new patient phone calls, including any dental assistants who might help out at the front desk from time to time. The goal of these meetings was simple: take the data from our calling tracking service and review each person's conversion rate on new patient phone calls and review the transcripts of why they were unable to schedule an appointment. We'd take out the calls they had no control over such as the ones mentioned above but we'd dive deeper into those they could by having them read the text or transcript of their calls that didn't lead to appointments. The recording of the phone call was there and available for us to use, but I've found that team members are very resistant to being recorded to start with and really don't like listening to recordings of their conversations. Fortunately, I got little resistance from them to read the text of their conversation. After reading these out loud to the group, I'd ask them a single question: "Reading this now and thinking back to this call, is there anything you can think of that you could have said differently that might have changed the outcome and led to the caller being scheduled an appointment?"

Sometimes there wasn't anything they could have said differently, so having them say no was an acceptable answer. Many times though, they could see where they bungled an opportunity and were pretty good about coming up with ideas on what they could have said differently. I would then put the question to the others in the group and ask for their insights. Did they have any ideas on what this person could have said differently? I'd then give them my thoughts if I had them. One by one we'd go around the room until every unscheduled new patient call was addressed. We left the meeting on a positive note and reconvened the following month. As a team, the office conversion rate rose from 24 to 55 percent, with no other formal phone training given. I made sure to celebrate that progress and success as a big win at that next meeting. The next month it rose to over 60 percent. Offices that make that commitment to meet once a month to report on their successes or challenges and work together to find solutions will always see significant improvements as a result.

The more phone calls I listened to and learned from, the more strategies I was able to teach them on how to continue their improvement. These were the strategies I've covered in this book and have proven to help dental teams around the world to make significant changes in their conversion rates, bringing each office more new patients, increasing their marketing ROI, but without them having to spend more money to attract them.

Chapter 10
Decreasing Costly No Shows

1. PATIENTS WHO DON'T SHOW UP FOR THEIR APPOINTMENTS

The cost to own and operate a dental practice in the United States has been steadily rising for years. If we have patients in our chairs, then we're most likely generating revenue to help us offset this overhead expense. If the chair had a new patient scheduled, but the person failed to show up for their appointment, this costs us on multiple levels.

First, that means that we were unable to produce any revenue during that time period. Since we can't have that time back, that means you'll need to produce more in the remaining time you do have to make up for this shortfall. Second, having a no-show from a new patient for their appointment means it will cost us more in marketing to replace them, decreasing our ROI in the process. For the purposes of this book, we'll define no-shows as appointments that were made by patients, new or existing, but those patients failed to attend that visit and they failed to notify your office of their intended absence.

A. Main Reasons for No-Shows Occurring

1. **They forget**: We've talked before about all of the distractions patients face daily as well as how many items they have on their to-do lists. In today's hectic world, it's not uncommon for someone to just forget that they've made an appointment with you.
2. **Fear and uncertainty**: Patient perceptions of the dental experience are not always as high as they should be, especially for those in the baby boomer generation who had traumatic experiences with dentistry as a child. I've heard countless horror stories from my own patients about how they were treated in their youth that surprised me that this person would ever return to a dental office again. It's because of this fear that practices that offer sedation dentistry have seen significant successes. Despite this, fear gets to us all and if that patient is afraid, then it's likely that they'll skip out on their visit with you.
3. **Pushed out appointments**: When making an appointment becomes top of mind for a patient, their general feeling is that they would like to be seen as soon as possible, not four to six weeks from when they called. If your practice is scheduling patients more than two days out to see the dentist for a tooth issue or four to six weeks out for a preventative cleaning appointment, then more no-shows can be expected. Many times the patient will take the appointment you give them so they have some guaranteed visit

scheduled and they will then call around to other offices to see if anyone can accommodate and see them sooner. If so, they don't usually take the time to call you back to cancel and thus choose to just to miss that appointment.

4. **Last minute conflicts**: Life happens sometimes. Emergencies come up, people get sick, they become injured, or maybe it becomes too difficult to leave work. Regardless, the more appointments you make for people, the more likely some will have to miss out because something else more pressing came up.
5. **The expense**: Dentistry is perceived by the public as being expensive. Especially by those who don't have dental insurance, but even for those who do, many times there is still a considerable amount of money that will be due that the patient is responsible for. We previously discussed this in the "Poor Phone Conversions" section and how quoting patients multiple fees over that initial phone call can cause more to skip out on the appointment that they made.
6. **There is no relationship**: We don't tend to make appointments to be with our friends or family members and then don't show up. Who would do that to someone they liked? So the fact that people do this very thing to us in the dental setting should be telling. This is a major reason why existing patients don't show up for their appointments. With new patients the risk is here as well because we haven't had a chance to meet them, connect with them, and influence them to like us and become part of our dental family.
7. **Lack of a commitment**: When people feel forced or intimated, they tend to say yes in that moment only to back out the first chance they can and when they feel safe to do so. Whether that was your intention or not, this tends to occur when people don't feel like they have a choice in the matter. If we're telling patients the times they can see us instead of giving them options to choose from, we tend to fall into this very trap.

Regardless of where you are in the world or why they didn't show up, it's costing you dearly. Most surveys report that patient no-shows across all medical practices and facilities in the UK costs that industry around 17 billion pounds in lost revenue each year. In the United States, that amount is estimated to cost the health care industry over $150 billion annually. A 2014 article in *Dental Economics* magazine reported that if a dental practice had one no-show a day for a year, the loss in revenue could range from $20,000 to $70,000. Across the dental industry in the United States it was reported that the average no-show rate of all appointments made is 15 percent. If you run the math, that means you could easily be missing out on one to two appointments per day and $100,000+ in lost revenue. In my own practices, the no-show rate between my two offices was 13 percent.

The good news is there is hope. There are measures you can take to reduce this percentage dramatically. Let's break these down into strategies for new and existing patients. These are strategies I used in my practices that took my overall no-show rate from 13 to less than 1 percent.

B. Strategies to Reduce No-Shows on Existing Patients

1. **Build the relationship**: You have to make a connection with them. People like to do business with people they like and they don't show up on people they don't like or those they don't feel they have a relationship with in some capacity. This applies for everyone in the office but especially for the dentist, hygienist, and dental assistant, who typically spend the most time with the patient. One way to build and reinforce your relationship with your patients is to leverage Dr. Cialdini's liking principle. Discover as many similarities and things you have in common as possible. Why? We tend to like those who are like us, those who have shared interests, hobbies, circumstances as we do. The more of these you and your team identify and point out to your patients, the more they will like about you.

   Another way to increase the connections to your patients are to show them that you like them. We tend to like those who like us and tell us or show us that they like us. If there is something genuine that you like about that person, tell them. Compliment them on their hair, watch, their clothes. If you know they do charity work and find that admirable, mention that to them. Whatever it is, if it's true and you really believe it, bring it up. The more connections we make with our patients, the more they will like us and will see us as a friend or family member. The more they like us, the less likely they will be to not show up for their next appointment.

2. **Give them a choice of appointment times**: In the influence section we talked about Dr. Cialdini's consistency principle and how people tend to live up to the commitments that they make. If your team is offering patient appointments one at a time, you're not really giving the person a choice in the matter. Not giving them a choice means they may feel forced or intimated into saying yes while not really being committed to it. Earlier in this book I discussed how we can avoid this potential issue altogether by offering patients a "this or that" framed choice. For example, "What works best for you? This week or next week? Morning or afternoon? 2 p.m. or 4 p.m.? This Wednesday or next Wednesday?" These are all examples of a "this or that" choice. Every time the person voluntarily makes a selection from those two options, they become more and more committed to the choices they have made. The more committed they are means they are more likely to show up for that appointment.

3. **Have them write down their appointment**: People tend to live up to what they write down. Writing it down signifies its importance and means we've made more of an active commitment to the task at hand. A study completed in a medical office setting showed when patients were asked to write down their own next appointment day and time, no-show rates deceased by 18 percent. This is why we ask our patients to fill out their next appointment card, which we call their reservation. We also ask our patients to fill out their name, address, and appointment information on their recall reminder card. In today's technology age, asking them to put their appointment into their own calendar on their smart phone serves the same purpose. If they write the information about their next appointment, they are more committed to showing.

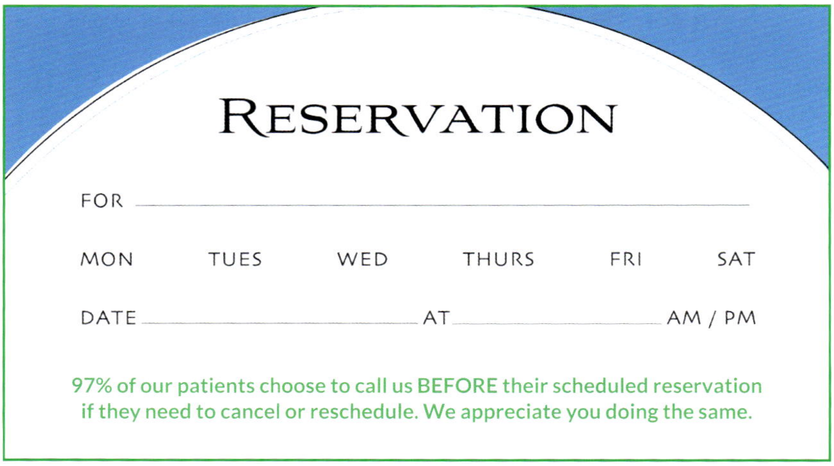
RESERVATION
FOR
MON TUES WED THURS FRI SAT
DATE AT AM / PM
97% of our patients choose to call us BEFORE their scheduled reservation if they need to cancel or reschedule. We appreciate you doing the same.

Figure 63. **Example of appointment card, which allows patient to write out the info of their name and next appointment day and time.**

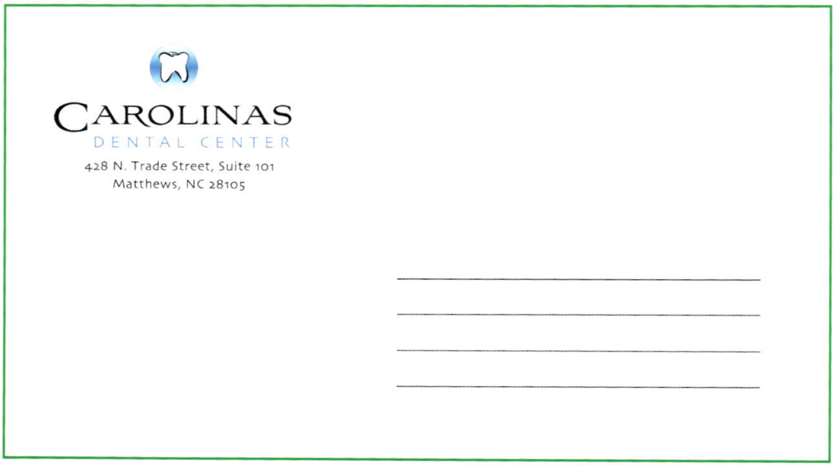
CAROLINAS
DENTAL CENTER
428 N. Trade Street, Suite 101
Matthews, NC 28105

Figure 64. **Example showing the front side of my recall card and the area we have the patient write in their own name and address to mail this reminder card.**

4. **Consider taking a deposit to hold the appointment**: Small commitments can help significantly decrease your no-shows. I worked with a practice that was a provider for the state-supported Medicaid program. Historically, because everything was covered for these patients, there was little value placed on the care they received. As a result, they had to schedule four patients for every available appointment time and hoped that one of the four patients showed. While overbooking is a potential solution to your no-show problem, it's not one I'd recommend as this practice experienced days when two or three patients all showed for the same appointment time. Imagine the chaos and havoc this would create on your schedule as it was assured to happen several times each day.

On my recommendation, I had my client's team ask patients to pay a $10 deposit before they were allowed to make any appointment at the practice. Any credit generated after all fees were collected was reimbursed to the patient, but everyone paid a $10 deposit to make an appointment. The result? Almost 100 percent of those who made this commitment showed up for their appointment, eliminating the need for overbooking and the chaos it was consistently creating. If you'd like more patients to show up, consider asking them to make a deposit to make an appointment.

5. **Remind them of the commitment they made**: Some more recent behavioral science studies show that when people don't follow through with a commitment they have made, it's not because they intended to be deceitful. Instead, they forgot or got distracted, having every intention of getting to the commitment they made at some point. To counter this possibility, you must remind them of the commitments they have made. That means having some type of confirmation system in place to remind them about their appointment, before it.

   The most influential way of doing this is to have a team member call the patient about three days before their scheduled time, getting that verbal commitment that they still plan to attend. I used an automated medium that recorded a confirmation message using my team member's voice. The program then called our patients on our behalf and confirmed those who answered into our scheduling software.

   You can also use a program that will send out an email and/or text message to confirm them as well. Some are hesitant to use this medium as they feel it's impersonal and could potentially lead to more no-shows, but as we mentioned in the unanswered call section, this action takes valuable time away from their capacity to answer potential new patient calls. The good news here is that we can still leverage this automated confirmation medium and add a simple strategy to reduce your no-show risk. One medical office study showed that when you use the patients first name in your messaging, this reduced no-shows by over 50 percent in this automated confirmation medium. Instead of them receiving a text that says, "Mr. Smith," or "John Smith, we're looking forward to seeing you on Tuesday, January 5th at 10 a.m. Respond with no if you can't make that time or yes if you plan on attending," it should read: "John, we're looking forward to seeing you on Tuesday, January 5th at 10 a.m."

   Despite leveraging the technology of these automated programs for confirmation, when there will be an extended amount of time between when the appointment is made and the actual appointment date, I recommend a more traditional confirmation approach be taken as well. At the chair, we'll give the patient a small clipboard and pen. We'll give them the two options, "this or that" series of choices until they make their next six-month cleaning appointment.

   Once decided, we ask the patient to fill out their name and address on one side of the recall reminder card (Fig. 65) and input the day and time on the opposite side. We then ask them to answer one important commitment question on the card: "Will you please call us if you need to cancel or reschedule?" asking them to write yes or no in that space. These cards are mailed in addition to using our automated confirmation reminders in five months' time, giving them four weeks' notice in case any changes to the appointment

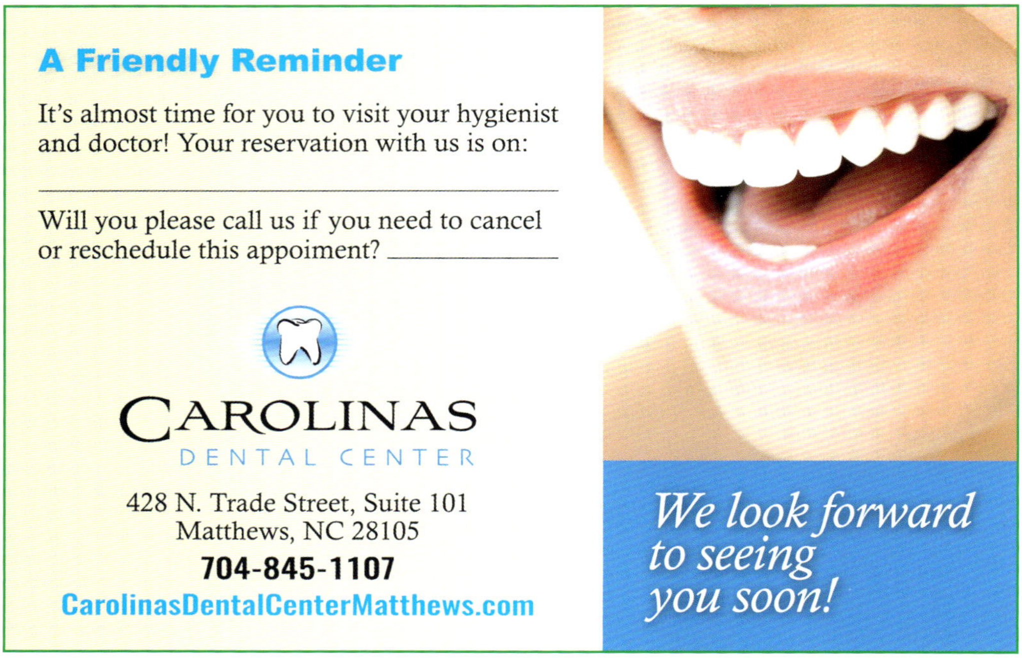
A Friendly Reminder
It's almost time for you to visit your hygienist and doctor! Your reservation with us is on:
Will you please call us if you need to cancel or reschedule this appoiment?
CAROLINAS
DENTAL CENTER
428 N. Trade Street, Suite 101
Matthews, NC 28105
704-845-1107
CarolinasDentalCenterMatthews.com
We look forward to seeing you soon!

Figure 65. Back side of a recall card, showing that the patient must write out the day and time of their next cleaning appointment and answer one commitment question for us with a yes or no answer.

need to be made and reminding them of the commitment they made to come to this appointment or at least call us to cancel or reschedule.

For those offices that are really struggling with higher than usual no-show rates, many have had success with two confirmation attempts, one five to seven days out from their appointment and one three days out, which leverages the principle of scarcity with their confirmations. For shorter time frames consider confirming three days out and then the day before their appointment.

If the patient didn't confirm via phone, text, or email on the first attempt, then three days out they'd receive this message: "John, we have you scheduled for Tuesday, January 5th at 10 a.m. We've tried to reach out to you to confirm your appointment, but we haven't heard from you. At this point, if we don't hear back from you to confirm in the next 24 hours, we will be canceling your appointment." Sharing that they stand to lose that appointment should motivate those truly interested in attending to make confirming this appointment a priority. Those not interested, the ones likely to miss their appointment will not call. At least now you'll have two days to try to fill that spot with another patient.

6. **Charge a broken appointment fee(?)**: Negative incentives are another way you could use to keep patients from not showing up for their appointment. By charging a $25–50 no-show fee, the assumption is that you may make your appointment more of a priority in their mind versus other activities they may choose to do instead. The reality in my experience is quite different. Instead of motivating them to come to their appointment,

oftentimes it upsets patients, especially those who had a legitimate reason for not attending. More often than not, the end result was a patient that left the practice, possibly providing a negative online review and never returned again.

7. **Influence them to show or at least call to reschedule**: My goal is to influence the patients to show up for their appointment. The more commitments they make, the more likely they are to show up. My secondary goal is that if they can't make it to their appointment, regardless of the reason, I want to influence them to let us know. In my practices, we have strategies to fill in any open appointment times that pop up but if the person doesn't shows up, then we have no chance to fill it and still make it a productive day. Notice the commitment language and messaging we use in our appointment scheduling: "Will you please call us if you need to cancel or reschedule?" Note in our reservation card the social proof messaging (Fig. 66) we use. At the time this card was presented, our no-show rate had been reduced down to 3 percent. That meant that 97 percent of those who made an appointment with us showed up for that appointment. That's a powerful message we can use to influence the person who made this appointment do the same or at a minimum, call us to let us know.

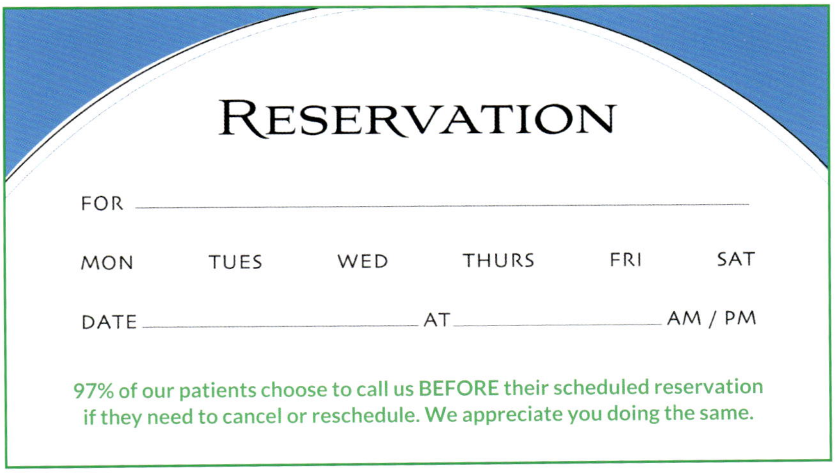
RESERVATION

FOR ______

MON TUES WED THURS FRI SAT

DATE ______ AT ______ AM / PM

97% of our patients choose to call us BEFORE their scheduled reservation if they need to cancel or reschedule. We appreciate you doing the same.

Figure 66. Reservation card showing example of social proof to decrease no shows.

C. Strategies to Reduce No-Shows for New Patients

1. **Make a connection**: It all starts with liking. When talking to a potential patient for the first time, your team's goal should be to establish some kind of connection with them. Connections open relationships and lead to liking. If possible, the team should try to find one thing in common with the caller before they attempt to schedule the appointment. For example, if they hear a dog barking in the background and they also have a dog or have an interest in dogs, they should bring up that fact when talking. "Oh, is that a dog in the background? I love dogs, tell me about your dog. What's their name?" Highlighting even a single point of interest can lead to the appointment being scheduled and ensuring that this person shows up to meet the person they connected with on the phone.

2. **Get more commitments**: Just like I discussed with existing patients, our goal with new patients should be to get them to make as many commitments as possible when making their appointment. We need to offer them voluntary commitments by giving them "this or that" choices of their appointment times. We need to get more of a verbal commitment out of them by asking them: "Will you please call us if you need to cancel or reschedule your appointment?" In a popular restaurant in Chicago, they were able to reduce their no-show rate on reservations by 75 percent just by asking this one verbal commitment question.
3. **Consider taking a deposit**: Remember, even though it may be a small deposit, they're actually making a large commitment to showing up. If asking every new patient to make a deposit to hold their reservation seems too extreme, consider using this technique more strategically, for high-demand times or days such as Saturdays where no-shows seem to be more prevalent or for patients scheduled from marketing media with higher no-show rates such as online advertising, sources that seem to generate interested people but not committed ones.
4. **Make it a public commitment**: If a group of people are aware of a commitment you've made, there is a lot of social pressure on you to follow through with what you've committed to. By adding more of a public nature to our scheduling attempt, we leverage this aspect of the consistency principle and can help decrease our no-shows. After scheduling the appointment, try adding in this statement: "Great, now that we have your appointment, I'll let the doctor and the other team members up front know that we're going to see you on January 5th at 10 a.m." It's another small commitment the patient can make to help ensure that they show up for their appointment.
5. **Remind them of the commitment they made**: New patients are no different than existing ones when it comes to the commitments they've made. The longer the time passes from when they make their appointment to when the appointment actually is, they too typically need some type of reminder. Use the same reminder strategies that I outlined for existing patients above. Another way you can remind patients of their commitment is to ask to repeat back the day and time of the appointment they just made. In a medical office study, asking patients to repeat back their appointment time reduced no-shows by 3 percent.

   What does it tell you if the person can't repeat back the day and time of the appointment they just made? Most likely it means that they really weren't planning to attend. Better to know that on the front end than after the no-show occurs.
6. **From 13 to 3 percent**: When I spent some time evaluating the no-show situation at my practices, I discovered our no-show rate was sitting at 13 percent, with new patients accounting for over 90 percent of them. At the time, the only thing we changed was that I asked my team to get more verbal commitments, to give the patients more of a voluntary choice of appointment times, and to remind them of the public commitment to our team they had just made. Doing so, our no-show rate dropped from 13 down to 3 percent.

   Here's an example of the language we'd use to do this: "Great, let's make you an appointment. What works best for you? This week or next week? Wednesday or Thursday? Morning or afternoon? 2 p.m. or 4 p.m.? Excellent, so I have you down for this Wednesday at 2 p.m. Do you have any dental insurance information we should know about? Thank you for providing me with that information. Looks like we have your appointment all set. Will you please call us if you need to cancel or reschedule your appointment? Thanks! I'll let the doctor and other team members know you'll call us if you can't make it. Before you go, would you mind repeating back the day and time of your appointment just so I make sure I have it right in my system? Thank you. That's what I have as well. We all look forward to seeing you then."

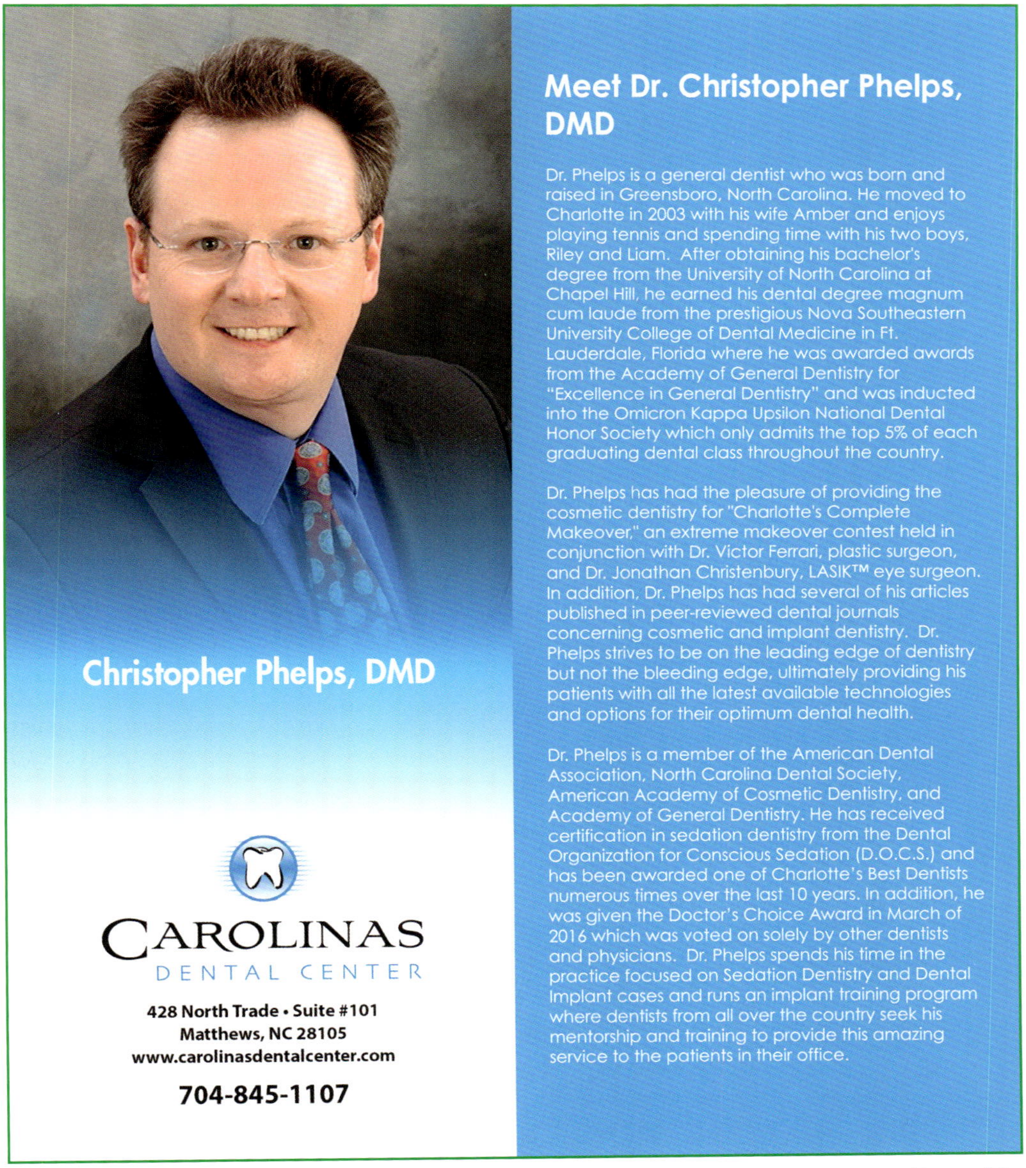

Figure 67. Example of authority card that you can use to introduce patients to you and have this promote your expertise and credentials, before they ever meet you.

7. **Authority cards**: The longer the time passes from when a new patient schedules their appointment to when they are due to show, sometimes some fear and uncertainty begin to build: "Will they like me? Will I like them? Did I make the right choice?" The more this anxiety builds, the greater the chance they won't show up at their appointment as a result. One way to counter this uncertainty is to introduce you and your team to the potential new patient before they actually meet you. As I like to say, from a behavioral science standpoint, "People want to meet you before they meet you!"

   At my practices we accomplished this task by creating "authority cards" (Fig. 67). These were designed as infographics that could be attached to an email sent after an appointment was made that welcomed the new patient to the practice, usually along with some new patient paperwork for them to fill out. With each email, we'd attach or embed the authority card for each of the team members that this person would meet that day. The first one they'd see would be the team member who would greet them and check them in. Then they'd see the hygienist or dental assistant card, depending on which chair they would be visiting that day. Next up would be the dentist's card, followed by our treatment/financial plan coordinator. By letting patients "meet us" before they actually met us, we were able to reduce our no-show rate from 3 to less than 1 percent.

   Plan for the worst, but hope for the best. Our primary goal is to influence existing and new patients to show up for their scheduled appointments. If they can't, our secondary goal should be to make them feel comfortable enough to call us up to cancel and hopefully reschedule their appointment. If they don't and don't show up, it's a lose-lose situation for us both. If we can influence them to call us, then we can use some of these strategies to fill that open-chair time so it doesn't cost the practice in productivity.

D. Strategies to Fill Newly Opened Appointments Times

1. **Same-day doctor treatment**: When a spot in the schedule opens up unexpectedly, look at who else is currently in the practice. Many times there will be a patient who is finishing up treatment in the doctor's chair that might want to stay a little longer and cross another thing off their to-do list. This could be a new patient seen in the doc's chair for the first time or an existing patient who came in for an immediate dental need that is overdue for their cleaning. If you find out about the opening with a day's or two's notice, you can reach out to the patients scheduled in the doc's column that day and ask them if they'd like to get their teeth cleaned as well while they are there. Offering them a chance to stay and further their oral health just may allow your team to turn an unproductive time into a productive one.

2. **Short call list**: Have your team create a list of patients who are interested in getting in on a short notice. This could be segmented by new patients and existing patients and should include whether they want to be seen in the hygiene or dentist's chair. It could comprise those who are scheduled to come in two to three weeks from today but expressed an interest in being seen sooner rather than later. These could be patients who came in on the doctor's schedule for emergency treatment that's completed and now need follow up on the hygiene side of things. This could also include patients who've missed, canceled, or rescheduled multiple prior appointments. Why do you keep rescheduling them when it's

obviously not a priority for them? Instead, let them know that there is limited availability in your schedule, that you'll put them on your short call list, and that you'll reach out to them when an appointment becomes open. Having this list handy gives your team quick access to those most likely to help you fill that spot today.

3. **Patients without insurance**: If we can influence our patients to notify us well in advance that they can't make their appointment, we have a chance to fill it. For hygiene chair openings, we have a choice of reaching out to patients with future appointments who don't have dental insurance. Usually these are patients who pay our full fee out of pocket, which we call "cash patients," or those who've prepaid their two cleanings for the year on our dental membership plan.

   Those who have dental insurance are not good candidates to reach out to as most of the plans require a certain time period expires before they'll pay for a new cleaning. Usually that time frame is six months and a day from their last appointment. In contrast, membership plan and cash patients have no time restrictions. As such, have your team look ahead two to three weeks in your hygiene schedule. Once these patients are identified, reach out to them and see whether they'd like to come in sooner for their cleaning appointment. If need be, offer some small incentive. A complimentary fluoride treatment or a free refill tube of whitening gel goes a long way here to say thank you. If they move up in the schedule, this now gives your team two to three weeks to fill their previous spot with a potential new patient or an existing patient overdue for their periodic cleaning.

   To get a return on your marketing investment you have to be able to convert these opportunities into actual appointments. That means answering your new patient calls, scheduling appointments, and influencing them to show. Mastering these steps in the process is no small endeavor, but they are all critical components to maximizing your marketing ROI. To accomplish this, it means getting the data you need to make smarter decisions, tracking out your unanswered new patient calls and identifying the pattern. It comes from knowing as much information about every new patient phone call that goes unscheduled. Why it happened and understanding if there was something different your team could have done to change that outcome.

   From there it means training and accountability, giving your team every tool they need to both answer and schedule more new patient phone calls, all the while teaching them how to influence more patients to show up for their visit, and focus on building relationships, getting more commitments, and reminding people of the commitments they've made to attend their office appointment. Neglect any of these areas and your new patient count will suffer and you will spend more money in marketing to get the desired result.

Chapter 11
Converting Them at the Chair

In the previous sections we've covered strategies to attract enough quantity and quality of new patients and to set the stage so that they attend the appointment they made. Having success in these areas can set the stage for a significant ROI, but if these patients don't spend any revenue with us, then the ROI will still suffer. That's why we must now turn our focus to one of the most important areas where lost opportunity is found, converting these opportunities at the chair.

In the dental world, this is commonly known as case acceptance. It is usually defined as a percentage of treatment presented compared to treatment performed. You can invest all of the time, money, and resources into creating patient opportunities, but if they don't accept the treatment you present to them, you're marketing ROI will suffer.

In 2018 *Dental Economics* magazine shared findings from thousands of dental offices across the United States indicating that the average dental case acceptance rate is 50 to 60 percent for established patients and 25 to 35 percent for new patients, highlighting just how much opportunity is present that is unfortunately wasted.

1. WHY DENTISTS STRUGGLE WITH CASE ACCEPTANCE

a. **Competition**: At first, you might have read this and assumed I meant competition with one another: that dentists struggle with their patients accepting treatment because other dentists are vying for their care as well. While I understand why many dentists may think this, the reality is that it's a misconception. There are more than enough patients in the world today to fill every dentist's chair, so dentists aren't really in competition with other dentists when it comes to their patients accepting treatment.

   What they are in competition with is what their patients are spending their money on, besides their oral health. As of November 2020, consumer debt is at $14.2 trillion, with Americans carrying an average personal debt of $92,727. The overall debt figure includes credit card balances, student loans, mortgages, and more. When making decisions about moving forward with dental treatment, a comparison will always be made to what other items they could spend their money on instead.

b. **Want vs. need**: Do people tend to spend money on what they want or what they need? Statistically speaking, numerous studies have shown that unless it's a life-or-death situation, one with grave potential consequences, then people tend to spend their money on what they want. Go to any Starbucks, anywhere in the world, and you'll see this to be true.

c. **Mindset**: If patients aren't even in the right mindset concerning their oral health, the door to getting a yes to your treatment recommendation has already been closed. For example, let's say a new patient has arrived early for her appointment, but before she comes in, she finishes having a terrible phone call with her spouse.

   Yelling, tears, a possible divorce on the horizon. The call does not end well. Now it's time for her to come in for her appointment. Now let's assume that she had a good experience. You were on time, nothing hurt her during her cleaning today, but when you come in to discuss her dental needs, where do you think her mind is right now? Concerned about your oral health findings or still stuck in that car and the fight she had with her spouse?

   You see, whether you realize it or not, when patients come into your practice, they are walking in with a mindset already established. Most of the time that mindset is in direct opposition to the dental needs you'll be presenting today. If you don't do anything to counter it, the door to a yes is already shut, and your case acceptance rates will suffer as a result.

d. **Absence of a relationship**: We typically say yes to people who we know and like, people we have some kind of connection or commonality with. If we don't take the time to foster and build the relationship with our patients, then we're more likely to hear some form of no to our request to schedule their next treatment. Maybe you asked them to schedule the crown they need done, and they respond with a direct no such as, "Not at this time" or "I need to wait on that." More often than not they respond with an indirect no such as, "Let me check my calendar and get back with you" or "Let me check with my spouse first." Ultimately in both examples, it ends with them not moving forward and accepting your treatment recommendations.

e. **Uncertainty**: If there are any questions or doubts in people's minds, they don't typically say yes and prefer to do nothing instead. When it comes to presenting treatment to patients, this doubt and uncertainty can be produced in one of two areas. Sometimes it's because the dentists themselves are not confident in the treatment options they are presenting. Given the patient looks to us as the authority or expert to guide them, if they feel like we're unsure about the treatment road ahead, how can they be confident in which path they should choose?

   Most of the time I find that uncertainty is created because we leave too many treatment options on the table for the patient to consider. While ethically we need to present all of the viable options to that patient, if we don't do anything to help guide them to one plan, then a weird paradox sets in. Barry Schwartz described it in his popular book *The Paradox of Choice*.

   In it, he describes how the more options a person has in front of them, the less likely they are to make a choice. It seems the more things a person has to focus on, the less ability they have to differentiate between the options at hand. Without being able to understand the differences, the uncertainty created prevents them from making a decision, and so they chose nothing. Studies now tell us that once you get past five choices, it becomes less and less likely a person will decide.

Let's bring this idea back to dentistry and how it relates to case presentation and ultimately acceptance. You come in and present three treatment options, for example the options to replace a single missing tooth. You cover the removable partial denture, a fixed bridge and a dental implant, and abutment and crown. Having presented these three options, you then turn it over to the financial specialist to come in and review the financial choices available, typically providing three financial options for each treatment option such as pay in full, pay over time, or use a financing company to assist in payments. When presented with three financial options for each of the three treatment options, the patient is left with nine things to consider, ultimately creating more questions and doubt that will likely result in no treatment being scheduled.

f. **Lack of urgency**: Let's say they like you, and because you've shown them their intraoral camera photo of their broken tooth, they've seen their x-ray that they understand and are certain that they need a crown to repair it. Yet they still leave without scheduling their appointment. Why is this? Oftentimes it's because there is a lack of motivation or sense of urgency regarding when they need to come back to get this tooth taken care of. I call this the "I got time" mindset. While they understand it's important, if there is no pain or discomfort to keep it top of mind in their thinking, then many will choose to wait. They possibly intend to call back and schedule that crown but ultimately get distracted by other things going on in their lives or other expenditures that come up that they'd rather spend their money on instead. If we don't take the time to emphasize the urgency required to keep their condition from worsening, then our case acceptance rates will be left wanting.

g. **Lack of anchoring**: Previously in this book, I discussed the contrast effect and how you can change people's perceptions about something by changing what they experience first. For example, if I wanted you to stick your hand into a bucket of room-temperature water, but I wanted you to perceive that water as feeling really hot, then all I'd have to do to change your perspective is have you stick your hand in a freezing cold bucket of water first and then place your hand in the room-temperature water.

The contrast between going from the cold water to the room-temperature water will make your brain perceive that water as being overly hot in comparison, even though that water really was at room temperature and not hot. It's this contrast and comparison that behavioral science studies teach us are the focal point of what we are using to make our decisions in any given moment, weighing out all that's been placed in front of us leading up and into that moment to compare and make our decision.

While we're contrasting everything that's led to this moment, we are also making comparisons to how this item will affect or fit into our future world, with the many items we want to spend our money on or that our budget allows. Remember this, whatever option you give to someone, whatever price you give them around that item, that person is always going to compare it to something in their life, many times being the things they prefer to spend their money on. If you do nothing and let the person control this

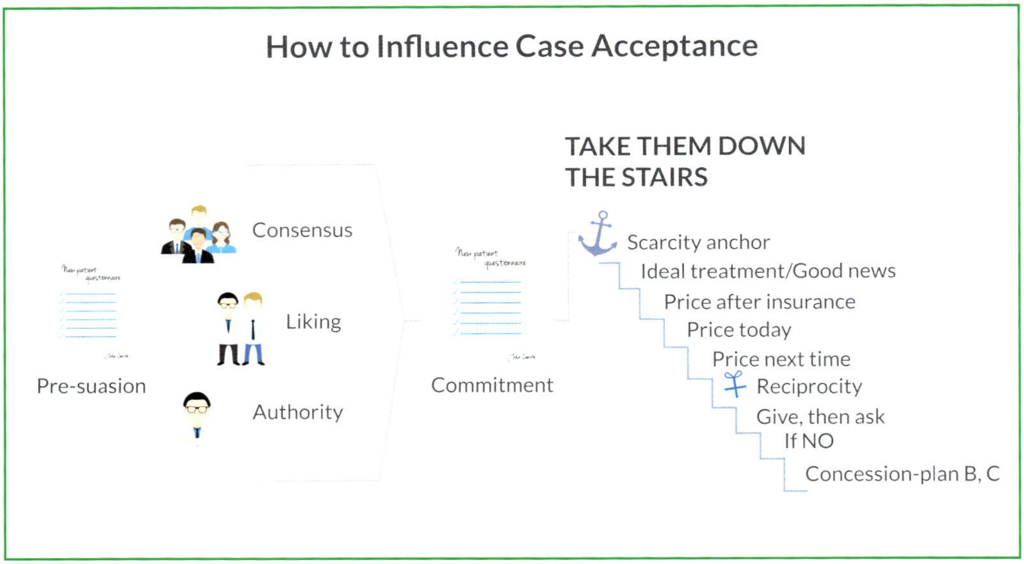

Figure 68. Sequence of where pre-suasion and the principles of persuasion can influence case acceptance.

comparison, the wants in their life tend to outweigh the dental needs you've placed before them. On the other hand, if you start your treatment and financial presentations by anchoring them to something else first, something of a higher value or cost and then go into the dental needs you'll present treatment for, then the contrast effect will start to work in your favor instead of working against you.

To combat these areas that lead more people to say no to our treatment recommendations we can once again lean on the research and findings of Robert Cialdini, PhD, and his six principles of influence and persuasion. As he described in his foundational book *Influence: The Science and Practice*, these principles act as triggers or shortcuts in our decision-making process. When these decision triggers are present, they tend to trigger a yes to the request at hand.

Let's stop for a second and define what true persuasion is really about. By definition, persuasion is when a recipient receives a message in some format, by seeing it or hearing it, for example. Once exposed, the message itself changes that person's perception about what they just experienced. Changing their perception changes that person's thinking in that moment, which then in turn leads to a change in their behavior, a change that doesn't reverse because that person chose to change their mindset and thinking. No one forced them into that position.

This is the complete opposite of negative influence factors such as coercion, intimidation, or someone in charge of you forcing you or telling you what to do. In these cases, you don't feel like you have a choice in the matter. Without a choice, when the threat has been removed, in this case once the patient leaves your office, their behavior reverts back to its original state.

Perhaps you've heard of the old adage, when the cat's away, the mice will play. What this speaks to is this aspect of human behavior that stays consistent throughout time. If people don't feel like they have a viable choice, they don't tend to say yes or return for more care. On the other hand, if we truly influence and persuade them, then they did have a choice in the matter, and it is now more likely than ever for them to say yes to our treatment recommendations and move forward with that care.

While these influence principles are extremely powerful and we lean on them heavily in our decision-making process, they are not a guarantee to having your patients say yes to your treatment recommendations. People still have a choice in the matter, and they could still choose to say no. The good news is that because my influence approach to case acceptance is based in the science of what people use to make their decision, I can guarantee you that more people will say yes to your requests than any other way you'd present it to them (Fig. 68).

2. REVIEW OF CIALDINI'S SIX PRINCIPLES OF PERSUASION

Before we get into that persuasion-based approach to increase your case acceptance, let's review and define these forces that have such an influence on our behavior and actions.

- **Reciprocity**: When a gift of value is given to you, there is an obligation that is created inside of us to give back in kind to the person who gave to us.
- **Liking**: We tend to say yes to people we know and like.
- **Consensus/social proof**: Many times we look to the behavior of others around us to decide what we should do.
- **Authority**: Since we don't have time to be an expert in everything, we look to credible experts to tell us what we should do.
- **Consistency**: When we make a commitment, there is an internal and external pressure on us to be consistent and follow through on what we said we'd do.
- **Scarcity**: When resources are dwindling or about to run out, it motivates us to want those resources more and be willing to do more to get them.
- **Contrast effect**: While not one of Cialdini's principles, it nonetheless has to be discussed in how it affects case acceptance because it's so central to our decision-making process. With contrast, what you say or do before your request is made sets the stage for a yes more so than the facts or merits of the request itself.
- **Ethics of persuasion**: Just because you can influence and persuade someone to a decision, how do you know that you should? Ethics for the most part are very subjective. Maybe you've heard the term "personal code of ethics," meaning that oftentimes what's right or wrong is up to that individual person. Objectively, we can be confident in using persuasion to guide our patients' decisions for several reasons.

  First, because they do have a choice in the matter. We're not holding a gun to their head and telling them to do this treatment. We're not forcing them or coercing them into moving forward. You'll see that we're just presenting options in a way they can make a more educated decision and fight their tendency to do nothing if they don't understand the options at hand. Second, we can feel confident in our actions because we are presenting the truth. Nothing in our presentation is made up or falsified.

Lastly, we should feel good about persuading our patients to say yes because it really is in both of our best interest to do so. Think about it, if people say no to the dental treatment they need, then we both lose in that scenario. We didn't get a yes today, we are missing out on needed production to help us achieve that marketing ROI, and the patient is ultimately left in a deteriorating condition, one that will worsen as time goes on. Yet if the patient really understood what we know will happen to them by doing nothing, that it will cost them more time, money, and potentially pain because of it, then most people would prefer to not let that happen. Instead, they'd choose to make it a priority today and find a way to make it happen.

If you're giving your patient choices, if you're telling them the truth about their dental condition and mapping out the costs if they do nothing, and if your intent is that every patient leave in better oral health than when they came in, then I can objectively tell you that you will be on the ethical side of the line in your persuasion attempts.

Now that we have more confidence of why we should use persuasion to guide our patients to yes and we have a better understanding of why patients tend to say no to us, let's turn our attention to the key areas we need to set the stage for a yes. When I sold my two best dental practices and took over the ownership and management of my two struggling offices, I spent over three years implanting Cialdini's principles into our everyday culture and communication, crafting and refining these decision triggers to the three critical areas where we need to set the stage for a yes.

3. THREE MAIN AREAS WE NEED TO SET THE STAGE FOR A YES

- **The plan**: While our natural tendency is to present multiple treatment options to patients, we have to be wary of the paradox of choice. Instead of leaving patients with too many items, which may confuse them, it's the job of the dentist to influence the patient and guide them to choose one treatment plan. Now, that plan could be all-encompassing, such as treating the whole mouth with a multidisciplinary approach. It could mean treating one arch vs. the other. The worst quadrant of teeth or simply starting with the most important tooth. Whatever that plan is, I leave to you. The key to remember is that we have to influence the patient to be committed to that one plan, not leave multiple plans and options for them to consider. In the next section I'll review my influence-based approach to present as many options as you feel ethically necessary while guiding them to choose one specific plan, all the while turning their dental need into a dental want.
- **The financial agreement**: For the majority of the people, when you turn their need into a want, suddenly it's not about the money or cost. Why? If they want it, they will find a way to make it happen. As such, we still need to have a persuasion strategy that helps us set the stage for the financial commitment we need to acquire before treatment can begin. Now this isn't to say that people won't consider the cost of treatment or in some cases truly can't afford the treatment presented. If your marketing has attracted the right quality new patient, then for the majority of them cost will not be the sole factor they use to make their decision. For those people who just can't financially make it work, I'll review how you can have some financial concessions available to give them and help them fit their dental treatment into their budget.

- **The appointment**: Just because you get a yes and commitment to the treatment plan and you get a yes to the financial agreement, it's still not a guarantee that they'll schedule and show up for the appointment to start. To aid, I'll review a strategy that can assist you in scheduling their appointment and influence them to attend.

A. An Overview of Where the Principles Influence Case Acceptance

1. Pre-Suasion

To set the stage for a yes to the treatment plan, it all starts with the science of "pre-suasion." While Cialdini's principles of persuasion are about how to influence a person to say yes to your requests when they are with you in that moment, Cialdini's research into "pre-suasion" tells us that there is a way you can prime the pump for a yes before that person is in your presence. In his 2016 best-selling book *Pre-suasion: A Revolutionary Way to Influence and Persuade*, Dr. Cialdini defines "Pre-suasion" as arranging for a recipient to be receptive to a message before they encounter it.

For the purposes of this book, I want to simplify this concept for you. Pre-suasion is about mindsets. It's about arranging for your patient to be in a mindset that makes them more likely to say yes to your main request when they hear it. Remember what I said earlier about mindset. Our patients enter our practice with some mindset already pre-established, a mindset that can either work in synergy with our treatment recommendations or one that can work against them. The problem before was that when you didn't do anything to change that mindset, the door to a yes was already closed and can be somewhat difficult to open back up during that patient experience. Knowing this, if we can somehow change their mindset, whatever it was, and focus it back on the importance of their oral health, now the door to the possibility of them saying yes to our treatment recommendations is open. Now we have a chance, and we're automatically more likely to get that yes than ever before.

2. Mindsets Affect Your Decisions

So what are mindsets? From a behavioral science standpoint, mindset is all about who you are in the moments leading up to and the moment you're about to make your decision. But who you are in those moments is really about where you are in those moments, where you are physically, meaning the sights, sounds, smells in the environment around you. These environmental cues surround us and shape our mindset. I know for me, when I smell fresh baked chocolate chip cookies, the kind that come right out of the oven, I instantly have a mindset of home and of family. In my house growing up, when that smell filled the air, you knew it was a special time as it often came as a real treat.

Mindsets are about where you are cognitively in that moment when you're about to make a decision, meaning what are the thoughts swirling around in your mind in those moments. Are they positive, are they negative? Regardless, your thoughts in those moments can shape your mindset and thus shape the decision you're about to make.

Mindsets are also about where you are emotionally in that moment. Remember the example of the new patient who had a terrible fight with her spouse. That emotional state she was in shaped her mindset, and despite the dental needs presented, it wasn't enough to refocus her attention away from that traumatizing phone call.

Right or wrong, when you put it altogether with the emotional state you're in, the thoughts you're occupied by and the environment surrounding you can all have a significant impact on the decisions you make.

Pre-suasion Creates Mindsets

Effective pre-suasion is about taking whatever mindset our patients come into our practice with and redirecting their focus and attention onto a new mindset, one centered on their oral health and its importance. While there are all kinds of factors you can use to create a mindset for someone, there are three that can have the largest effect. Changing the environmental cues people experience can change their mindset. Want to create a mindset of home or family for your patients? Instead of having your reception area look like a traditional medical or dental office waiting area, what if you made it look like a living room that someone might have in their own home? Instead of the traditional "dental smell" that patients have come to experience at the dental office, which used to consist of a combo of x-ray film fixer and developer, eugenol-based intermediate restorative material (IRM) and prophy paste aerosol, what if they came in and were greeted by the smell of fresh baked chocolate chip cookies? Remember in the internal marketing section how effective this was for a dentist in Canada that I spoke with who grew three of his practices through internal referrals using this very method.

People often say that pictures are worth 1000 words. Studies today actually show that they can be worth over a million. Pictures and other images are powerful tools that create mindsets. The image of the sun rising, for instance, has been shown to create a mindset of change. Why? Because a new day is dawning, fresh with possibility. What better time to make a change than that? In my influence process, I'm going to show you other images you can use to create a synergistic mindset in your patients.

Our last tool to help us comes from asking people questions. The words or phrases we use in those questions will create a mindset in our patients. The danger is we have to be careful of the questions we ask. Sometimes those questions can create a mindset that works against us.

I remember early in my career I struggled guiding patients to say yes to more elective procedures such as tooth whitening, veneers, or clear aligner therapy to straighten their teeth. hovering around a 30 percent acceptance rate for these cases. Magically, after a few years' time I noticed a sharp increase in my acceptance after presenting these procedures. At the time I couldn't put my finger on what had changed, other than I was a few years older. Perhaps having more experience made the difference? The reality was that the improvement happened after I had made a change in our new patient paperwork. An important question that used to be asked and was ultimately creating a barrier to yes by creating the wrong mindset had been eliminated on the new form.

On the original form the question read: Rate your smile from 1–10, 1 being you are completely dissatisfied with your smile, and 10 meaning that you absolutely love it. Over that three-year period, I noticed a pattern emerged when I reviewed the answers to this question. The overwhelming majority of people would rate their smile a 7, in essence committing to a mindset in that moment that their smile wasn't the worst thing ever, a 1, and it wasn't the best thing ever, a 10, but it was better than average. Once this "better than average" mindset was created, it was difficult for them to see the value of enhancing that smile cosmetically with the options I'd present. Why would they want these cosmetic changes when in their mind, their smile is well above average? Once I changed my new patient questionnaire and realized that this question had been omitted on the new form, I then realized why the door to yes on my cosmetic recommendations was open and why people were suddenly more inclined to say yes to my requests for these elective treatments.

Mindsets to Increase Case Acceptance

To create a mindset in our patient, we first have to identify what mindset you want to create, a mindset that if established in this patient would make them more likely to say yes to our persuasive request they'll soon hear from us. When looking at the traditional dental practice model and studying the behavior of the patients in my own practice, I realized that there were two main mindsets present.

My patients were either reactive in their behavior or they took a more proactive stance. Reactive patients are those who did not move forward with the treatment recommendations presented to them today and they were okay with the fact that delaying treatment would likely cost them more time, money, and potentially pain down the road as a result. On the other end of the spectrum were my proactive patients, those who consistently came in for their cleanings twice a year, who wanted to move forward with the fillings or crowns they needed today in order to avoid having to have a root canal or extraction down the road. They didn't want it to cost them more time, money, or pain because they waited.

When it comes to your oral health, do you prefer to be proactive, someone who likes to avoid complications, who'd rather take care of an issue today instead of letting it worsen over time, which might cost more time, visits, money, and/or pain to fix down the road?

○ Yes ○ No ____________________

Do you consider yourself more of a reactive person, someone who would rather wait to deal with any issues after they develop, even if that means costing you more time, visits, money, and/or pain to fix down the road?

○ Yes ○ No ____________________

Figure 69. Example of question to ask in new patient questionnaire to create a new patient mindset.

Once I discovered these were the inherent mindsets present, I could then set about in some pre-suasive efforts to get my patients to actively choose which one they preferred to be, a choice that would be made when they answered the questions from my Influence-based patient questionnaire (Fig. 69) before they saw me at the chair. Plus, regardless of whatever mindset they came in with, by asking this and the other questions in this form, you're able to refocus their attention back on to their oral health, overriding whatever mindset they came in with. This is now who they are in this moment before you begin discussing their dental needs.

Mindsets to Reduce Uncertainty

With his research into the core motive's model, Dr. Gregory Niedert, PhD, discovered that the principle of social proof and authority could be used to decrease people's uncertainty about their given situation. Note in the picture below (Fig. 70) the use of social proof from this patient's viewpoint and perspective from the dental chair. By displaying before and after photos and full-face photos of actual patient smiles, patients are able to see evidence that you've done this procedure before and that you've done it on many people before them. That evidence of what others have done will then make them more certain about their choice to have you as their provider, and if cosmetic dentistry is of interest to them, they're now more likely than ever to say yes and move forward with that treatment.

By putting up your credentials, degrees, any awards you've received, and any patient testimonials, you're letting these items present you as an authority, someone with expertise and training in this subject matter as well as someone they can trust. Since we look to credible experts to tell us what we should do, the evidence that this is you is overwhelming, and now the patient is more likely to say yes to your treatment requests once you enter the room.

In the center area you'll note some distinctive pictures or images on the wall as well as a popular TV show here in the United States called *Fixer Upper*. Remember, images create mindsets, good or bad, so you have to be very cognizant of what the patient is exposed to. The last thing you want is the patient watching a news program that spouts negativity, having them watch the stock market losses of the day, thinking about how that has affected their retirement fund, and then you come in to discuss the dental treatment that they need. Being in that negative, loss mindset oftentimes will influence them toward a no and away from a yes.

In contrast, if you have a show like *Fixer Upper* playing, a different mindset could be generated. In this show, homeowners are faced with a dilemma. At first, they feel like their home

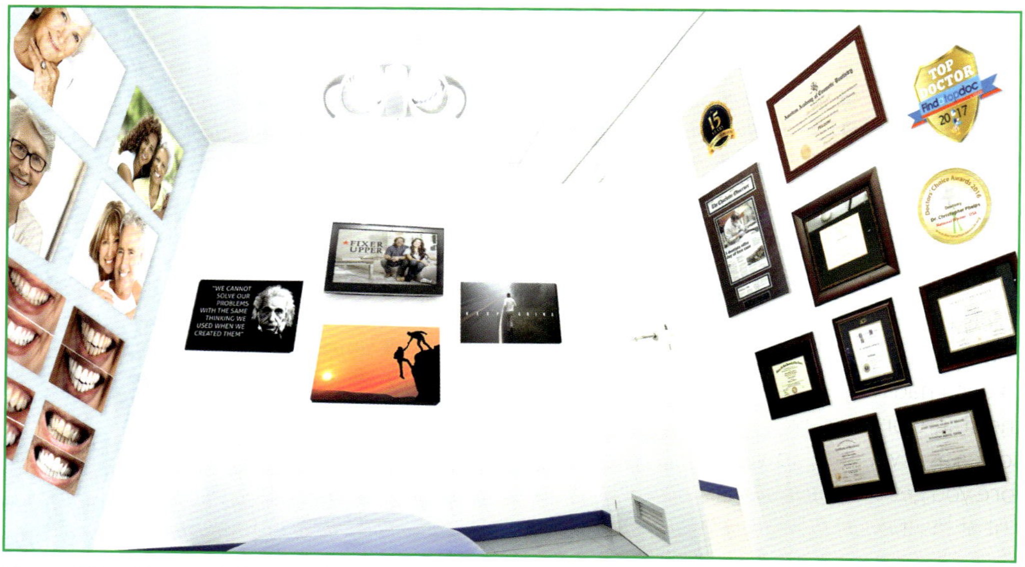
"WE CANNOT SOLVE OUR PROBLEMS WITH THE SAME THINKING WE USED WHEN WE CREATED THEM"
FIXER UPPER
TOP DOCTOR
Find a topdoc
2017
Doctors' Choice Awards 2016

Figure 70. Influence triggers of social proof, authority, and mindset from the patient's perspective in the operatory.

has little value or is too far gone to be saved. Wait, don't our patients have that same mindset sometimes about their own teeth? Then, with the help of some expert advice from the hosts and an investment of time, money, and effort, the home is radically transformed into something beautiful and amazing. Isn't this similar to what we do for patients? I love for my patients to be watching television shows like this because they create mindsets of renovation, rehabilitation, and metamorphosis. Having the patient in this mindset before I come in will automatically make them more receptive and likely to say yes if our discussion turns to elective cosmetic dental treatment.

3. Persuasion: The Principle of Liking

Now that we've established some pre-suasive strategies to get our patients into the ideal mindset to be more receptive to our treatment recommendations, it's time to directly interact with that patient and leverage our persuasion principles. For this, it all starts with liking. People tend to say yes to people they know and like. That's why this principle is key to building relationships with your patients. If they like you, they are more likely to say yes to your treatment recommendations than if they don't.

To leverage this principle properly, I want you to accomplish these two tasks before you get down to reviewing the patient's medical history, reviewing their dental questionnaire, or beginning your examination. First I want you to find at least one thing in common with the patient. One commonality, a shared interest, or something you share with them. Why? Because we like those who are like us, those who have some connection to us. When we see ourselves or something about our self in them, we can't help but like them more.

I remember a new patient who had checked in at our front desk area. On the surface, it didn't appear that I would have had anything in common with this patient. Determined, I set about trying to find some connection between us. When walking toward the operatory to start her new patient exam, I briefly reviewed her medical history and instantly discovered the commonality. After being introduced to the patient by my hygienist, I started by asking her about her birthday. "Is your birthday October 14, 1976?" She confirmed that it was, and I replied, "Well, you know what? We're birthday buddies! I was also born on October 14, 1976!" What are the odds? We were both born not only in the same month but also on the same day and year. Given that we were both about to turn 40 years of age, a monumental day for us both, we had lots to discuss. We spent the next 20 minutes talking about our birthdays.

While this connection may not seem that big of a deal for you, what if I told you that my birthday buddy left the appointment, scheduled to start her $12,000 treatment plan. Was it solely because of this connection? Given the treatment costs, I'd say probably not, but don't you see now how that similarity could have played a part, making her more likely to say yes than if I had not found that connection? That's what these principles do and why I say it sets the stage for a yes. Not a guarantee, but the more of these things you tap into, the more the scales are weighted toward you receiving a yes to your treatment recommendations. So before you get started, find at least one thing in common with that person. The more the better, but at least one similarity will build your relationship with that person.

Once you've found that commonality, if there is something you genuinely like about that person, then don't hide that fact. Tell them. Why? Because we like to do business with those who like us or those who tell us that they like us. If people know you like them, then they are naturally inclined to reciprocate and like you back. Giving people praise and compliments is an easy way to accomplish this.

To leverage liking, talk to your patients and ask questions about their family, where they grew up, their hobbies or interests, their job, any pets they have, and so forth. If you have something in common with them, don't hide that fact—bring it up. If there is something you genuinely like about the person, then tell them. Liking is probably the most overlooked and bungled of the six principles in dentistry. No one has "time" to do it, or they're "too busy." The fact of the matter is by not showing your patients that you like them, you're missing out on hundreds of thousands of dollars in treatment.

4. Creating Consistency and Reinforcing the Mindset

After you've established some kind of connection with the patient, now you can go and review their medical history with them. Review any x-rays taken and complete your extraoral and intraoral exams, acquiring as much diagnostic data as needed to craft one or several treatment plan options. Once you have a good idea of what those options will be, there is an important step you must complete before you begin your treatment presentation. This step involves Dr. Cialdini's principle of consistency.

The consistency principle states that once people make a commitment to something, there is a significant amount of external and internal pressure on them to stay consistent with the ideals of the commitment that they've made. On the external pressure side, let's look at what society calls people who are inconsistent in their actions, words, or beliefs, those who don't do what they say they would do. Typically, we call them flakes, wishy-washy, or oftentimes we call them liars. So there is social pressure created when we commit to something as we don't want others to view us or our actions in that light. At the same time, there is an internal pressure created because we don't want to view ourselves in that light either. So the key to remember with this principle is this: People tend to live up to what they commit to.

When you look at this example of a new-patient questionnaire (Fig. 71) that we had them fill out to help create an ideal mindset, you'll also notice that we asked questions that got people committed to what they value most when it concerns their oral health. By having the patient fill this out before they get in front of you, you've used this as a pre-suasive tool to create an ideal mindset. Now that they are in front of you and you've gone through the medical history, acquired your diagnostic data, and have formulated some type of treatment plan, you can use this tool again in a persuasive manner to reinforce the commitments they have made.

CUSTOMIZED TREATMENT AND PRESENTATION QUESTIONNAIRE

CAROLINAS DENTAL CENTER

Patient Name:	
Reason for visit:	Approximate date of last dental visit:

Do you consider yourself to be a Proactive person? Someone who likes to avoid complications. Who'd rather take care of an issue today instead of letting it worsen over time which might cost more time, visits, money and/or pain to fix down the road?

◯ Yes ◯ No ______________________________

Do you consider yourself more of a Reactive person? Someone who would rather wait and deal with any issues as they develop. Even if that means costing you more time, visits, money and/or pain to fix down the road? ◯ Yes ◯ No

____

If we were sitting here together a year from now, what needs to happen for you to consider our office an excellent choice for you? Examples might be: Being pain free, in great dental health, having whiter teeth, no more silver fillings, cost, etc.
Please write answer below:

____

____

What do you value most in a dental office? **Please write answer below.**

Cosmetic - You most value how your teeth look. Want them straight. Want them white.
Function - You most value an ability to enjoy your favorite foods and drinks. Don't want to be limited to just eating on one side or area. No food or drink should be off limits to you.
Comfort - You most value NOT being in pain or having any tooth or gum sensitivities. Example: I can't eat this anymore because it hurts or is sensitive.
Longevity - You most value the ability to have your natural teeth forever. You wish to have the work you have done in the chair to last as long as possible.

____

____

What is the most import ant objection or obstacle you have to visiting a dental office? **Please write answer below.**

No objections or obstacles - I come faithfully every 6 months and value my dental health. Fear-Of pain. Noises. Environment. Past experiences.
Time - Night schedule. Getting appointments to suit your schedule. Not able to take off work, etc. Getting in and out of office quickly.
Have NOT had a sense of urgency - Nothing really hurts so haven't seen need to go to dentist in years or something has been hurting at some level for a while but I've been able to live with it.
Budget - Knew I needed a lot of work, didn't have money to address any issues found.
No Trust - Felt you were told you needed treatment you didn't need. Felt ripped off. Bad previous experience. Didn't give me any data to support treatment they recommended.

____

____

When the Dentist or Dental Team Member needs to talk to you about options to restore your dental health (such as crowns, dentures, implants, etc.), do you prefer: **Please write answer below.**

1. A simplified oral explanation and description of dental treatment needed.
2. Both detailed oral and visual explanations which could include video animations demonstrating the procedure recommended and or photographs of the procedure or photos of other patients' mouths that had similar treatment.
3. Have physical models on hand to hold and feel to aid in visualizing the work needed to be performed.

____

Do you prefer to break your appointments up into smaller visit s and schedule out over time? ______________

Do you prefer to get any necessary treatment done today, if possible, as getting into the office is a challenge for you? ______________

____

Figure 71. Example of influence-based new patient questionnaire. Each question is designed to create a new mindset and commitment on what the patient values.

Go through each question, read back what the patient wrote, and get the patient to verbally commit that these answers are important to them:

***Doctor*: So I see here that when it comes to your oral health, you prefer to be proactive, someone who wants to avoid dental issues getting worse and costing you more time, money, and potential pain because you waited. Is that true? (Then let them confirm this is what they value.)**

Patient: That's right, doctor, I don't like for things to fester or worsen.

***Doctor (If you believe the same, invoke some liking and similarity here)*: Great, I feel exactly the same. I hate for things to worsen when they don't have to. Okay, I see here that you value comfort, so you don't want to have any kind of sensitivity or pain. Is that correct?**

Patient: That's correct, doctor. I don't want my mouth or teeth to hurt.

***Doctor*: Nor do I. Okay, it seems here that a big objection you have to getting dental treatment performed is time. So if we had to schedule a lot of treatment visits, this would be a challenge for you?**

Patient: That's correct. My work situation is tough right now. They really need me there and aren't very forgiving for those who take a lot of time off work.

***Doctor*: Okay, good to know. I see here that if I find several issues or problems with your teeth, you'd prefer that I create a plan to address everything and not just a single-tooth issue. Is that correct?**

Patient: That's right, doctor. I'd rather have a plan to fix it all if you can do that for me.

The new patient questionnaire I have provided for you here is just an example of some types of commitment questions you can ask your patients. There are many more possibilities you could ask here or substitute in as well. I leave the questions themselves up to you, but pose them in this manner. In fact, while I've been referencing this form for new patients, you can also have your existing patients fill it out for you so you know what they value and are committed to as well. This is best done when they fill out their annual medical history update for you. When doing so, have them fill this form out as well because understanding what they value is just as important as knowing it for your new patients. In both scenarios, your case acceptance will increase.

Probably the #1 mistake I find dentists make when presenting their treatment recommendations is that they assume that they know what the patient values. They assume it's all about the price or cost of treatment. They assume that they'd want to get it done today instead of waiting and it getting worse.

When we are correct and we tie our treatment recommendations back to what they value, we tend to get a yes to those requests. When we're wrong and we've tied it to something they don't value, it tends to trigger a no. The goal of using this questionnaire is to help you stop guessing, to get the patient to take a stand and commit right here and now as to what they really value, what means the most to them, and what kind of patient they will be in your practice moving forward. With this information in hand, along with the commitments we've received from them at the chair, more people will say yes when they see how our treatment recommendations will affect their stated values and beliefs.

B. Getting a Yes to One Treatment Plan

1. Reactive Mindset Case Acceptance Strategy

At this point in our case presentation strategy, you've used the new-patient questionnaire as pre-suasive tool to help change whatever mindset your patients came in with and have refocused it back onto their oral health. You've established some kind of connection with them, some kind of commonality to create a shared bond. You've also gone through and identified exactly what it is the patient really values when it comes to matters in their mouth, what I call value anchors, vocally, reinforcing the commitments they made to these value statements before being in your chair. Lastly, you've presented all of your diagnostic findings to the patient, showing them their x-rays, intraoral camera photos, extraoral photos, and so forth, to justify there are dental issues that are concerning.

Now it's time to present your treatment recommendations. To accomplish this, I have two main strategies I employ, each designed for the main mindset the patient has chosen. Let's start with the most challenging mindset: the patient who states that when it comes to their oral health, they prefer to be reactive.

Right off the bat you should realize that the door to a yes has already been closed. They've made a commitment that if they are not really in any real pain or discomfort, then they don't want to move forward with any treatment. They are good with waiting and fully understand and are okay with the fact that it's going to cost them more time, money, pain, and so forth, because they waited. Remember, once people make a commitment, it's hard to reverse it. That's who they are and what they believe in that moment with you. So instead of trying to win an uphill battle and reverse this mindset, my strategy is to work with it. To communicate with a reactive mindset patient, I'm going to focus my efforts in two areas:

1. Make myself and my treatment plan the scarce resource.
2. Focus on the relationship. "I got your back."

One of the only ways to reverse this type of commitment is to use the principle of scarcity. That principle states that when resources are dwindling or about to disappear, suddenly we're more motivated to want that item and do more to get it, even if we didn't want it before. So in this moment, I will attempt to make myself and my treatment plan the scarce resource.

Ethically, I'm required to let my patient know that they have dental issues. I'm required to let them know that I have a plan to address all of those issues today so that they won't worsen. I'm going to document all of those issues in my chart notes as well as the plan I came up with to address them.

What I'm ethically not required to do is to present my detailed plan to someone who does not want to hear it and has committed to not moving forward with any treatment as long as they are in this pain free, "out of sight, out of mind" mindset. So I'm going to inform the patient that I see dental issues present. I will let them know that today is the best day to address those issues as it will save them more time, money, and potential pain versus waiting. I'm going to tell them that I have a plan that addresses all of the issues I see, but then I'm going to take that plan away, making it and myself the scarce resource.

***Doctor*: Mr. Jones, I see here that when it comes to your oral health, you prefer to be reactive, someone who isn't concerned with issues today, even though it might worsen over time. Is that correct?**

Patient: That's right, doctor. If I'm not in pain, then I'm okay waiting and don't want to discuss it today.

***Doctor*: Okay, I understand. But ethically I do have to let you know that you have several dental issues going on. Time bombs in your mouth, if you will. While I know those bombs will explode at some point, the problem is I can't see the timer and don't know when it will occur. Now the good news is that today is the best time to address the issues as it will cost you the least amount of time, money, and potential pain versus waiting. In fact, I have a complete plan here that I could review with you that addresses these issues, but it sounds as if you don't want to hear it. So I tell you what, if you ever change your mind and want to discuss my plan, you come back in and let me know, and we'll go through it together.**

At this point, I pause and wait to see how the patient reacts. I've given them all of the information I'm ethically bound to do but at the same time honored their request to not talk about it today as it's not a concern. I've taken my treatment plan to address their issues, put it in front of them, and then took that plan away. Making it scarce by not discussing it, one of two things will occur. Either they will stand firm in their commitment and leave or the scarcity of not hearing the plan will motivate them to change their mindset and want to have me go through it. Usually the patient will say something like: "Okay, okay, doctor. You're right. I probably should hear what you have to say. Let's go through your plan."

If they change their mind and ask you to review the plan, the door to a yes to your treatment recommendations is now open and the possibility is there whereas before, their commitment had shut that door before you even began. Now you would proceed and use the influence presentation approach I'll soon cover for the proactive mindset patient.

If they don't change their mind and are steadfast in their commitment to wait it out, then I shift my strategy to focusing on the relationship. I want the patient to know that there will be no judgment from my standpoint because of this path they've chosen, but I want them to know that when their oral condition does take that turn for the worse and they need me, I've got their back and will do everything I can to get them into the office that same day to address that problem.

Doctor: Okay, I understand. But ethically I do have to let you know that you have several dental issues going on. Time bombs in your mouth, if you will. While I know those bombs will explode at some point, the problem is I can't see the timer and don't know when it will occur. Now the good news is that today is the best time to address the issues as it will cost you the least amount of time, money, and potential pain versus waiting. In fact, I have a complete plan here that I could review with you that addresses these issues, but it sounds as if you don't want to hear it. So I tell you what, if you ever change your mind and want to discuss my plan, you come back in and let me know, and we'll go through it together.

Patient: Okay, sounds good; thanks, doc.

Doctor: You're very welcome. Before you go, just remember this. When the time bomb does go off, please don't hesitate to call us. You won't hear any judgment on our end, but I promise we'll do our best to get you in that day and take care of the problem at hand. We got your back. Does that work for you?

Patient: Thank you, doctor. I really appreciate that and you understanding my needs.

When the dental issue does become a top-of-mind concern for this patient, we try to stay true to our word. We attempt to schedule them the same day to evaluate the issue. If we have time, we'll start or complete the treatment needed or worst case, manage their symptoms until we can get them back in to complete the treatment. Case acceptance rates on these patients are extremely high because you've built trust with this patient at your last encounter. At this point, I keep the presentation simple as they knew this day was coming, they knew it was going to potentially hurt, and that it's going to cost them more in treatment and fees because they waited. The difference here is now they are motivated and want a solution. So don't waste any time with a grand presentation. Keep it simple:

Doctor: Well, Mr. Jones, I guess we knew this day was coming, right? Okay. Let's get down to it. Here's where we are today and what it's going to take to address this issue and get you out of pain. (Then go through your treatment plan). Let me get the financial team to come in and review that with you, and if you're ready, we can get started today.

The point of this influence questionnaire is to get the patient in front of you to declare what they value, instead of us having to guess it. Once you know what they really value and are committed to, then your goal is to tie your treatment presentation and the pros and cons of those recommendations back to these value anchor statements. Just like what we did for this reactive mindset patient. Truthfully, I don't care what choice they make for these questions. I just want to be ready to communicate with them and present the issues at hand as they relate to the choices they've made.

2. Proactive Mindset Case Acceptance Strategy

If your practice model is that of an emergency clinic, then you'd want the majority of your patients to have that reactive mindset, and you'd direct all of your marketing efforts to target them accordingly. For the majority of you reading this book, you'll want those who prefer to be proactive with their oral health, those who come in for their preventative cleaning visits and who move forward with the fillings and crowns that you've planned so as to avoid having to have root canals, extractions, or dental implants. These are the patients who should be filling 80–90 percent of our chair time and support the traditional dental model of practice, leaving 10–20 percent of your chair time to fit in those reactive patients with emergent needs.

Now that I've covered my system for presenting to patients who prefer to be reactive, let's turn our attention to the other side of the coin: those who prefer to be proactive. Statistically, when presented with this choice on what they prefer when it comes to their oral health, the vast majority of people choose to be proactive. Let's go into the two main strategies you'll need to use when presenting treatment to these patients.

The first main strategy applies when there is really only one treatment option, for example, if they need a crown. The second route we'll cover will teach you how to ethically present multiple treatment options but get them dialed in and committed to one of your plans, whether that be a series of choices like a removable partial denture vs. a bridge vs. a dental implant, abutment and crown, or a series of comprehensive care options such as completing the whole mouth of treatment, half of the mouth of treatment, a single quadrant, or the worst tooth. The good news is that the structure in how you present single options compared to more complicated treatment plans is exactly the same.

3. Proactive Mindset Case Acceptance Strategy: Single Treatment Option

Let's use a crown as an example of a single treatment option. You've reviewed the x-ray and completed your intraoral examination and are confident in this treatment that you'll propose. Normally, you would start your presentation by educating your patients about your findings and then telling them about the crown that's needed. There's just one problem with this scenario. You didn't give them a choice. In fact, you took the decision-making process completely out of their hands and are now at the mercy of what I call "the remote control phenomenon."

A 2009 study at Oregon State University found that men are more likely to dominate the use of the remote control and dictate what is being watched on television in that moment. In my household, I can relate as the TV remote stays with me at all times. If my wife borrows the remote for any reason, then an uneasiness creeps in the longer she holds onto it. In that moment, I can't explain why I'm nervous or bothered by this, only that I am until the remote returns back to me. What this effect alludes to is a deeper desire to control the environment around us. Yet little in our world is actually under our direct control. So the more out of our control things around us seem, the more we strive to control something. For men in this case, it's that television remote.

Now imagine you have a male patient in your chair and you tell them that they need a crown. By dictating this treatment need to them, in essence you've taken away their control of the situation. You've taken the remote. When people do that, our tendency is then to hold out or take that control back. Thoughts begin to creep into the patient's mind: "Who are you to tell me I need a crown? It doesn't hurt right now, so I'll be the judge of if or when I need this crown." The end result is that the patient doesn't schedule for the crown they need. Women are not immune to this "remote control phenomenon" either. Everyone in the world desires to be in control of their destiny.

So how do we get away from telling our patients about the treatment they need, taking away their control, and instead move to influence them to make a decision? We do so by giving them a choice. When they have a choice, they have control. When they have control, they're much more likely to make a decision and act vs. when they are not in control. The other great thing about giving people a choice is that once they choose, they are now more committed than ever to following through with the choice they made. We're tapping into the power of the consistency principle by offering people this voluntary choice so they are in control of where they want their oral health to go from here.

Anchor with Scarcity and Then Present Your Single Treatment Option

Let's go back to our example with the crown treatment plan. We need to structure our presentation into a "this or that" style choice (Fig. 72). The first option, or "this", will always be to anchor them to the scarcity of what will occur if they do nothing. Scarcity, as I've mentioned before, is a powerful influence tool to motivate people to say yes and take action today. That's why we're going to anchor them to what they stand to lose by doing nothing in three categories:

1. **Treatment consequence**: If they do nothing today, then what additional treatment will be required in the future, to help them get back to their current tooth condition? For the crown, doing nothing could lead to the tooth requiring a root canal, core buildup, and crown.
2. **Value consequence**: If they do nothing today, then what will it cost them with the value statements they committed to in the new-patient questionnaire? If they value comfort, not being in pain, then by waiting, the tooth very well may become symptomatic from the invading bacteria or an infection that begins to spread from the tooth and into the body.
3. **Financial consequence**: We have to put a financial cost to the additional treatment they will need because they waited: that root canal, core buildup, and crown now costing them a total of $3600 to treat down the road.

Behavioral science studies on scarcity tell us that people care more about what they stand to lose than what they stand to gain in your proposal. So by anchoring them to the ethical consequences of any additional treatment that will be needed, the financial cost of that treatment, and how it affects what they value, we're maximizing the scarcity effect. By presenting a viable alternative choice or path they can take to avoid those consequences, we're putting the control back in the patient's hands, motivating them to make a choice and stay consistent to move forward with the choice they've made.

Scarcity Anchor: Option 1, do nothing outlines ethical consequences of not moving forward with treatment. Sets a $ value to that cost (RCT/BU/CRN $3600)		
Ideal Crown Option		
The *bad* news is...	BUT...	The *good* news is...

Figure 72. **Example of how to structure your influence presentation when only one viable treatment option is present.**

Now let's put it together, using our example of the crown. Before you start your case presentation, you still need to justify why the patient needs any treatment at all. This means showing them their x-ray, sharing with them the intraoral camera photo showing their current tooth state, and pointing out any deterioration seen. In this example, we'll assume that the patient has committed to being proactive, that they value comfort and not being in pain, and that time is a concern for them.

***Doctor*: So, Mr. Jones, I see here that when it comes to your oral health, you prefer to be proactive. You value comfort and not being in pain, and if multiple visits were required to treat you, this would be a problem. Is this correct?**

Patient: That's correct, doctor.

***Doctor*: Okay, if that's true, then I know you'll see why I'm concerned when I saw this with your tooth. (Show them the x-ray and point out any decay seen, show them the intraoral camera photo and point out any issues identified as well).**

***Doctor*: So your first option here is to do nothing. The good news is that it will cost you nothing, but the bad news is that at some point, the bacteria in this tooth will continue until they reach the nerve chamber. Once there, they'll kill off the nerve and the tooth will die, typically causing pain or discomfort and a spreading infection. Once that happens, we'll have to spend three to four visits and perform a root canal, core buildup, and crown, and that treatment will cost you around $3600. But hey, we're not there yet, if we get to it today, we're just looking at repairing the tooth with a full coverage crown. The bad news about the crown is that it might seem expensive, but the good news is that we can avoid the added expense, visits, and potential pain you'd be in for by waiting and doing nothing. So what would you like to do? Do nothing and we'll plan on that additional root canal work and expense in the future or take care of it with a crown today?**

Patient: Oh, I don't like that idea of doing nothing and needing a root canal and such later. We better move forward with the crown today.

***Doctor*: Great, you've made a smart choice. I'll get my financial team to come in and review details on that crown option you've chosen.**

By showing the patient their x-ray and intraoral camera photo and pointing out the issues we see, we've justified to them that there is a legitimate dental issue present. Notice how I tied the cost of doing nothing back to their proactive mindset, wanting to avoid conditions worsening, and what their stated values were: avoiding being in pain, taking multiple visits to treat, requiring more complicated dental treatments and then anchoring them to financial cost of delay. I then simply contrasted this future scenario to the treatment option available today and asked them to make a "this or that" choice, giving them the remote control so they are free to make the decision accordingly.

Also note that the doctor did report a cost to the patient. Not the cost of the ideal treatment today, which the financial team will be discussing, but the $3600 cost of doing nothing, adding in what it would also require in the future to get back to where they are today. A tooth without pain, infection, present in their mouth, and so forth. The last thing I want to point out is how I not only described the pros and cons of each treatment option in terms of good news and bad news, but also note that the order in which I presented them for each choice was different. Each choice presented pivoted around the word "but." I'll go into more detail on the rationale of contrasting the pros and cons in this specific sequence and why we leverage the power of the word "but" in the next section.

Regardless of the treatment option you have to present, there is almost always something else you can anchor the patient to first: an ethical consequence or something of a higher value and cost, which then allows you to frame your ideal treatment choice today. Let's look at another example. Let's say your treatment plan was for scaling and root planing. Imagine what would happen if they did nothing today. Then after some time period, a year, 5 years, 10 years, or some other time period, they return seeking treatment. What would it cost them using those anchors we discussed?

Most likely, their periodontal condition would have deteriorated to the point that they may need to have all of their teeth extracted and a full set of complete dentures fabricated. Since these appliances won't let them chew and function like the natural teeth they have today, perhaps they'll need dental implants and screw-retained appliances to engage them.

So what do you think the patient might prefer? Losing all of their teeth and getting dentures, only to discover that they can't eat or chew well with them? Requiring dental implants on both arches and fabrication of new fixed appliances, costing upwards of $60,000 for the whole mouth of treatment? Or would they prefer to not let that happen and move forward with the scaling and root planing needed today, which comes at a significantly reduced cost? When framed with a "this or that" scenario, the brain will always put more emphasis and value on "that" and oftentimes choose this outcome as a result.

4. Proactive Mindset Case Acceptance Strategy: Multiple Treatment Options

Anchor with Scarcity and Then Present Multiple Treatment Options

When it comes to presenting multiple treatment options, we have some challenges to face. The first is that we have to help the patient overcome the paradox of choice, where the more options we give them means the less likely they'll be to pick any of them. At the same time, we still need to give them some choices to get them more committed to one of the treatment options we'll present. Next, we need to establish some type of trust with them.

Trust is typically something that isn't established quickly with someone, and it's rarely on your first encounter with them. Trust is usually built over time and after multiple experiences with someone. Our problem is we'd like our patients to trust us and say yes today, not two or three visits from now. So for this presentation format we'll need something that will help us build trust quickly, even with someone we've just met for the first time.

Lastly, we need to present their treatment options in a way that they can make an educated decision about their care. Even though they are not a dental expert and we're asking them to make a decision as if they were. In doing so and guiding them down to one treatment option or plan, our presentation will change their perspective about their options at hand and turn their dental need into a desired want, setting the stage for a yes to one of our treatment options. This is the worksheet (Fig. 73) I've designed to help you structure your multi-option presentations. For this example, we'll use the single missing maxillary first molar tooth as our multiple option treatment scenario.

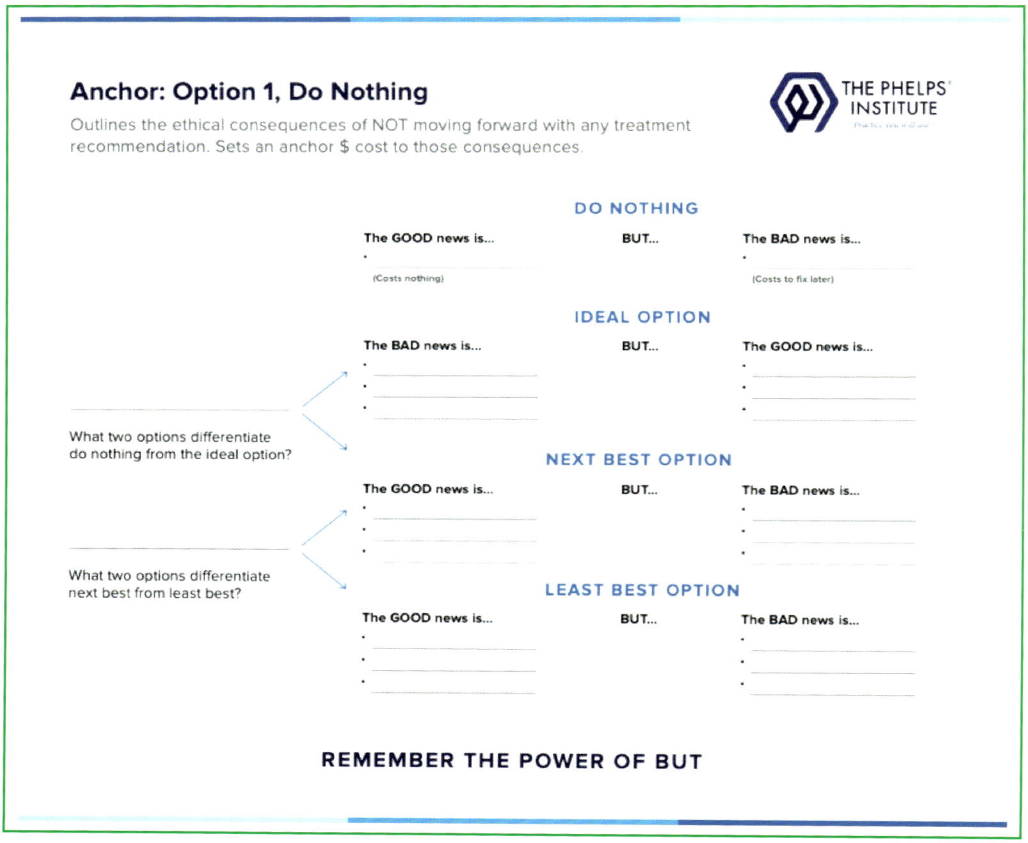

Figure 73. How to structure your treatment presentation when there are multiple treatment options available.

Doctor: So, Mrs. Jones, I see here that when it comes to your oral health, you prefer to be proactive. You value longevity, wanting your teeth to stay around for the long run, and if multiple visits were required to treat you, then this would be a problem. Is this correct?

Patient: That's correct, doctor.

Doctor: Okay, then you see why I'm concerned by this area where you are missing a tooth. Did you know that the only thing that keeps the bone in your jaw are your teeth? Without the teeth, you begin to lose the bone in that area, compromising the teeth next to them. Did you know that the only thing that keeps your teeth in place are your other teeth? When they lose the tooth next to them or the one they connect with on chewing they then erupt out of the bone or shift positions until they find something to connect with. You have a large sinus cavity here that we call the maxillary sinus. Did you know that without the tooth roots present, your sinus cavity will grow in volume, taking up the available space, which will lead to more sinusitis, potentially causing more sinus infections?

Doctor: Now your first option to treat this area is to do nothing. The good news about this option is that it costs you nothing, but the bad news about this option is that you'll continue to lose more bone in this area, compromising the teeth next to them, which could lead to more potential tooth loss in the future. If we wait to treat this down the road, you'll most likely need to have orthodontics to move the teeth back into their original position and create space to put your missing tooth back. You'll need to have a sinus lift, bone graft, and then have a dental implant, abutment, and crown placed, costing you over $10,000 and approximately two years of treatment.

Doctor: Your second option is to not let that happen and move forward with a dental implant abutment and crown. Here's a picture or model of what this option looks like. The bad news about this option is that it's the most expensive option and takes the most time, but the good news about this option is that you won't lose bone around that area, which should protect you from losing those other teeth around it.

Doctor: Your next option is to do what we call a dental bridge. Here's a picture or model of what this option looks like. The good news about this option is that it typically costs a little less than the implant option and takes less time to complete, but the bad news about this option is that you may have to replace this bridge three or four more times in your lifetime. You see, dental insurance companies are paying for a new bridge every seven years on average, telling us that this is what they see are the current life expectancies of this option.

Doctor: Your last option is what we call a removable partial denture. Here's a picture or model of what this option looks like. The good

news about this option is that it's the least expensive of the options and doesn't require a lot of time, but the bad news about this option is that for it to stay in position, it requires placing damaging forces on the teeth around the space, which studies show usually leads to the loss of one or both teeth around the space present within 10 years.

By framing our presentation using this influence-based structure, we've accomplished a lot of critical items that will help us set the stage to the patient saying yes to one of our treatment options. First, we got their attention by anchoring them to all three of our scarcity anchors, or what they stood to lose by doing nothing, tying that loss back to additional treatment that will be needed to fix the problem in the future, a cost to the longevity they said they valued about keeping as many teeth for as long as possible, and by putting a financial and time cost to it of $10,000+ and two years of treatment time. By anchoring them in this way, our message of these costs will be perceived as of higher importance because they came in with a proactive mindset, one who preferred to avoid these very type of things.

The next thing we accomplished is that we've instantly built trust with this person. Why? Because we leveraged an authority shortcut. Notice how we start the presentation of our ideal treatment option, in this case the dental implant, abutment, and crown with why this might not be such a great thing. It's expensive and takes the most time of the other options. Why did we do this? Isn't it better to hide the elephant in the room and not bring it up at all?

Not if you want that person to trust you sooner than later. Behavioral science studies show that if you start your presentation off with a weakness in your case, some negative aspect of your ideal option early on and then go into its positive aspects, this instantly builds trust with someone you meet for the first time. If you think about it, it makes sense. Why would you ever start out talking about the negatives of what you're presenting unless you were someone who could be trusted? You're not trying to hide anything from that person, but instead you're being open, honest, and transparent. You're not hiding the elephant in the room, you're starting with it.

Now we come to that pivotal word, "but." "But" is an important word. That's why it's emphasized here. "But" is a word that wakes the brain up, telling it that something important is coming, so it is better to pay attention to what comes next. Studies show that when we are presented options around this pivot word, people don't really remember what was said or how they felt before the word "but." All they remember is what was said and how they felt about your option from the descriptors used after the word "but."

Remember I said earlier that our patients are not really dental experts. That means unless they've had a crown in their mouth, they've had an implant, or had some type of personal experience with the treatment you're talking about, they have very little actual understanding about the treatment options you've presented. Yet, they still need to compare and contrast something they do understand so they can make a decision. Using this pivot word, we've helped them do just that. While they don't really understand what a dental implant is, they will remember that it's a "good" option. While they don't really understand what a dental bridge or removable partial denture are, they will remember the "bad" aspects about them. So when it comes down to making their choice, which do you think they would prefer for themselves? The bad treatment options or the good one?

By structuring our presentation in this format, we've now alerted them to the dangers of doing nothing, motivating them to want to do something. We've built trust with someone we've just met for the first time, avoiding the normal three to four encounters it would have taken. We've given them viable choices to the problem at hand but presented it in a way that they can make a real educated choice, influencing them to desire your ideal option over the other two, turning that dental need into a dental want for them. But we're still not done. We still have to address that paradox of choice as there are too many options left on the table. Remember, the job of the doctor is to guide the patient to commit fully to one of these options. So let's review how we finish this sequence out.

I mentioned before that the problem with too many choices is that the person loses the ability to differentiate between them. If they can't tell the difference between the options, then it's that uncertainty or doubt that leads them to do nothing in contrast. So it's our job to help the patient understand the biggest or most significant differences of our options. Now we'll go from the bottom of the choices, as it relates back to their value statement, in our example, longevity, and then present those differences in a "this or that" format as we work our way back up the options list until the patient has chosen the plan that's best for them. So think to yourself, what is the biggest difference between the removable partial denture vs. the fixed bridge? What's the biggest difference you can think of between the bridge compared to the dental implant option?

***Doctor*: Okay, Mrs. Jones. We've now gone through all of the treatment options. Let's go through them again and figure out which one is best for you. Now, we talked about this removable partial denture and this dental bridge. Remember, that partial is that plastic tooth appliance that comes in and out of your mouth and may cause you to lose an additional tooth in the future the longer you wear it. That bridge option is bonded into place and doesn't come out at all. So which would you prefer? Do you want to have to take your teeth in and out or would you prefer something that stays in place and doesn't ever come out?**

Patient: Oh, I don't want to take my teeth out, that sounds terrible.

***Doctor*: I agree. Okay, let's look at your next choice. This dental bridge vs. the dental implant option. Now based on estimates from dental insurance companies, you'll have to replace this bridge every seven years or so, paying for three or more teeth each time you replace it. This dental implant option, if you take care of it and we see you for your preventative treatments, is one of the few things we could put in your mouth that could last the rest of your life, preserving the bone and the teeth around them. So which would you prefer? Do you want to take the risk of having to replace this bridge three or four more times in your life or would you prefer a longer-term option like the implant?**

Patient: I don't want to have to keep messing with this thing, so I think I'll take the implant option.

Cont'd

***Doctor*: Great! You've made an excellent decision, one I'd hope my own family members might make in your situation. Now let me introduce you to Shelley. She is our expert financial coordinator and will come in to discuss how we can fit this implant option into your budget.**

Now we've completed the sequence. We've educated the patient on the pros and cons of all of the treatment options we were ethically obligated to cover but have guided them into choosing and committing to one of our treatment options. With each voluntary choice they made in the "this or that" approach, they became more committed and more likely to moving forward with that treatment option. Sometimes the patients are satisfied with your least ideal option. Sometimes they choose the option in the middle, but the majority of the time they choose to want your ideal option. If they now want it, then usually it won't be solely about the cost, and they'll be more motivated to find a way to fit it into their budget. Ultimately, by using this influence-based approach to case presentation, more people will leave saying yes to one of your treatment options, instead of doing nothing, increasing your case acceptance and setting the stage for you to achieve a higher marketing ROI.

What Do You Do If There Are No Ethical Consequences of Saying No Today?

In all of these examples, we've discussed the real ethical consequences of doing nothing. Tooth decay doesn't improve over time by doing nothing, it worsens. Mild to moderate teeth crowding doesn't spontaneously resolve over time, teeth continue to shift and get worse. Periodontal disease doesn't take time off; it continues to be the silent killer that costs people the bony foundation around their teeth. But what about situations such as getting cosmetic veneers where there doesn't appear to be any ethical consequences of tooth destruction, erosion, pain, infection, and so forth, from doing nothing?

In these situations, we still need to anchor the patient to something else first before we go into our presentation of the ideal option available today. Our challenge now is figuring out what that anchor should be. The solution to the problem is this: When you don't know what to anchor that person to, you must go to prior patients that have said yes to this elective treatment and ask them a simple question: "Why did you do it?"

Remember when I talked before about the contrast effect that whatever that first option or price you give to someone, they will always compare it to something in their life, the other things they're spending their money on. Usually when you let that person control this comparison, we tend to lose, and the other things they are spending their money on win out. For the patients who have said yes to your elective treatment, something is different.

Here is a situation where they compared it to something in their life, and because of this comparison, you won and they decided to move forward with treatment. The problem is, you don't know what they anchored themselves to, but you can be sure it was of a high enough value that your treatment recommendations seemed much more favorable as a result. So the next time these patients are in your chair, see if you can ask that question and find out what they anchored themselves to and what value they put in that anchor. Then you can use that anchor and value to start your presentation with future patients interested in this procedure.

C. Getting a Yes to the Financial Plan

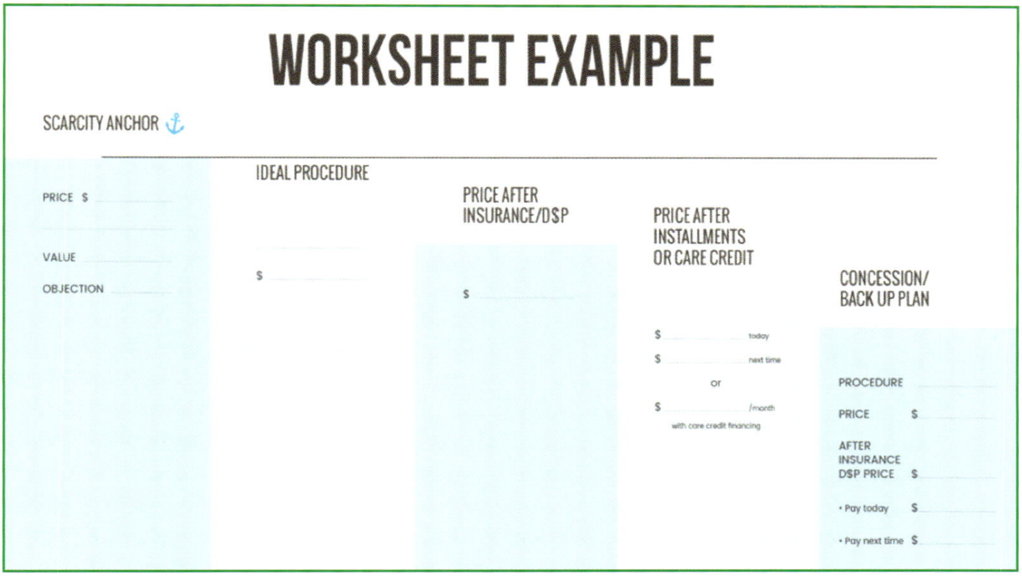

Figure 74. Financial "take them down the price stairs" worksheet.

Once the dentist has worked with the patient and influenced them to commit to one treatment plan, it's now time for the financial team to come in and present the options at hand. Using the above worksheet (Fig. 74) to successfully set the stage for a yes to the financial plan, the team must come prepared with the following:

1. Know what scarcity anchors the dentist presented to the patients;
2. Understand this idea of contrast and the power of taking people down the price stairs;
3. Leverage the principle of reciprocity and have alternative financial options available to present in case the main choice won't work for that patient's budget;
4. Be prepared to fall back to the next treatment option if the finances for the main option just won't work.

1. Scarcity Anchor

Before the financial plan can be presented for the main option selected by the patient, the financial team will need to find out what anchors the dentist used in their presentation and what the viable backup treatment options would be if they can't make the finances work for the ideal choice. Typically, once I've influenced the patient down to one treatment option, I'll go to my financial coordinator and review the patient's mindset, value statements, the consequences of doing nothing, and the financial cost I gave the patient as a result. I'd then review the ideal option, which is the one treatment option the patient ended up choosing.

2. Contrast: Take Them Down the Price Stairs on Simple Treatments

Once the scarcity anchors have been identified, the team will continue to fill out this worksheet. Next, moving to the right, they will fill out the ideal treatment today and what that cost will be. When patients ask us how much our treatment is, they aren't really asking about the total. Instead, they are asking for what they really want to know. How much are they paying out of their own pocket. How much are they writing us a check for or how much will they be putting on their credit card?

In the columns to the right of the ideal treatment, I want them to see if there is any way they can get the price to look smaller in contrast to the anchor amount already given and the price of the ideal treatment they've chosen. Usually you can deduct any funds that the patient's dental insurance plan might put toward this treatment. If the patient doesn't have dental insurance, then perhaps you can show them the cost difference after their dental membership plan discount or maybe a discount for being a senior citizen or because they prepaid for their treatment in its entirety. There are many ways to make that total treatment amount seem less in contrast. Let's use a crown as an example of our treatment option of choice.

Financial coordinator: Okay, Mrs. Jones. Now, Dr. Phelps has reviewed all of your options with you and let you know your first option was to do nothing, but in doing so, this most likely will lead to a root canal, post and core buildup, and a crown, causing more time off work, potential pain, and infection, and that will cost you around $3600 in additional expense. The good news is that if you move forward with that crown today, then it's only $1200, and after your dental insurance pays its part, it's really only $800. Does that work for you?

At this point in the process, I want you to ask for what you really want: for them to pay the full amount of their portion of the treatment, whatever that amount is because for the majority of your patients, you'll get them to agree to your request in doing so. Why? Now look at this from a contrast standpoint. Remember we make our decisions in the moment based on the comparisons available to us in that moment. After anchoring them to the $3600 fee, how does $800 sound? A whole lot more favorable than if we would have started by telling them the cost of the crown was $1200.

Had we started by telling them about the $1200 crown fee, you would have let them control the comparison, and they would have compared that to the other things they were spending their money on: maybe their car payment, house payment, or utilities, perhaps a vacation they want to go on. Ultimately hearing that $1200 and then comparing this to what they'd rather spend their money on will lead to a no, and they'll leave without scheduling treatment. By anchoring them to the $3600, they'll realize that this amount definitely won't work within their budget, but by the time we get to the real amount they'd pay of $800, this now seems more favorable and manageable in contrast. It's still not a guarantee of a yes, but it makes it statistically more likely.

Reciprocity: Be Ready for Rejection

We've talked before about the principle of reciprocity and how if we're the first to give a gift of value, people tend to reciprocate in kind. Reciprocity also plays a part when it comes to us being rejected. While it's human nature to be afraid of rejection, studies show that people actually hate to say no to you. In fact, they hate it so much that they really hate to say no to you multiple times in the same moment.

So in a situation like this where we're asking for them to pay the full out-of-pocket portion for their treatment, if the patient is unable to accommodate this request and rejects it, then we should be ready to fall back to our next best alternative option. If after we get a no, we immediately ask for something else, studies show we're even more likely to get a yes to this second request. Receive another no and ask for something else, and then we're even more likely to get a yes. Why? Well, after we receive a no, if we're the first to offer some type of compromise or alternative, people tend to want to reciprocate and compromise back by agreeing with our next request.

When it comes to simple treatment, say for amounts less than $3000 in total, my team has been authorized to offer them three fallback positions to help them fit this treatment into their budget:

1. Offer the treatment over two payments, half down to start and the remaining one half when the case is delivered the following month, planning the treatment steps out monthly to coincide with their monthly payments.
2. If two payments won't work, then we offer three payments, a down payment of one third today, and we'll schedule to start the treatment next month, getting a powerful active commitment in the process. The second third we'll collect the following month when we start the treatment. The final third is collected when we deliver the case the following month.
3. If the patient genuinely can't get the finances to work at this level, then our last option is to give them our "as low as" price, meaning the price they would get if they were approved for some third-party patient financing such as CareCredit, which we use in my practices. Budgeting out the longest possible term we'd offer of 60 months.

Here's how it might play out:

***Financial coordinator*: Okay, Mrs. Jones. Now, Dr. Phelps has reviewed all of your options with you and let you know your first option was to do nothing, but in doing so, this most likely will lead to a root canal, post and core buildup, and a crown, causing more time off work, potential pain, and infection, and that will cost you around $3600 in additional expense. The good news is that if you move forward with that crown today, then it's only $1200, and after your dental insurance pays its part, it's really only $800. Does that work for you?**

Patient: No, unfortunately I can't pay that amount today.

***Financial coordinator*: Okay, I understand. How about this? What if we broke this up into two payments? Could you do half, or $400, today, and then we'll collect the remaining $400 when we deliver the crown next month?**

Patient: I can't do that either.

***Financial coordinator*: Okay, what about this? What if we broke it up into three payments? We'll do one third today. We'll start it next month and collect another third. Then we'll finish it up the next month and collect the last third?**

Patient: Well, that sounds better, but I still can't do that right now.

***Financial coordinator*: Okay, well, what if I can get it down as low as $20 per month? Would that work for you?**

Patient: "Oh wow, that would be amazing. I can do that.

***Financial coordinator*: Okay, great. Let me go over how we can do that with CareCredit and see if we can get you approved.**

I ask the financial team to hold off on offering financing at all until we're sure one of our other prepayment options just won't work for them. I also don't want them going into too many details of how the financing plan works because if we can't get them committed to that monthly amount that will fit into their budget, then there really is no point of wasting time discussing the payment plan details.

If all else fails and none of the financial concessions work, then the team jumps to the last column on the right and goes through the next best available treatment option and takes them down the price stairs from there:

***Financial coordinator*: Okay. Well, what if I can get that crown price down as low as $20 per month. Would that work for you?**

Patient: Oh, wow, that would be amazing. I can do that.

***Financial coordinator*: Okay, great. Let me go over how we can do that with CareCredit and see if we can get you approved.**

Patient: Oh, I'll stop you right there. I won't get approved for any financing. My credit isn't really that good right now.

***Financial coordinator*: Okay. Well, since we can't make the crown fit into your budget, let's look at the next best option. Dr. Phelps told me that if the crown won't work, then the next best thing to do would be to just do a core buildup. The tooth won't be as protected as if it had the crown on it, but this way you'll be cavity free and eliminate the risk of infection that would come by doing nothing. Now, that price is**

$340, but after your insurance pays its part, it's only $100. Does that work for you?

Patient: I can't really do that right now.

***Financial coordinator*: Okay, what if we did two payments: $50 now, and we'll schedule your appointment for next month where we'll collect the final $50 due. Does that work?**

Patient: You know, you've been so nice and understanding with me, let's do that. I'll make that work.

By being prepared and having fallback positions to jump to after a no is received, you'll set the stage to hear a yes to one of the financial options you'll present.

3. Contrast: Take Them Down the Price Stairs on More Complex Treatments

Now, the structure of how my financial team presents treatment cases over $3000 is exactly the same as I've showed you before. They still need to repeat the scarcity anchors the doctor presented to the patient. They need to then go into the price today and the price after any insurance payment, dental membership plan discount or prepayment discount and then ask the patient if they are prepared to pay that today. What changes is what comes next if we get a no at this point. Given the amount of consumer debt across the United States, it's rare for patients to pay in full when their out-of-pocket costs are above $3000. For the majority of these cases, we use some type of third-party financing aid such as CareCredit. As such, I want my team to be prepared with at least two fallback positions utilizing this type of financing. One will be the two-year interest-free option, or 24 months of payments, and the other will be the "as low as" amount if they need to extend the financing term to, say, 60 months. Let's do an example using a total treatment amount of $20,000 for six dental implants and some type of fixed appliance.

***Financial coordinator*: Okay, Mrs. Jones. Now, Dr. Phelps has reviewed all of your options with you and let you know your first option was to do nothing, but in doing so, this most likely will lead to more bone loss in your jaws, which will make placing dental implants nearly impossible. To counter this effect, he'll have to refer you to the oral surgeon to perform extensive bone grafting to try to get back some of the bone you've lost, bone that could come from a rib, your leg, or other areas. That will result in a more major surgery, healing time, and a treatment cost that could easily be above $50,000. That's why it's great that you're not there yet and you have bone he can work with today. Given his plan of six dental implants and teeth that are attached and would not come out of your mouth, that treatment package is only $20,000. After your insurance pays its part, you're looking at around $18,000. Does that work for you?**

Patient: Well, I can't write a check for $18,000. That much is for sure.

***Financial coordinator*: Okay. What if I could break those payments out to $750/month. Would that work for you?**

Patient: Well, that's starting to sound a whole lot more manageable, but I can't quite spend that amount per month.

***Financial coordinator*: Okay. Well, I can get this down as low as $300 per month. Would that amount work for you?**

Patient: Yes, I can definitely make $300 per month work. Tell me more.

By utilizing the power of scarcity and contrast, more people will say yes and pay their full out-of-pocket portion due. For those people for whom finances generally are a concern and issue, by being the first to give financial alternatives and showing a general interest in helping them fit their treatment into their budget, more of them are likely to say yes to one of your financial fallback positions, avoiding the worst-case scenario for us all by them choosing to do nothing.

D. Getting a Yes to Scheduling the Appointment

Using the above influence approach, we've outlined a behavioral science–based protocol to help you present all of the options you feel should be presented but provided you a path to help guide the patient down to one treatment option or plan. By being committed to that one plan, you reduce the uncertainty that having too many options to choose from creates and have turned their dental need into something they want. With the scarcity anchors and taking them down the contrast price stairs, you've reduced their sensitivity to the price of the option they've selected, and if needed, you have offered multiple concessions to help them fit this desired treatment into their budget.

The last piece of our case acceptance puzzle comes with influencing the patient to schedule and show up for their treatment appointment. While it's not a necessity to take this extra step, I do recommend it. As I've mentioned before, when patients leave your practice, life tends to get in their way. They get bombarded with new challenges and get distracted by other wants that arise, potentially pushing their dental treatment further and further down on their priority scale.

To offset this risk, we can lean on the principle of reciprocity to set the stage for them to not only schedule to start their treatment but also that they'll show up for this visit. To accomplish this, we'll use the same method that can help influence more referrals to come into your office and offer patients a choice of gift cards. Two gift cards to no more than four options should be presented once the patient has accepted one of your financial options. These gift cards should be to places that the patient really values, places where they are already spending their money such as Amazon, Target, Starbucks, and iTunes. Once the choice of gift cards is given and the patient genuinely thanks you, that is your moment to ask them to schedule their appointment, and they'll likely reciprocate in agreement. If they use that gift card, then the internal obligation rises, and they'll be even more likely to show up for the appointment they've scheduled.

***Financial coordinator*: Mrs. Jones. I'm glad we were able to find a financial option that works best for you. Before you go, Dr. Phelps and I wanted to give you a small gift to say thank you. We know you had a choice of dental offices in the area, but you chose us, and we appreciate that. Here are a couple of gift cards. Why don't you pick one for yourself.**

Patient: Really? Wow. Well, I was going to Target right after my appointment here, so this is perfect. Thank you very much.

***Financial coordinator*: You're most welcome. Before you go, let's get you scheduled for your first visit to start this treatment. What works best for you? (Then schedule their appointment.)**

E. Amplify Your Case Acceptance Results

The more you present your treatment options using the influence structure I laid out above, the greater the increase in case acceptance you'll see. The more people come back for treatment, the higher the likelihood that you'll see a positive ROI for the marketing dollars you invested to attract that patient. To help you amplify your success rates even more, consider putting the influence presentation for your most popular procedures into an informational flyer to give to your patients. Below (Figs. 75 and 76) are some examples of ones that I use to present crowns and to present the options for the single missing tooth.

Having your team put these flyers into your patients' hands before you enter the room creates a great pre-suasive tool to help shape their mindset. You can then use these as a persuasive visual guide at the chair when explaining the treatment options at hand. For those who don't move forward with treatment today, taking this home creates a powerful "post-suasive" tool to remind them that they have a dental issue that will continue to worsen until they act. Combined, by using these influence flyers your case acceptance rates are sure to be magnified.

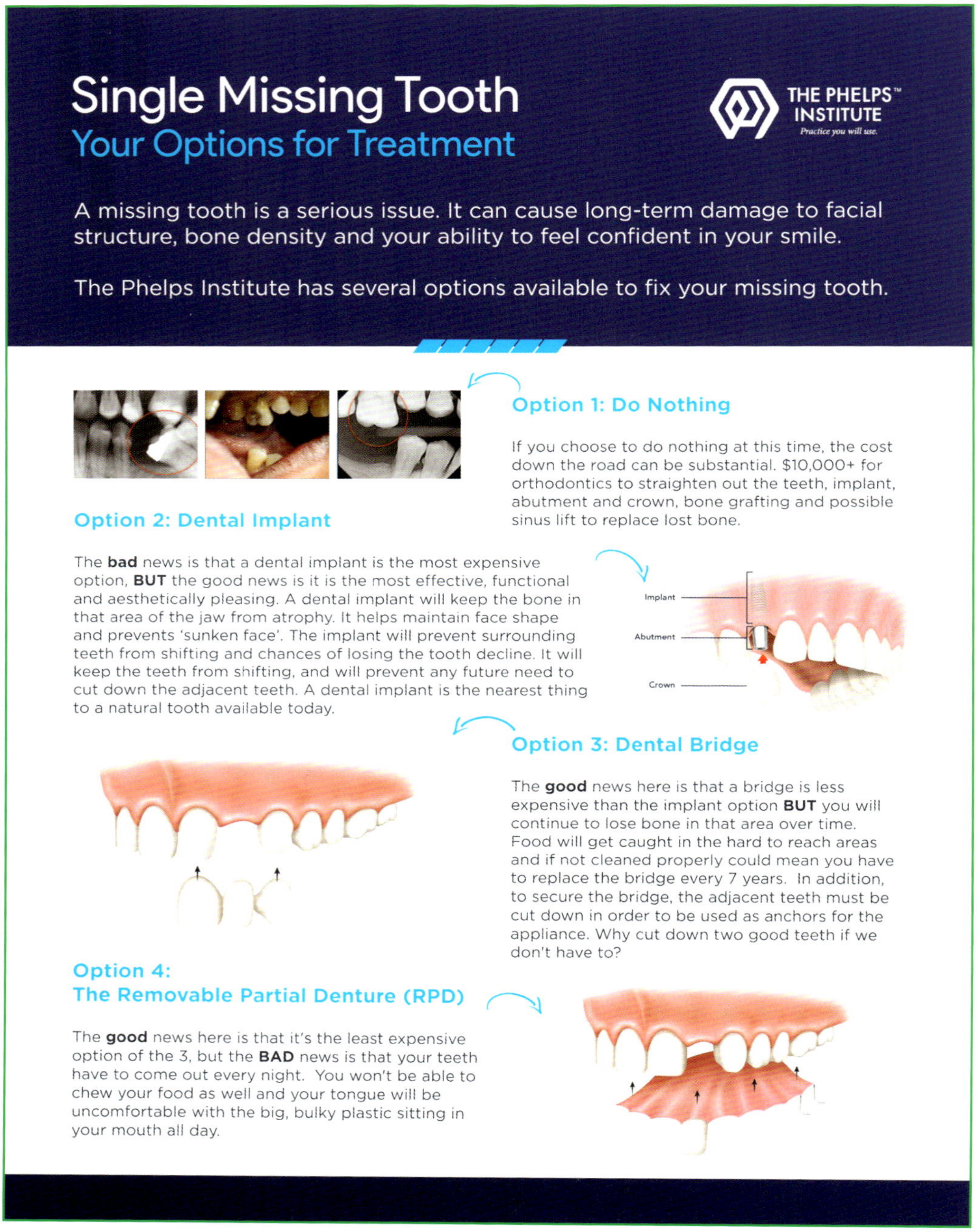

Figure 75. Pre-suasive, persuasive, post-suasive single missing tooth options flyer.

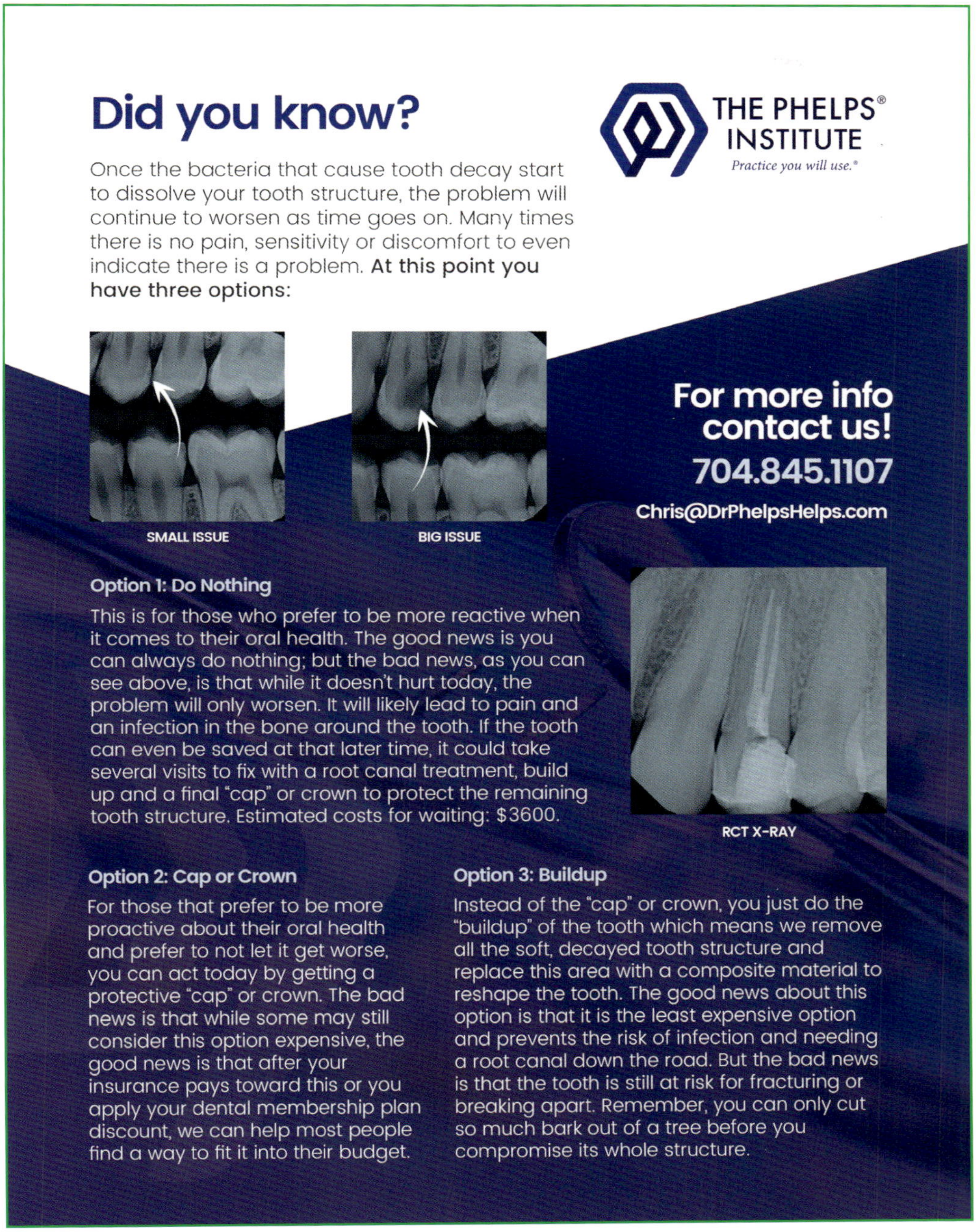

Figure 76. Pre-suasive, persuasive, and post-suasive crown presentation flyer.

Part 4

Maintaining the Patient Relationship

Chapter 12
Confronting Attrition and Uncertainty

If you've reached this stage of the book, then you've no doubt invested a lot of time and energy into creating strategies to attract more new patients, to influence them to schedule and show for their appointments while persuading them to say yes to your treatment recommendations.

Maximizing the number you attract while minimizing the lost opportunity that could have presented means the revenue you collect at this point should more than offset the money you invested in your marketing campaigns, giving you an ROI larger than 1:1 and allowing you to grow your practice. Unfortunately, we're not done. There are two other areas where lost opportunity can sabotage our success and ROI: patient attrition and when they're in uncertain times.

1. PATIENT ATTRITION

Patient attrition is the gradual loss of patients who fail to return to your practice for preventative or restorative care over some period of time. If you don't turn your focus onto keeping the patients you've attracted through your marketing efforts, you essentially have just wasted the money you spent to acquire them as you will need to spend more marketing dollars to replace them and the production they provided you.

A. The Cost of Attrition

Across the United States, the average patient attrition rate (PAR) for dental offices has been reported to range between 17 and 25 percent. Let's look at an example of what this could mean for a practice with 2000 active patients, which we'll define in this moment as those who have been seen at the dental office in some capacity within the last 18 months.

If 17 percent of those 2000 patients do not return to the office for care over a period of one year, that means your attrition was 340 patients, or 28 patients per month on average. Let's now assume that each one of those patients might have spent an average of $1000 with you over their first year as a patient. By losing 340 patients per year, you've now lost $340,000 in revenue you could have produced that year. Compound that over a five-year period, and your practice has just missed out on $1,700,000 in revenue.

Now consider that the total lifetime value (LTV) of a patient: the amount they might have spent at your practice over a longer period of time. Most experts put the average LTV of a patient above $10,000. Using our prior example, not only did you miss out on $1,700,000 over a five-year period, but you're missing out on $11,700,000 over the lifetime they could have spent in your practice. The higher your attrition rate becomes, the more it will cost you in lost revenue over time.

Patient attrition not only affects your revenue over time, but it also stifles your growth and profitability today. That's why we have to factor in your patient attrition rate when it comes to reaching your ideal new patient number for growth. Gaining 30 new patients a month may sound healthy on the surface, but if you factor in that you're losing 28 patients per month through attrition, you'll quickly realize why your overall revenue numbers aren't changing from year to year.

It's why most practices in the US can barely muster a 3–4 percent revenue growth rate year over year. For each patient they've lost through attrition comes the revenue they would have spent in your practice in the coming year. To counter this, you will have to replace them with a new patient, one who's revenue collected will be needed to offset that which was lost.

B. The Benefit of Reducing Attrition

While the average attrition rate is between 17 and 25 percent, those practices considered to be in the top 10 percent of dental practices in the US have rates that range between 7 and 8 percent. As these practices can probably attest, reducing your patient attrition rate will have several positive outcomes for your practice. Let's look at a few examples:

1. **Accelerates your growth**: A practice that gained 722 new patients over one year and only lost 254 patients has a net gain of 468 new patients, or 39 per month on average. This practice will have an easier time reaching their production and financial goals than one who acquired 848 new patients that year but had an attrition of 1021 patients, leading to a net patient loss of 173.
2. **Recoup lost revenue**: We talked earlier about the short- and long-term value of a patient. By decreasing your attrition rate, you will see revenue increases the longer they stay active in your practice.
3. **Saves your marketing budget**: Studies show that it will cost practices an average of four times more in new marketing efforts to replace lost patients versus just retaining them in the first place. So by decreasing your attrition, you're not having to overspend in marketing to replace them.
4. **Adds to your practice value**: Even a small change in your attrition rate can have a large impact on your practice value. By improving your PAR by 2–3 percent for three years you will increase the asset value of your practice by $100,000.

C. Calculating PAR

Now that we've covered the costs of ignoring your PAR and the benefits of focusing your attention to reducing it, let's dive into how you might calculate this rate of patient attrition.

The general consensus in the United States is that the PAR is dependent on your total active patient count. Most of the dental software metric companies used today consider your total active patient count to be the total number of patients seen, either in the doctor's chair or the hygienist's chair, over an 18-month period.

To calculate your annual PAR, you will take your total active patient count from 24 months ago and subtract from that your total active patient count during the last 12 months. Once you have that number, you'll then divide it by your total active patient count during the last 12 months. This will give you that year's percentage attrition rate. For example, if a practice had 1200 active patients over the last 24 months and they have had 1000 active patients over the last 12 months, that means they had a net difference of 200 patients, which divided by the original 1200 active patient count gives you an approximate 17 percent patient attrition rate over the last year.

D. Reducing PAR

Once you understand how big of an impact your PAR has on your practice growth and you've identified what your current PAR is, it's now time to turn your focus on ways to make improvements in this part of the dental marketing cycle.

Prevent It from Happening

Many times the best defense is a good offense, so the ideal way to reduce your patient attrition is to prevent it from ever happening, to plug the leaks in your boat that are allowing these patients to slip away. Let's look at some ways we can accomplish this:

1. **Build better relationships**: One of the main reasons patients leave your dental practice is because they didn't really make a connection with anyone at the office. Remember from the influence section when I said people typically don't do business with those they don't really know or like. By building better relationships with our patients, by telling them or showing them that we like them, we're more likely to see them return.
2. **Focus on the patient experience**: Creating a positive and friendly environment is key to promoting a great patient experience. The happier they are visiting your practice means the more likely they'll be to return. Another way you can promote a positive experience for them is to focus on their wait times. In dental offices across the US, patients can find themselves waiting 10–20 minutes past their appointed time to be seen, only to follow that with another 10–20 minutes of wait time needed while they attempt to check out and leave. The more they have to wait, the more their overall experience is tarnished. In today's fast-paced world, staying on time and being on time is key. By ensuring that you reduce or eliminate your patients wait times, you're improving their experience and setting the stage for them to happily return.
3. **Convenience**: Expanding the hours of your practice is another way you can help prevent attrition from occurring in your practice. By providing before work, after work, and/or weekend hours, you're giving your patients an opportunity to return but at their convenience. I can't tell you how many of my existing patients thanked me when we expanded the hours and days we were open in my practice, many telling me how hard it was getting to take off work or pull their kids out of school to come to the dentist whereas now they didn't have to make that difficult choice.

4. **Anchor them to your practice**: The more anchored they are to your practice, the less likely they are to leave you. Anchors come in many different forms. Building better relationships with you and your team members is a powerful way to anchor them to your practice. Giving them a great patient experience and making it convenient for them to attend are other great anchoring examples.

   In addition to these, you can anchor them by providing services that few in your community offer such as a dental membership plan. Not only do patients with a membership plan spend more than insurance or cash-paying patients, but they stay longer as well, with average attrition rates ranging between 17 and 24 percent; those at Dental Membership Direct cite that less than 5 percent of those with a dental membership plan cancel their subscription, significantly decreasing patient attrition rates as a result.

5. **Schedule their next appointment before they leave the office**: In my practice, our first attempt was to schedule their next appointment at the chair, either by the hygienist or the dental assistant they were working with. If that attempt failed or the team was running behind, then we'd make our second attempt at the front desk as the patient was checking out. Scheduling the patient before they leave is one of the most important ways to prevent attrition, but at the same time is the one that is most often bungled in dental offices around the US. In one nationwide study it was shown that those offices that fail to schedule their patients' next appointment before they leave the office lose 15–18 percent more patients than those who do.

6. **Free up the team's time**: For many practices, the patient's next appointment is scheduled at the front desk. In the "Attendance" section of this book we discussed how the team's focus is constantly being shifted and pulled into different directions at any given time. By outsourcing some of their duties such as appointment confirmations, insurance verification, and new patient calls, we can free up the team's time to focus on this important task, making sure the patient had a great experience, followed by making sure they leave with their next appointment scheduled. If the team is distracted or being pulled in multiple directions during this patient's checkout, the patient will very likely leave without making that next appointment, promising to call us back and schedule but all too likely meaning we'll never see that patient again.

7. **Make scheduling convenient**: Offer multiple ways for your patients to make their appointments. If you didn't make their next appointment while they were at your office, then you need to give them more options to schedule than just calling you up and getting a busy signal or having their call go to voicemail time and time again. Instead, make it easy and convenient for them to schedule. Let them chat with you on your website, send you a text or email, or embed an online scheduling software into your website so they can pick their own appointment day and time on their own.

8. **Communicate between appointments**: A popular nationwide survey of patients found that 30 percent will leave a dental office over time because of changes in their job, they move to a different area, or some other important life event that occurred. Seventy percent will do so because of the indifference they felt by the dental team. Think about it. You see them today, schedule their next cleaning appointment for 6 months out, and then never talk to them again. By engaging with your patients in between their scheduled

visits, you're showing them that you care and want them to be closer to you and your team as result. That's why I'm a big advocate of patient newsletters, things that can be emailed and mailed out to them at least once between now and their next hygiene visit in 6 months. The more you communicate with them, the more you show you care and the more likely they'll be to return.

E. After It's Occurred, Focus on Reactivation

If you've dropped the ball on any or all of the above ways to prevent patients from leaving your practice, then you need to redirect your attention to ways that can influence those who did slip through the cracks and never returned. Here are some ways you attempt to reactivate those thought to be lost:

1. **Automated reactivation system**: In previous sections we've discussed the power of leveraging automated technology in your practice. Having an automated appointment confirmation system has been shown to increase confirmations from patients by 200 percent, while having an automated appointment reminder system can reduce no-shows by 71 percent. By having an automated program reach out to all of your overdue patients simultaneously, you can leverage technology and save valuable time that your team doesn't really have to spare.
2. **Dedicate someone to this position (hygiene and doc Tx)**: One of the best decisions I ever made was when I hired someone to be our recall reactivation manager, a person's whose sole job was to make sure the hygienists schedules at my two offices stayed full.

   As part of their daily routine, this person would create a list of those overdue for their next hygiene appointment and segment them based on the highest probability of success for reactivation. Those overdue from one day to 6 months, followed by those overdue 6–18 months, and followed lastly by those overdue over 18 months. Within each of these three categories, she created a schedule of when and how she'd communicate with them as well as what messages she'd use in her reactivation attempts, rotating her communication efforts between calling the patients, sending them emails, texting them, and mailing them reactivation postcards.

   While her primary role was to get more of these patients back on the schedule, her secondary goal was to identify why they hadn't returned to date. Was it because of some life change, a move, or a new job position—things you can't really do much about—or was it something more in our control to change? With one of my dental coaching clients, I had his team focused on discovering why those patients who were overdue for a cleaning hadn't returned. To their surprise, a good percentage of those patients surveyed reported that they had not come back to the dental office because at some point they had lost their dental insurance benefit.

   Given this practice had just implemented a dental membership plan (DMP), a great option for patients who don't have dental insurance, it then gave them a great message to share with these patients. With a simple email that talked about the benefits of the DMP and how it was a solution for those without insurance, the data from their Dental Membership Direct database tracking and billing software showed that the office was able to schedule 80 of those patients over a three-month time frame, generating an additional $29,200 in hygiene revenue that year from a series of emails. This didn't count any of the revenue generated from the restorative needs of these patients. Overall, this effort had an excellent ROI.

The larger your office grows, the more you stand to benefit by freeing up the team's time to work on reactivating overdue patients or ideally dedicating a team member to this critical job. For my team member, I hired her at a salary of $35,000 per year. Her main assignment was to keep our hygiene chairs fully scheduled at both of my practice locations. Two days a week she'd focus on one practice, and two days a week she'd focus on the other. Over a 6-month period, we collected over $350,000 in revenue that was generated in hygiene and restorative care from the patients she was able to reactivate, a 10:1 return for my investment in her and this position.

3. **Outsource the role**: If you don't have the means to dedicate a team member's time to reactivating lost patients, then consider outsourcing the task: someone who can identify and categorize your overdue patients, who can dedicate the time to emailing, mailing, texting, and calling them on your behalf but still provides you a great return for your investment. Dr. Peter Bowman who practices in Walpole, New Hampshire, recently hired Golden Goose Scheduling (GGS) to take over his hygiene recall reactivation program. In the first month, GGS was able to schedule 12 patients overdue in the one-day-to-6-month category, 12 patients in the 6–18-month category, and 4 patients in the 18-plus-month category. Because each patient will spend a minimum of $300 in hygiene care this year, that's $8400 in additional revenue they were able to add back to his practice, all for an investment in their services of only $800, giving him a 10.5:1 ROI. When done properly, outsourcing can be a productive way to help decrease your patient attrition rate.

2. CONFRONTING UNCERTAINTY

Our last area of lost opportunity occurs when our existing and potential new patients are uncertain about the events unfolding around them. These events could be local in origin or worldwide, but the end result is the same. When people are uncertain, when there are major doubts or questions in their minds, they don't move, usually staying stationary until the situation around them becomes clearer. In our world, that means that they stop coming to our practices, stop moving forward with treatment, and we see all of our marketing messages fall on deaf ears. Having recently lived through a major time of uncertainty, one that will leave its mark on the dental profession for generations to come, I feel strongly that the lessons I learned during this event can help your practice when other such events take place, giving you a path to follow to keep your practice successful and your marketing ROI strong, regardless of what's happening in the world around you.

In 2019 the world was forever changed by the discovery of a new type of coronavirus called SARS-CoV-2. This virus manifests as a respiratory disease called COVID-19 and was thought to spread mainly from person to person through respiratory droplets produced when an infected person coughs, sneezes, or talks. Symptoms of COVID-19 can range from mild to its most severe form causing death. Because this virus was previously undiscovered, there was little understanding of it and no real accurate way to test or screen for it. To compound the problem, a large percentage of those infected with the virus did not present with any symptoms. As these silent carriers and those with mild, cold-like symptoms continued their daily routines, the virus began to spread around the world at an alarming rate.

On January 30, 2020, the World Health Organization (WHO) declared the COVID-19 outbreak a global health emergency. On March 11, 2020, the WHO declared COVID-19 a global pandemic. This was the first time they'd done so since the H1N1 influenza virus of 2009. As of this writing, there have been over 29.9 million recorded cases in the United States with the virus claiming the lives of over 532,000 Americans. Worldwide the toll has been 119 million reported cases and 2.64 million deaths. On March 13, 2020, the president of the United States declared COVID-19 a national emergency. On March 19, 2020, California became the first state to issue a stay-at-home order, mandating that all residents should stay at home except to go to an essential job or to go out for essential supplies. Within days, other states followed with similar warnings and mandates. For two to three months, the world seemed to be on hold during this time of apprehension.

As time progressed, businesses began to reopen. People started returning to work and attempting to adapt to the new normal of living in a COVID-19 world. But as life began to re-emerge, there was a fundamental shift in the mindsets of the masses. We talked in the acceptance stage of this book about the two main patient mindsets we would encounter in our practices before the COVID-19 pandemic. The majority were those who preferred to be proactive with their oral health, who wanted preventative care and to address things such as crowns and fillings when they are relatively small in nature, not wanting them to progress and worsen, costing them more time, money, and potential pain because they waited. On the flip side, the minority of our patients had a different mindset. Instead of being proactive, they preferred to be reactive with their oral health, ignoring the small problem today and choosing to wait until it became an issue tomorrow.

In times of apprehension, when there is a great uncertainty present, two other mindsets have evolved, affecting the behavior of our patients in ways we could not have predicted before COVID-19. That's why I'm taking the time to address it here. If your reading this and find yourself living through one of those times, as we are now, you will need to adapt your attraction, attendance, acceptance, and attrition strategies to be successful. Otherwise you might find yourself stuck in a gap that could be extremely detrimental to your practice.

A. Pre- and Post-COVID Mindsets

Before COVID-19, the predominate mindsets were proactive and reactive, 80 percent of our daily schedules being filled with the proactive patients, who want to get their cleanings, fillings, and crowns completed so that things don't get worse down the road, and the remaining 20 percent of schedules with the reactive mindset patients, the ones who need the extraction, the implant, the root canal—people who knew the problem was present but were not ready to deal with it at that time, preferring to wait until the problem escalated before addressing it.

After COVID-19, those two mindsets took on a totally new form: the risk tolerant and the risk averse mindsets. Someone who is risk tolerant is willing to make a calculated risk. For them, the benefit of action outweighs the potential consequences. Someone who is risk averse sees things as just the opposite. They see the consequences of action outweighing its benefits, and thus choose to remain static until the situation around them becomes more favorable.

When it comes to the pre-COVID-19 mindsets of proactive and reactive, we can see their evolution into these post-COVID-19 mindsets of being risk tolerant and risk averse. Patients who led with a reactive mindset before COVID tended to develop a risk tolerant mindset during a time of uncertainty. Those with a proactive mindset developed more of a risk averse mindset during these times. This is not to say that risk averse patients can't also be reactive in nature or that risk tolerant patients can't be proactive. Of course they can, but what I want you to understand is what you will find the majority of the time. Once you know what to expect for the masses, then you can give your strategies for practice growth the best chance of success, even during trying and uncertain times.

B. Dental Offices Reopening

Within two to three months of the nationwide shutdown, the majority of states in the US started lifting their stay-at-home orders, allowing businesses to reopen and people to freely go out and about again as long as they took certain precautions such as social distancing at least 6 feet apart from one another and wearing some type of mask over their faces, limiting the respiratory droplets released into the environment and hopefully decreasing the risk of contracting COVID-19.

As dental practices began to reopen, there were recommendations from the Centers for Disease Control (CDC), the American Dental Association (ADA), and other local and state government leaders on what precautions we as health care providers should take to keep our patients safe and to help limit the spread of this disease. Offices invested in air purifiers and medical-grade air scrubbers, and they got fitted to wear air respirators, called N95 masks, during dental treatments. They stopped using ultrasonic units during cleaning visits to limit the spread of potentially harmful aerosols. They limited the number of patients that could be seen in their office at any given time and eliminated the use of their waiting or reception areas, instead requiring patients to wait in their cars until the office sent them a text message to let them know it was okay for them to come in for their appointment. Not since the AIDS epidemic in the 1980s had dentistry made such sweeping changes to the personal protective equipment (PPE) we wore and how we provided care to our patients.

But all of this was done with one goal in mind: to keep our patients safe, to allow them to receive the dental care they needed but without fear of contracting the virus as a result. It was an unsure time indeed. Even with these additional precautions taken, there was no guarantee that our patients would return. Dentists everywhere were concerned that the economic effects from the nationwide shutdown could have spelled the end for their dental practice, just as it had for so many other businesses, both large and small. The good news for us was that because of these new mindsets, it wouldn't be the end at all. In fact, for most, it would be just the opposite. Let's look at these two mindsets in more detail.

C. Risk Tolerant Mindset

Someone with a risk tolerant mindset is willing to take action in a time of uncertainty. For them, the benefit of action outweighs the risk. When businesses and restaurants began to reopen, these were the first ones you'd find out and about. With daily COVID-19 cases still very much a concern and rising, these people were out there trying to live their new normal.

In our dental offices, this was no different. I remember spending an entire day with our team the day before we reopened our office to the public. We reviewed all of the precautions we'd taken to keep our employees and our patients safe. We reviewed all of the PPE, air filtration equipment, and other new policies we had enacted to keep everyone safe. On the day we reopened, the team huddled up and again reviewed our new check-in policy, trying to limit the number of patients in the office and asking patients to wait for us to send them a text before they physically came inside. The idea of doing this made sense, yet when we broke from our huddle, we were all surprised to find five patients standing in our reception area, none of them wearing masks, despite a state mandate to do so. Not one of them followed our instructions and waited to receive a text message from us before entering. While shocked, we quickly sat them and began our day.

Afterward, I interviewed my team members and discovered that none of these patients had asked about new PPE and other precautions we had taken. Ultimately, they just didn't seem that concerned and were definitely not afraid of catching the virus from this visit.

What they were concerned about was the immediate dental need they had. You see, the majority of them were our reactive patients, those who knew they had a dental issue but always felt like if that issue ever manifested as a real problem, they had plenty of time to address it, without much inconvenience. What the COVID-19 shutdown taught them was that this is not always the case. When their dental issue started to become more pressing, they couldn't get into a dental office to get it taken care of, and now had to manage any pain or discomfort this caused as a result. This is why when the shutdown was over and dental offices reopened, they were the first ones filling up our chairs and the vast majority that continued to do so over the next six to eighteen months we were open.

D. Risk Averse Mindset

For someone with a risk averse mindset, their focus is on safety and minimizing risk. If the potential consequences for action outweigh the benefits to them, they don't tend to move. In a time of uncertainty, you won't find them out and about, going to restaurants, bars, or any other place where people might be congregating. Unless they have an immediate dental need, one that usually involves pain, you won't be seeing them in your dental practice either, not until they feel safe and the risk of catching the virus has been minimized or neutralized altogether. From a treatment standpoint, these patients tend to be our more proactive mindset patients, which makes sense. People who prefer to be proactive are ultimately trying to avert or diminish risk. That's why they seek treatment today instead of letting it get worse by doing nothing.

I remember talking with one of my proactive patients around the age of 65 who had come in on one of the first couple of days after we reopened the office due to a toothache. She and her older husband have been longtime patients of mine, and I could tell that she was very concerned sitting in our chair that day. When I asked her about it, she told me that she was very nervous about coming in because of her age, her husband's age and health status, and the fact that her elderly parents were currently living with them. If not for the toothache, she said, she would not be in our office. I told her that I completely understood and reviewed with her all of the precautions we had taken to keep our patients safe. When I mentioned that we had invested in a few medical-grade air filters that were able to capture the COVID-19 virus despite its small particle size, the patient perked up with interest. I then mentioned that we were due to receive more units in the coming days so that every square inch of air in the practice would be scrubbed every 5–10 minutes. Without hesitation the patient told me to call her as soon as we had those up and running. Once we had, then she'd feel safe coming back in with her husband and parents to get their teeth cleaned.

When your market speaks, you should listen. Many times they will give you valuable insights into what mindset they are in, what barriers are keeping them from taking action, and possibly give you solutions or ideas on how to solve the problem. The more of these proactive, risk averse patients I talked to, the more I realized that their desire to be safe trumped their desire to be proactive. Thus, until they felt safe, they had no plans to return to our office. When looking at our future schedule, I could see the evidence of their absence and noticed a gap in patient care that was sure to follow.

E. The Gap

I define the gap (Fig. 77) as the period of time when you'll see a significant amount of open chair time for both the dentist and hygienist. Open chair time refers to a lack of patients scheduled or seen during that time. It's created because of the mindset shift that occurs in our patient base in times of apprehension such as what COVID-19 has caused. Without direct action to counter this effect, it's not likely to resolve naturally for some time.

When dental offices reopened, they were instantly flooded with patients, most of which were of the risk tolerant mindset, who'd put off dental care for too long and now had pressing dental issues. Fueled by the scarcity of not being able to see a dentist during the shutdown,

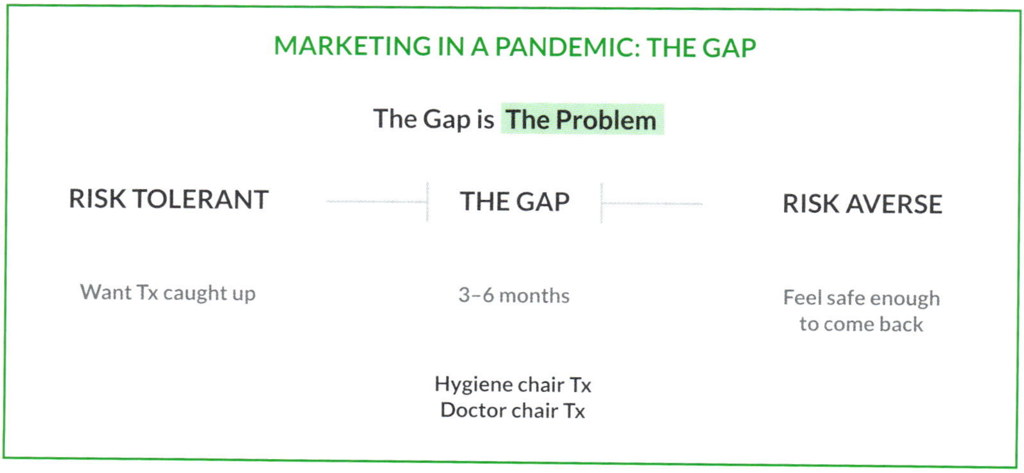

Figure 77. The gap.

a massive desire was created within them to find a dentist somewhere to take care of their dental needs. If they had a relationship with a dental office already established, they'd go there; if not, then they'd search until they found one. At my office, during the first several months after reopening, the new patient count increased by 120 percent. Everything geared toward filling the doctor's chair with treatment to be performed.

Unfortunately, a problem was brewing in the hygiene chair, one that would create a gap in hygiene treatment because of a significant amount of open chair time. Normally, after you received your cleaning today, a patient would make an appointment to return for their next cleaning in six months. When offices across the country were shut down during March, April, and part of May, there were no patients seen in hygiene. That meant those patients weren't rescheduled in six months. Come September and October, our entire hygiene schedule was wide open, not a single patient scheduled as a result.

With the hygiene chair gap looming, several offices were also starting to see a large decrease in patients scheduled for the doctor. This gap in the dentist's chair resulted for several reasons. First, it meant that the practice was running out of the risk tolerant mindset patients who were already a part of their patient base. If a doctor had been practicing for over 15 years, then it might take them six to eighteen months to cycle through all of the risk tolerant patients they had built up over the years. For those practicing only a few years and who didn't have a large patient base to draw from, they would very quickly start to see that gap occurring in their chairs. In addition to their existing patient pool drying up, it also meant that they weren't marketing enough to attract more risk tolerant patients to their practice. Compound this with the fact that their risk averse patient base, who pre-COVID far outnumbered the others, didn't feel safe enough yet to come in for any type of care, routine or otherwise. Thus, a gap in patient care was occurring.

F. Closing the Gap

To close this gap in patient care, you'll need to modify the strategies we discussed in the previous stages of this book. In short, it's going to require an increase in your external marketing

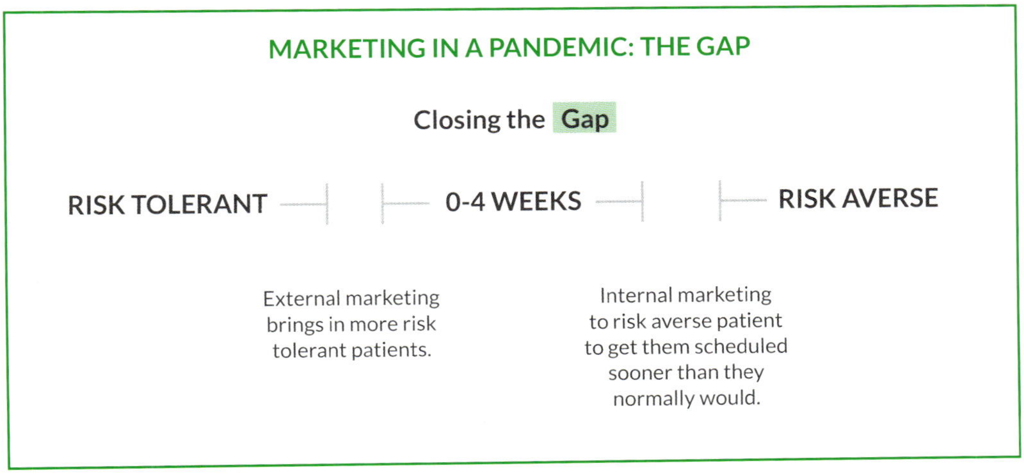

Figure 78. Closing the gap.

efforts to try to attract more risk tolerant patients to your practice, increasing their numbers and extending the amount of time your chairs will be full as a result. At the same time, you will need to increase your internal marketing efforts to your risk averse patient base. Left to their own accord, it could be six months to a year before they will feel safe enough to return to your office for care. By communicating all of the ways you're keeping them safe and focusing your messaging on how you've minimized their COVID-19 risk, you will influence more of them to return sooner to your office.

By extending the time you're able to fill your chairs with risk tolerant patients, along with shortening the time the risk averse patients delay their care, you can effectively close or eliminate any gaps in patient care and keep your chairs full and productive. For those in my dental coaching program, I advised them about these two mindsets and the gap in patient care I foresaw coming. By following the advice I'll lay out below, these offices were able to avoid that gap for both the hygienist and dentist. Most of them had significant increases in new patients as well as case acceptance and were able to produce enough in the last six months of the year to make up for the lack of production they had during the two-month shutdown, effectively producing the same in 2020 as they had in 2019.

G. Actions in Times of Uncertainty

One of the lessons the COVID-19 pandemic showed us was that we need to be prepared to adapt our actions for whatever crisis comes our way. Whether that crisis stems from biological, economic, political, environmental, or financial sources, there will always be uncertainty and thus apprehension in our patients' mindsets that result. Regardless of its cause, when present, you can count on the two predominant mindsets I discussed to reappear, each with its own unique set of blessings and challenges, but both effecting a change in our patients' and potential new patients' actions.

If your practice doesn't understand or have a plan to address these mindsets, you will see a gap in patient care, more open chair time, and loss in practice revenue. If you use the strategies above and increase your external marketing efforts to attract more patients with the risk tolerant mindset, you'll not only be more productive and help recoup any lost revenues the uncertain situation created, but you'll also be able to maintain that productivity for a longer period of time, keeping both doctor and hygiene chairs full of willing patients. At the same time, if you can increase your efforts on marketing and communicating with your existing risk averse–minded patients, focusing your messaging and content on how you'll keep them safe, you'll be able to shorten the amount of time it would take to attract them back into your office, minimizing or eliminating the gap in patient care that otherwise would have been created.

Conclusion

1. PUTTING IT ALL TOGETHER

In this book I've identified the two macro areas that affect dental marketing and your successful return on investment: creating new patient leads and minimizing the lost opportunity that can sabotage your ROI. I've dissected these macro areas into the smaller areas that comprise them.

When you think of creating new patient leads, you now understand that means having a solid foundation or brand to build from. You also need to understand your target market and who you want more of at your practice. With that in mind you will be able to craft differentiating messages and create content with call-to-action offers that not only grab your target market's attention but also motivate and influence them to want to respond. I've also provided you with worksheets that you can use to communicate these important areas to anyone you've hired for your dental marketing purposes, giving them the info they need to set the stage to provide you and your practice with the best quantity and quality of new patients.

With these new patient leads now coming in, you have a better understanding of how bungling them can cripple your marketing ROI. To minimize these areas of lost opportunities, you learned how to answer more new patient calls, what language you can use to schedule more appointments, and how to influence those patients to show up to your practice. Ignoring any of these areas means less new patient opportunities and wasted marketing efforts.

Once present in your chair, you now know how to add pre-suasive elements to erase whatever mindset the patient comes into your office with and replace it with a mindset more conducive to discussing their oral health. In the right mindset, you've learned how to persuasively anchor them to the consequences of what can happen if they choose to do nothing and how that choice will cost them in what they value as a result. I discussed how to build trust with someone upon your initial encounter but help frame their treatment options in a way they can truly understand, modifying their perspective from listening to their dental needs to now choosing treatment that they want. I've covered how to take the commitment they've made toward one of your treatment options and shown you how your financial team can help the patient find a way to fit this plan into their budget, all of which can help you significantly increase the acceptance of the treatment you're presenting.

I reviewed the various reasons why patients don't return to our office and the costs we incur as a result. I talked about how to prevent this attrition or loss from occurring and given you ways to reverse the process, attracting back those thought lost. Lastly, I covered how to protect your practice from the gap in patient care that inevitably occur during times of nationwide or global apprehension, listing out specifics you can do to reduce or eliminate that gap altogether.

Taken together, when you attract an unlimited number of new patients, when the majority schedule and show for their appointments, accept your treatment recommendations, and return for future visits, you can be confident that you will have the seeds to grow to whatever production or collection levels your practice has the capacity to achieve. Moving forward, successful marketing is no longer a mystery but a tool you can consistently invest in to grow without fear or remorse.

2. GLOSSARY OF MARKETING TERMS

Actual return on investment (aROI): The ratio between the actual revenue collected from all of the new patients your marketing endeavor delivered to your office over a period of time and the cost of said marketing investment. For our purposes, we're using the shorter patient lifetime value (PLV) time period for our calculation. This could be the amount those patients spend after their first visit, within six months, or the amount they spend within the first year. A high aROI means the investment's gains compare favorably to its cost in a shorter amount of time. That's more money back into the practice's bank account in a shorter period of time. The aROI is the preferred metric to evaluate over the eROI when measuring a marketing campaign's effectiveness. For example, if a direct mail marketing campaign attracted 50 new patients who spent an average of $300 in their first visit, the total revenue collected after their combined first visits was $15,000, which divided by your marketing campaign cost of $5000 gives you an aROI of 3:1. A 3:1 aROI is the minimum recommended ratio I like to see within the first six months of any marketing spend.

Advertising: Activity or profession of producing advertisements for commercial products or services, advertisements that describe or draw attention (to a product, service, or event) in a public medium in order to promote sales or attendance.

aROI = ROI: For the purposes of this book, ROI actually refers to the aROI calculation.

Authority: Since we don't have time to be an expert in everything, we look to credible experts to tell us what we should do.

Cialdini's six principles of persuasion: In the book *Influence: The Science and Practice*, Dr. Robert Cialdini introduced the world to his research on the six principles of persuasion. These universal principles are shortcuts that we use to help make our decisions. They are:

Consensus / social proof: Many times we look to the behavior of what others around us are doing to decide what we should do.

Consistency: When we make a commitment, there is an internal and external pressure on us to be consistent and follow through on what we said we'd do.

Estimated return on investment (eROI): The ratio between an estimated revenue amount one might collect from all of the potential new patients who came in from your marketing endeavor spent over a period of time and the cost of said marketing investment. Typically, the PLV is factored into this equation. For example, let's say a PLV is estimated to be $5000 that they'll spend over the course of time they are your patient. If a marketing campaign produced 20 new patients and we know their PLV spend is typically $5000 each, that gives a total estimated revenue spend of $100,000, which divided by $5000 marketing cost to attract those 20 new patients gives us an eROI of 20:1. The downside of using this calculation is that it's purely an estimate. The reality of what is actually spent by these patients and when they spend it can change the calculation and your bottom line dramatically.

Liking: We tend to say yes to people we know and like.

Marketing: Activities a company undertakes to promote the buying or selling of a product or service. It includes advertising, selling, and delivering products to consumers or other businesses. For the purposes of this book, we'll use marketing and advertising interchangeably.

Patient acquisition cost (PAC): The cost of acquiring a new patient and dividing that by the number of patients acquired over some defined period of time. From our previous direct mail example, $5000 was spent to attract a total of 50 new patients in the first month. This amount divided by 50 new patients gives as a PAC of $100. This number can be used to help estimate how much you'd need to spend to reach your new patient goals. For instance, if your goal was to reach 100 new patients in a month and we know we can expect a PAC of $100 per new patient we attract, then it can be estimated that it will cost $10,000 to reach that goal of 100 new patients that month.

Patient lifetime value (PLV): The amount of money a patient spends at your practice over a defined period of time. PLV normally refers to their entire lifetime spent at your practice, but for the purposes of calculating the marketing return on investment, I prefer to look at this over a shorter period of time: amount spent at the first visit, second visit, or within the first year.

Reciprocity: When a gift of value is given to you, there is an obligation that is created inside of us to give back in kind to the person who gave to us.

Scarcity: When resources are dwindling or about to run out, it motivates us to want those resources more and be willing to do more to get them.

Acknowledgments

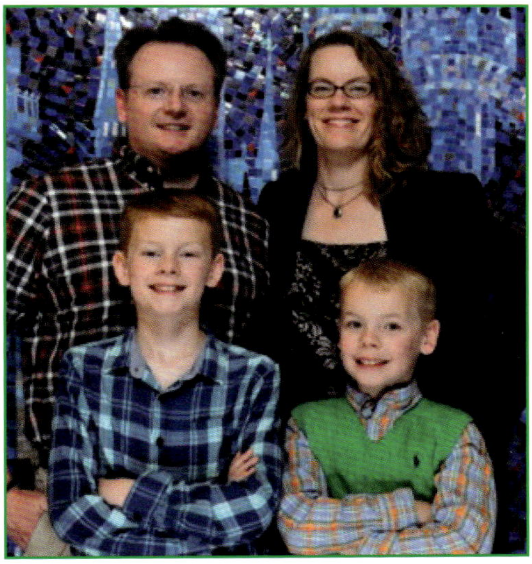

My family.

This book is the culmination of what I've learned and experienced in the world of dental marketing for more than 17 years. Without those who accompanied me on this journey, this book could have never become a reality.

My wife, Amber, has always supported me in whatever idea or opportunity I wanted to create, even if it seemed crazy or unattainable. Without her love and support, there is no way I would have had the successes that I've had.

My sons, Riley and Liam, have shown incredible patience and understanding while I was writing this book. Many a Saturday and Sunday went by when I knew they wanted to hang out with me. Like their mom, they are the reasons why I do what I do.

I've had many mentors that have helped guide my path. Dr. Robert Cialdini has been the most significant. I truly feel blessed to be a certified trainer in his method of influence and persuasion. His research completely changed how I view the world. What I have learned from him is now a part of me at my core and shapes every interaction I have with people.

Mark Ferber, I am grateful to be a part of the circle of influence and the community that you've built. To watch you in action, to see the big picture of things that I never saw before, in all its moving parts, is like looking at a masterful production. Thank you for your coaching, your mentorship, and for this opportunity. Without your guidance, this book would have never come to fruition.

In the world of dental marketing, I have a met few kindred spirits. Some had a profound understanding of what it takes to get quality new patients in the door of our dental practices. All of them care deeply for helping us attain real results. Karen Galley at Patient News Marketing, Sean Hamel at the Art of Dental Marketing, Shad and Brian at TinyRhino, thank you all for your unique input into this tome on marketing.

My colleagues in the dental world Dr. Nate Jeal, Dr. Michael Grossman, Dr. Michael Ling, Dr. Eric Jones, Dr. Travis Campbell, Dr. Ritchie Wyne, Dr. Peter Bowman, thank you for your specific contributions to the case studies in this book and, most importantly, for your friendship. Dr. Duc Tang, thank you for hosting me in your practice while I was pecking away at my keyboard, working on this book, in between patients.

Finally, Dr. Reza Ardalan, Dr. Nate Jeal, Dr. Amanda Matsuhara, you have made this book better because you cared enough to offer your diligent comments on my drafts. Thank you.

Yet, for all of the help I've received from my colleagues and friends to bring the best version of dental marketing to you, my readers, any omissions and errors are strictly my own.

Chris